Health and Cultures

Volume I

Policies, Professional Practice and Education

Health and Cultures

Volume I

Policies, Professional Practice and Education

Editors
Ralph Masi
Lynette Mensah
Keith A. McLeod

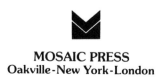

MOSAIC PRESS
Oakville-New York-London

CANADIAN CATALOGUING IN PUBLICATION DATA

Health and Cultures : exploring the relationships
ISBN 0-88962-549-2 (v.I)
ISBN 0-88962-550-6 (v.2)

1.Minorities - Medical care. I. Masi, Ralph. II. Mensah, Lynette Loleta. III. McLeod, Keith A., 1935-

RA 563.M56H43 1993   362.1'08693   C93-095005-4

Published by MOSAIC PRESS, P.O. box 1032, Oakville, Ontario, L6J 5E9, Canada. Offices and warehouse at 1252 Speers Road, units #1&2, Oakville, Ontario, L6L 5N9, Canada.

Mosaic Press acknowledges the assistance of the Canada Council and the Ontario Arts Council in support fo its publishing programme.

ISBN 0-88962-508-5   PB

MOSAIC PRESS:
In Canada:
      MOSAIC PRESS, 1252 Speers Road, Units #1&2, Oakville, Ontario, L6L 5N9, P.O. Box 1032, Oakville, Ontario, L6J 5E9, Canada.

In the U.K. and Europe by:
      John Calder (Publishers) Ltd., 9-15 Neal St., London, WCZH9TU, England.

Table of Contents

Acknowledgements vii

Section 1 - Introductory Chapters

Introduction 3
Ralph Masi, Keith A. McLeod, Lynette Mensah

Multiculturalism In Health Care:
Understanding and Implementation 11
Ralph Masi

Transcultural, Cross-Cultural and Multicultural
Health Perspectives in Focus 33
Lynette Mensah

Section 2 - Policies & Theory

Introduction 45

The Montreal Children's Hospital, A Hospital Response
To Cultural Diversity, ... 47
Heather Clarke

A Changing City: The Response of the City of Toronto
Department of Public Health 63
Maria Lee, Maria Herrera

First Nations Peoples in Urban Settings:
Health Issues 71
Chandrakant P. Shah, Gloria Dubeski

The Universal Right to Health: An Ideological
Discourse 95
Audrey L. Kobayashi, Mark W. Rosenberg

Section 3 - Professional Practice & Education

Introduction 111

General Theory & Approaches

Multicultural Health Care: An Introductory Course for
  Health Professionals 113
  Hope Toumishey

Education for Self-Reflection: Teaching About Culture,
  Health & Illness 139
  Margaret Lock

What is Experiential Learning? 159
  Basanti Majumdar

Specific Issues & Foci

Cultural Perspectives In Chronic Illness 169
  Enid Collins

Acculturation of Food Habits 187
  M.M. Krondl, D. Lau

Lay Health and Self-Care Beliefs and Practices: Responses of the
  Elderly to Illness in Four Cultural Settings in Canada in the
  United States 197
  Amarjit Singh, Barry Kinsey, Ph.D.

Cultural Factors Affecting Self-Assessment of Health
  Satisfaction of Asian Canadian Elderly 229
  K. Victor Ujimoto, Harry K. Nishio, Paul T.P. Wong, Lawrence Lam

The Semiotic Representation of "Health"
  and "Disease" 243
  Marcel Danesi

Ethics in Cross-Cultural Health 255
  John R. Williams.

Cancer and Cultural Attitudes 271
  Marion Poliakoff

Seniors, Culture and Institutionalization 291
  Milada Disman, Ph.D., Miroslav Disman, Ph.D.

Section 4 - Research

Introduction 317

Ethnocultural Communities as Partners in Research 319
  Joan M. Anderson, Ph.D.

Contributors 329

Index 333

Acknowledgements

The publication of these two volumes was made possible by the support of the Canadian Council for Multicultural Health. The support of Multiculturalism and Citizenship, Canada is also gratefully acknowledged.

The editors would like to thank those who have contributed articles; their material reflects the development of Multicultural Health. We also thank Victoria Grant for her professional editorial assistance. Finally, we thank John Dow and Marilyn Cap for their assistance throughout the production of the publication.

Ralph Masi
Lynette Mensah
Keith A. McLeod

The views expressed in these volumes are those of the authors and are not to be construed as those of their institutions, agencies or organizations.

Section 1

Introductory Chapters

- 1 -

Introduction

Ralph Masi
Lynette Mensah
Keith A. McLeod

The shift in state policy to a multicultural policy in 1971 has been slow in affecting health policy, perspectives and practices. Several reasons have been advanced - the sheer cost of health care and of change; the lack of political and community control of health policy, institutions and organizations; the resistance of the health professions; the ineffectiveness of health ministries, their political leaders and the bureaucracies; and the domination of health by science and technology. However, there have been some changes in the direction of health policies and practices and these changes seem likely to continue and even accelerate as society contends with health issues related to ethnic, racial and cultural diversity and as the demography of Canada continues to change.

As outlined in the text as well as in the twenty-seven recommendations of the 1988 Report of the Canadian Task Force on Mental Health Issues Affecting Immigrants and Refugees, *After The Door Has Been Opened*, a great deal can be done to accommodate the ethnic, linguistic, racial and cultural backgrounds of Canadians in the health policy and practices. This Task Force and the Report marked a greater awareness of multicultural issues in health, in this instance mental health. Similarly, the 1991 Report of the Multicultural Health Curriculum Project Committee, *Cultural and Racial Sensitivity: Implications for Health Curricula*, identified a multitude of ways in which multicultural issues not only might but should be included in the education of health professionals. Among the specific areas it outlined that are crucial to care were knowledge, skills, and dispositions related to cultures and cultural values, intercultural communication, health behaviour, professional health care and racism and race relations. In introducing the discussion of these in relation to pluralism the report stated:

> The core concepts identified as essential components of any theoretical framework for multicultural health education, reflect primarily on the similarities and differences in perspectives and interpretation of relationships, interaction and communication patterns, and lifestyle and behavioral norms of people as cultural beings. A focus on political and socio-economic power, discrimination, racism, inequality, and stereotyping, must also be addressed as they capture many of the realities of living in Canadian Society.
>   ...The sole intent was to highlight the critical cultural factors which influence health and illness behaviour, and current approaches for the delivery of professional health care. (p. 47)

The above reports are but two current indicators of the awareness of the needs and the necessity of implementing multicultural health in the 20th century. This is not new. One of the editors of this volume, Dr. Ralph Masi, often quotes Hippocrates: "Observe the nature of each country; diet; customs; the age of the patient; speech; manners; fashion; even his silence ... one has to study all these signs and analyze what they portent."

BACKGROUND - DEMOGRAPHIC CHANGES

The immigration patterns to Canada have been changing gradually over the last century or so. From the 1860s to the 1960s Canada's immigration rate remained relatively constant in that one in six Canadians identified themselves as immigrants. The sources were primarily European.

However, the places from which people emigrated changed considerably starting in the mid-1950s. Whereas earlier 90 percent of the annual immigration to Canada had come from European sources, by the late 1980s 70 percent came from non-European or globally diverse origins such as South Asia, Southeast Asia, Central and South America, Africa and China.

The result is a society that is more racially, ethnically and culturally plural. For example, and to cite another dimension of the diversity, the percentage of Canadians that identify neither British nor French as their mother tongue has increased to approximately one-third. When the statistics are examined, there is no ethnic group that constitutes a majority.

The very real diversity that exists requires a better understanding of care issues in a pluralistic society.

DEVELOPMENT OF MULTICULTURAL CARE

The concept of multicultural health has been receiving increasing attention as health professionals and institutions seek to better address the needs of racial and cultural communities. Although there have been some significant developments and a better understanding of the issues now exists, there has often been insufficient information. There has also been some resistance by professionals, administrators, organizations, institutions and their boards to adjust to the pluralistic realities of the nineties even though the policy of multiculturalism was adopted in Canada some thirty year earlier, in October 1971 (see Canada, House of Commons Debates, October 8, 1971).

Since its founding in 1986-87, the Canadian Council on Multicultural Health/Conseil Canadien de la santé multiculturelle (CCMH/CSSM) has been instrumental in promoting a better understanding of the impact of cultures on health. In 1989 it sponsored the first national conference on *Multiculturalism and Health Care: Realities and Needs,* and in 1992 the second national conference, *Towards Equity in Health.* In addition it has:

- Established and published the newsletter entitled *The Multicultural Health Bulletin.*
- Published the proceedings of the first national conference; these have served as a resource guide to health professionals and community groups.
- Held many provincial workshops on such diverse topics as mental health and cultural communities, substance abuse and cultural communities, policy development, equity, seniors, and refugee and immigrant adjustments.
- Held a national consultation on AIDS and cultural communities.

There has been widespread influence upon other organizations as well among the institutions and agencies who have participated or whose employees have taken part. In addition, CCMH/CSSM has contributed substantially to or participated in other national initiatives in the area of multicultural health care. Some of these initiatives include:

- The 1988 National Workshop on Ethnicity and Aging.

- Active participation from 1988 to 1992 in the Multicultural Aging and Seniors Coordinating Committee which was formed subsequent to the Ethnicity and Aging Workshop.
- The Immigration and Refugee Health Needs pre-conference workshop held prior to the Canadian Public Health Association National Conference on "Cultures and Health" (1990).
- Participation in areas such as oral health, prevention issues for physicians, family violence, prescription drug use and the education of health professionals.

The work has been done nationally through the national organization, and provincially through the affiliates in each province.

There have been many general developments as well as specific initiatives across the country to identify, understand and develop changes that particularly address the racial and cultural diversity in our country. Organizations such as the Multiculturalism, Aging and Seniors, Coordinating Committee have been examining issues of ethnicity and aging; and the AIDS Cultural Network has been addressing diversity within the AIDS field. Community Health Clinics have developed which take a particular interest in the welfare of the diverse people in their community. Some provincial governments have taken steps to adjust policies and programs. And some institutions such as hospitals have developed a better relationship with all segments of their communities. There is more extensive research being done on diversity, prevention and care and there is a greater awareness of cultural needs, human rights, linguistic needs and equity issues.

For example, in Ontario, policy guidelines on the integration of racial and cultural awareness were adopted in 1991 by the Ontario Ministry of Health. Other provinces have undertaken similar initiatives. In Quebec, they have developed the ACCESSS Report, which is a policy framework governing equity of care for racial and cultural communities. In Newfoundland, the first compulsory component on pluralism and care has been incorporated in the nursing program at Memorial University. From British Columbia, the significant publication *Cross-Cultural Caring - A Handbook For Health Professionals in Western Canada* edited by Waxler-Morrison, Anderson, and Richardson has become a best seller for the University of British Columbia Press. A consultation on educational objectives on racial and cultural sensitivity for the health disciplines was successfully undertaken and the 1991 report on that consultation has been completed by the Canadian Council on Multicultural Health. The report of the Canadian Task Force on Mental Health Issues Affecting Immigrants and Refugees, *After The Door Has Been Opened*, (1988) mentioned earlier, has been a milestone in drawing attention to the needs of diverse people in the area of mental health.

GENERAL PURPOSE OF THESE VOLUMES

There has been a beginning but there is much that remains to be done, and much left to be accomplished. In these two books we are attempting to look at a number of issues from the diverse vantage points, disciplines, research, and experience of people from across Canada. Our primary focus is on health care for a pluralistic society; in other words, we are most interested in looking at health and care which is sensitive to the cultural, racial, and linguistic communities.

There are several terms used in the field that we define below in a generic manner. We have encouraged contributors to be consistent; however, the reader must always be prepared for variations regarding their use. The terms are outlined below.

TERMS AND QUALIFICATIONS

Terms

Multicultural health is defined as health care which is culturally, racially and linguistically sensitive and responsive. The definition includes concepts of ethnic and race relations, cross-cultural or transcultural health care; it also includes issues related to human rights and to equity.

The term **community** is used in reference to the group of people for whom the program or service is intended. From the context you will see whether the community is ethnically and racially or linguistically diverse or whether the text is focusing primarily upon a particular group.

Cultural refers to the way of life developed by a group of people and which members acquire. Cultural refers to that which is totally learned and it includes language, concepts, beliefs, and values, symbols, structures, institutions and patterns of behaviour. A person's culture may or may not be the same as his or her ethnic origin or identity. In a complex pluralistic world and in Canadian society, a person may have encountered a variety of cultural influences or perhaps, be the product of a mixed marriage.

An **ethnic group** is a group of people who share a common ancestry or history, and who have distinctive patterns of family life, language, values and social norms; above all they feel they are one people different from all other people. A person's ethnic origin, therefore, identifies him or her as having come from a particular group background; however, as we have indicated, he or she may have a somewhat different cultural identify as a result of having acquiring other cultural attributes.

Qualifications

Three important qualifications should be noted:

1. References to ethnocultural groups such as "Chinese" are intended to identify an ethnocultural background, not citizenship. Also, it must constantly be remembered that there is as much or more variation within a cultural group as there may be between groups or communities. Identity is complex. Within Canada we refer not only to ethnic groups but also to linguistic groups such as "the Spanish-speaking people," or to racial groups, such as "the Black community." A member of either of the specific aforementioned collectives could come from anywhere in the world and have a complex identity. Similarly, a collective group such as the Southeast Asians are diverse not only ethnically and culturally but also linguistically.

2. To allow for the discussion of issues, generalizations must be made. Generalizations should not be interpreted as representing characteristics applicable to all or, in some instances, even to most of the individuals within a group. Generalizations may, in fact, be completely inappropriate when applied to the individual or the circumstance. The application of generalizations in this manner constitutes stereotyping because they are over-generalizations.

3. There may be more similarities between the health beliefs or practices of different ethnocultural groups at the same socioeconomic level than there are among the people within the same ethnocultural groups who are from different socioeconomic levels. Although socio-economic factors contribute significantly to health beliefs and practices, they are largely outside the scope of these volumes.

ORGANIZATION OF VOLUMES

In organizing these publications we have divided the articles into eight sections. The divisions are functional and were established to give focus to the content.

The two volumes are as follows:

Volume I: Multicultural Health: Policy, Professional Practice and Education

1. Introductory Chapters
2. Policies and Theory
3. Professional Practice and Education
4. Research

Volume II: Multicultural Health: Programs, Services and Care

1. Introductory Chapters
2. Care
3. Programs and Services
4. Immigrants, Refugees and Health

The content of the sections are outlined below:

I-1) Introductory Chapters

These chapters introduce readers to the background of multicultural health in Canada and to its' concepts, principles, and applications.

I-2) Policies and Theory

The articles emphasize the broad institutional, organizational, and systemic changes which have been developed at the policy level to encourage better participation, access, or involvement of the racial, linguistic, and cultural communities within the health care delivery system.

I-3) Professional Practice and Education

This section will focus primarily on knowledge, skills and dispositions related to teaching and learning multicultural awareness and understanding within the health disciplines. It also includes chapters on the application of cross-cultural skills or knowledge in a variety of clinical settings.

I-4) Research

In this section the author highlights important research questions. However, the whole book points out the need for further research as it also demonstrates how research can assist practice.

II-1) Introductory Chapters

In this section the introduction in the first volume is re-printed for the benefit of readers who do not have access to both volumes. The section also contains a chapter which develops a paradigm for multicultural health care.

II-2) Care

The authors in this section focus on specific care issues within the context of health care directed primarily to cultural communities or other specific groups in a multicultural context.

II-3) Programs and Services

In this section the authors examine various programs, services and resources that have been developed by or within cultural communities directed towards improving health care.

II-4) Immigrants, Refugees and Health

In this section the authors look at various issues that immigrants, newcomers and refugees face upon arrival in this country and within the first years of settlement.

CONCLUDING COMMENTS

In Canada and other countries, including the United States, an elaborate literature on change and how it can be facilitated is developing. The need for the implementation of multicultural health is still great—there are human barriers to implementation, to equity and to providing more appropriate and better health care for all. In some instances the barriers present outright opposition. We suggest that you consult the literature on facilitating change. It is important that people within the health care sector—whether in government, the professions or the community—be part of the solution, not part of the problem.

- 2 -

Multicultural Health: Principles and Policies

Ralph Masi

The past decade has seen a significant growth in the awareness of and response to racial and cultural dimensions of health care. This growth has occurred as a result of an increased emphasis on various factors such as client-based care, community-based health concepts, and concern about the accessibility and availability of health care. It has also been influenced by Canada's changing demographics. Understanding the principles of multicultural health is a necessity if we are to address effective health care in our increasingly pluralistic society.

This chapter will contain an overview of the demographic changes of Canada's population, as well as of the principles and applications of multicultural health care. It will identify some of the racial and cultural factors that need to be considered within health programs and services. It will also examine some of the misconceptions or misunderstandings that reduce the effectiveness of interventions and the policy developments that have taken place.

THE CHANGING FACE OF OUR COUNTRY

Confederation was built on the concept of cultural plurality, and from the outset diversity was acknowledged to be integral to its continuation. "In our Federation," wrote Sir George Cartier, "We shall have Catholic and Protestant, English and French, Irish and Scotch. They are of different races, not for the purposes of warring against each other, but in order to compete and emulate for the general welfare" (Monet, 1992). This fact is often forgotten by many Canadians, who appear to believe that immigration and multiculturalism are relatively new concepts in Canada. The changes that we witness now are simply an accumulation of patterns that have long existed, but have only become more recognizable because they are affecting a larger percentage of our population.

The percentage of Canadians that identify themselves as foreign-born has not changed to any great degree since the time of Confederation (Canadian Task Force, 1988). During the years 1900-15, one in five Canadians identified themselves in this manner, a significantly higher ratio than today. Nor, as some believe, has there been a recent sudden shift in the percentage of individuals whose ethnic background is neither British nor French. There has been a gradual but steady increase in this percentage over the past 100 years, to the point where as of 1991, approximately one-third of the Canadian population identify their background as other than English or French (Statistics Canada, 1992).

All of the provinces in Canada are affected by these demographic changes. In 1991, a mother tongue other than English or French was reported by 13 percent of the general population (Statistics Canada, 1992). In some cities, this figure was significantly higher: Toronto reported 32 percent, Vancouver, 27 percent and Winnipeg, 21 percent (ibid.). Moreover, it is important to note that the sources of immigration to Canada have changed substantially. Prior to the 1950s, some 85 percent of immigrants came from European countries. Since the 1950s, this percentage has been decreasing to the point where it is now less than 15 percent. At present, the majority of immigrants to Canada come from various global locations such as Central and South America, East Africa, and South and Southeast Asia (Canadian Task Force, 1988). The net result is a global diversity of inhabitants whose cultural, socio-economic, linguistic and political backgrounds are substantially different from each other. Such diversity presents a significant challenge to anyone working within the health care field.

Canada is not alone in addressing these issues. Studies in England have been undertaken to examine the interaction of racial and cultural dimensions on health (Mares et al., 1985). The same is true of the United States, where the Task Force on Minority and Black Health was commissioned in 1985. Australia has established an Office of Migrant Health, which has been creating policies and encouraging the development of programs and services to respond to the diversity of the Australian population (South Australian Health Commission, 1988).

Interestingly, the findings of these international experiences coincide very well with the Canadian studies that have been done, such as the reports of the Canadian Task Force on Mental Health Issues Affecting Immigrants and Refugees (1988) and of the National Workshop on Ethnicity and Aging (Canadian Public Health Association, 1988), as well as of many other provincial reports and studies. There is a consistency in the findings of these diverse initiatives, which include the following:

- a stronger emphasis on community-based services
- greater representation of racial and cultural communities within the decision-making and planning levels of administration as well as within the health disciplines
- multicultural and cross-cultural components to health disciplines training
- programs and policies on qualified interpretation between client and professional
- information that is linguistically and culturally appropriate
- greater emphasis on participatory research related to issues involving ethnoracial communities
- recognition of the stresses involved in immigration or migration as significant factors in the health of individuals

MULTICULTURAL HEALTH: WHAT IS IT?

Health professionals will at times remark that they treat all client groups the same. Hence, they may further argue that there is no need for multicultural health because all people receive similar care. However treating people in the same manner does not mean that they are necessarily being treated equally. If we are to treat people equally, we must acknowledge the differences and respond to them appropriately.

This is the challenge of multicultural health care. How do we develop heath care that acknowledges racial and cultural diversities, yet still maintain a coordinated approach to overall health planning and services? To do so, we must examine the issues. They can be divided into two categories: individual and community (Masi,1988).

Individual multicultural health issues are those that primarily affect interactions between an individual client and a health
professional. Community issues are those that affect programs
and services for groups of people at a community level.

Individual Issues

a) Risk of genetically inherited disorders

Ethnic groups have differing predispositions to a variety of
conditions or traits that are genetically inherited. For example, sickle cell anaemia is more common among some
Black communities, thalassaemia among people of the Mediterranean area and Tay-Sach's disease among those of
Jewish background. Such conditions represent genetic traits
that are not common in the general population and tend to
be overlooked. Therefore it is important to understand
differing predispositions to some conditions among different populations.

b) Biological Variations

Eighty percent of the Southeast Asian population is lactose
intolerant as is a substantial percentage of the Black population. A lesser, but significant, percentage of the Native
Canadian and South European populations is similarly
affected (Bayless et al., 1975). Lactose intolerance is an
example of biological variations that health professionals
must consider when working with diverse ethnic groups.

There are also differences of height and weight (Leung,
1987), as well as of metabolism (Task Force, 1988) that
could affect the administration of some medications. For
example, Southeast Asian populations metabolize anti-
depressants at a different rate than do other groups (Task
Force, 1988). Failure to take into account such biological
variations might result in the administration of an inappropriate dosage of medication.

c) Mortality and Morbidity Risks

Differing populations may have a substantially different risk of some disorders and illnesses. For example, the risk for ear, nose and throat cancer among the Chinese community is substantially greater than in the white population (Harwood, 1981). Similarly the risk of cervical cancer is substantially higher for the Aboriginal populations (Freeman, 1989). The risk of hypertension in the Black community is twice that of a corresponding group from the white community (Spector,1985). If such factors are not sufficiently considered, it is possible that the needs of groups at higher risk for some diseases might be overlooked.

d) Verbal and Non-Verbal Cues

Clinical/professional interactions depend not only on the spoken word but also on body language. The issue is not simply one of translation: different cultures express themselves differently. Characteristics and mannerisms, if misinterpreted, may lead to difficulties in interaction. For example, some populations may, as a sign of respect, be more reserved. Others may be more expressive, and as a result may be considered angry or aggressive. Even simple gestures such as a handshake may be interpreted differently by a variety of groups. Non-verbal cues are strongly affected by cultural values and norms, and are an important consideration in the client/professional relationship.

Community Issues

a) Culturally Sensitive Health Information

There is a significant lack of health information available in languages other than English or French. Moreover, other considerations are also important. Materials must be acculturated in order to reflect the dietary and cultural norms of the communities. For example, their content must reflect vegetarian diets or diets for those who have specific food prohibitions such as pork or beef. Simple translation without acculturation severely restricts the usefulness of educational materials. Distribution is also an important consideration. Many health information distribution systems fail to recognize that the principle sources of information for racial/cultural groups include ethnic media, or immigrant serving agencies.

b) Hours of Operations

Many services operate during what are commonly considered "normal" working hours, that is Monday to Friday, 9 a.m. to 5 p.m.. For many immigrants/refugees who arrive in Canada, accessing services during these hours is prohibitive. Newer immigrants are often unable to leave work because of financial or job security. Similarly they may be unable to accompany other members of their family during these hours who require translation or other assistance to receive health care. Failure to provide more flexible working hours can thus result in barriers that inhibit access to programs and services.

c) Community Norms and Values

Culture is not static: it adapts over time to changing circumstances and situations. Norms and values that are acceptable in one decade may not be so in the next. For example, the spanking of children that was considered important earlier in this decade could now be considered child abuse. Similarly the treatment of women and the acknowledgement of womens' rights has substantially changed in our society over the past century.

Some members of cultural communities arriving in Canada have not had sufficient opportunity to understand the patterns of acceptable behaviour in Canada. What may be considered normal patterns of family life in their own culture may be totally inappropriate in Canada. While their motivation may be to maintain the quality of their family life and values, their disciplinary practices may come into conflict with what is acceptable in Canada. They often require a greater opportunity to understand and change.

d) Community and Individual Interactions

It is the norm in North America that the community is considered linked to, but distinct from, the family or individual. This means that health services may be focused on the individual, the family or the community. In contrast to this, many cultural communities consider the norm to be more analogous to concentric circles: the individual is not distinct but rather integrally connected to the family and even the community. For such groups, programs focused on the individual that do not acknowledge the family and the community may be disruptive and even destabilizing.

MULTICULTURAL HEALTH POLICY DEVELOPMENT

In 1991, the Ontario Ministry of Health passed policy guidelines that address racial and cultural diversity in health programs and services (Ontario, 1991). The guidelines were developed through a series of community consultations. More than simply stating policy, these guidelines provide specific considerations for making the concepts operational.

Since the acceptance of the guidelines by the Ontario Ministry of Health, they have been well received by many different groups. They are seen as providing a good basis for the development of pluralistic health care systems. The policy guidelines are appended at the end of this chapter as a guide for health planning for a racially and culturally pluralistic society.

COMMON MISUNDERSTANDINGS AND MISCONCEPTIONS

In recent years there has been an increased awareness and understanding of multicultural health. At the same time misunderstandings and misconceptions have arisen that hinder its development and that must be addressed (Masi, 1992). Some of the more common of these are outlined below.

Like Should Treat Like

It is occasionally stated (and perhaps more frequently thought) that a health professional ought to be of the same racial or cultural group as the client in order to be able to provide appropriate care. While health professionals of the same cultural group as the client may better understand the cultural norms, values and issues of the client, there are some inherent dangers in this argument. For example, there are many components that make up a client-professional interaction, of which racial or cultural background is only one. There are also others that significantly impact on the interaction, such as socio-economic status, education and religion. The professional should have an understanding of cross-cultural care and the client's needs. His or her personal identity should not be the primary consideration.

It should also be recognized that there is a subtle form of racism inherent in such an argument. It suggests that individuals should work primarily with those of their own ethnicity. This leads to the sort of belief that Caucasians should only be treated by Caucasians, Natives by Natives, Blacks by Blacks and so forth. This is not multiculturalism; this is stereotyping and racism. It suggests that the colour of one's skin is the principle consideration, rather than the knowledge, abilities and interests of the individual.

All or Nothing

It has been said that, given the more than 100 cultural groups in Canada, it will be impossible to learn enough about all of them to make multicultural care practical. Such a knowledge base is not required. The principles of multicultural health care call for a willingness to learn the particulars of a culture within the context of the needs of the location. The issue is not that the health professional should know everything about everyone.

Knowledge, Not Process

In recent years there has been an increasing demand by health organizations and professionals for information on cultural norms and values of specific groups. While such information is helpful, it can also encourage stereotyping.

Multicultural health calls for understanding the process of obtaining information rather than simply accessing sources of information. Professionals must understand how to obtain required information while interacting with individuals. They must be sensitive to the tremendous variations that exist between individuals of any one cultural group.

Cultural Differences Are a Problem

It has been stated by some that multicultural health is problematic for many professionals, that it is not needed or that it is an unwelcome burden. Multicultural care should be seen as a solution rather than a problem. At times we as professionals tend to overlook the purpose of our interventions. We are more likely to be able to help ease the suffering of individuals if we are aware of cultural influences on the healing process. A better understanding of cultural issues is therefore indicated.

All Behaviours Must Be Acceptable

Some cultures have norms and values that are simply unacceptable to Canadian society. Practices such as female circumcision, wife abuse and others that are accepted by some cultures become difficult management issues for Canadian health professionals. Within the context of multicultural health care, must professionals accept such behaviour? The answer is emphatically no! However, the question still remains whether or not the health professionals have really understood the difference between behaviour that is morally unacceptable according to the norms and values of one individual and that which is legally unacceptable within the context of human rights in Canada.

Consider, for example, the issue of blood transfusions. In the past, some health professionals have argued that it is their responsibility to provide blood transfusions in order to save a life, even if it is against the wishes of the adult client. Is the refusal to accept blood in this situation morally unacceptable, or is it legally unacceptable? Similar questions are involved in the provision of abortion services.

As well, there is the issue of whether or not the health professionals sufficiently understand the specific practices or behaviours. For example there have been instances where children have been referred to the Children's Aid Society because of a misinterpretation of marks and scratches that result from the harmless Southeast Asian practice called "Scratching The Wind." Scratching The Wind is a benign cultural practice in which a cup is heated and gently applied with its rim to the skin. As the cup cools it create a vacuum and suction on the skin, resulting in a small bruise. Often a coin may also be used to lightly scratch the skin to allow for the exit of harmful spirits or toxicants. The marks of other similar North American practices such as the use of a mustard plaster are more recognizable by health professionals. It is highly unlikely that the Children's Aid Society would be called in such instances. Understanding the practices is thus the key to successful treatment.

It's All Up to the Health Professional

At times health professionals complain of the difficulties that they must overcome when they have to work with clients of different racial or cultural backgrounds: for example, they may complain of difficulty in obtaining interpreter services, or in getting sufficient information from clients. What such profes-

sionals often overlook are the difficulties that the clients themselves have had to overcome in simply presenting themselves
for assistance. Many of the client groups are in lower socio-
economic income brackets and can ill afford to take time off
work or to encounter significant problems negotiating such
things as registration processes simply because of lack of flu-
ency in one of the national languages. While it is true that an
effort is required on the part of the health professionals, there is
also an equal or greater effort that is necessary on the part of the
client to access the services, programs or care.

One Culture, One Group

There are those who would argue that the racial or cultural
background of clients is the most significant factor in understanding the health needs of individuals of differing ethnoracial
backgrounds. This argument overlooks the fact that there are
probably greater similarities between different cultures at similar socio-economic levels than there are within the same cultural
group at different socio-economic levels. Racial background and
cultural norms and values are simply some of the aspects of a
person that are likely to have a greater impact on a person's
overall health status than is his or her ethnic identity. Issues of
age, gender, time of migration, education, and others are similarly important variables that have a significant influence on the
health of an individual.

Cultural Sensitivity: Either You Have It or You Don't

Some faculties of health disciplines have commented that
cultural sensitivity relates to a student's personal character; that
is, it is more an inherited quality than it is a teachable skill. While
it is undoubtably true that some students are more empathic or
have greater communication skills than others, it is also true that
we can facilitate the cross-cultural skills development of any
student through a properly structured educational process. It is
important that we set standards of care and educational objectives in order to provide the framework for multicultural health
for students and professionals in the health disciplines.

Generalizations Are Unacceptable

Some are concerned that applying generalizations to groups
is equivalent to labelling the characteristics of all individuals
within a particular group. To suggest that no generalizations can
be made within cultures is also to suggest that there is no such

thing as culture. Culture is generally defined as shared values or norms; there are some characteristics that can be identified with particular groups. At the same time we must be very sensitive that generalizations must not be not applied to individuals without careful consideration of the other dimensions relating to that individual. Otherwise, generalizations become stereotyping, which is unacceptable.

It is also important to recognize what factors we are trying to address when we apply descriptive statements to particular groups. For example, if we comment on "Southeast Asians," the only commonality is a geographic one. Within what is commonly described as the Southeast Asian area, there are many cultural and linguistic groups that are substantially different from each other.

Many individuals identified as "Black" come from diverse backgrounds, ranging from fifth- or sixth-generation Canadians to New Canadians from the Caribbean, East Africa, including Somalia, Kenya and other diverse global locations. These individual groups may have very little in common other than skin colour.

Generalizations must thus be used with caution and sensitivity; at the same time some generalizations are necessary if we are to provide a structured understanding and approach to common issues, concerns and needs.

CONCLUSION

The purpose of this chapter has been to provide an overview of the issues, principles, and policies of multicultural health. Understanding multicultural health care will simplify the task of health professionals as they attempt to provide effective health care within a pluralistic context. Multicultural health should be a fundamental concern of any health professional working within the Canadian context.

REFERENCES

Bayless T.M., Rothfeld B., & Massc, et al. (1975). Lactose and Milk Intolerance: Clinical Indications. *New England Journal of Medicine, 292,*1156-9

Canadian Public Health Association. (1988). *Ethnicity and Aging: The Report of the National Workshop on Ethnicity and Aging.* Ottawa

Canadian Task Force on Mental Health Issues Affecting Immigrants and Refugees. (1988). *After The Door Has Been
Opened*. Ottawa: Multiculturalism and Citzenship.

Freeman, H.P. (1989). Cancer in a socio-economically disadvantaged. *CA. -A Cancer Journal for Clinicians, 39*(5), 266-87.

Harwood A. (1981). *Ethicity and Medical Care*. Cambridge, Mass.:
Harvard University Press.

Leung, A.K.C., Siu, T.O., Lai, P.C.W., Gabos, S., & Robson,
W.L.M. (1987). Physical Growth Parameters of Chinese
Children in Calgary. *Canadian Family Physician, 33*; 396-
400.

Mares, P., Henley, A., Baxter, C. (1985). *Health Care in Multiracial
Britain* Cambridge: Health Education Council & National
Extension College Trust Ltd.

Masi, R. (1988a). Multiculturalism, Medicine and Health: Part II:
Individual Considerations. *Canadian Family Physician , 34*,
69-73.

— —. (1988b). Multiculturalism, Medicine and Health: Part II:
Community Considerations. *Canadian Family Physician,
35*, 251-54.

— —. (Ed.) (1989). *Multiculturalism and Health Care: Realities and
Needs*. Toronto: Canadian Council on Multicultural Health.

— —. (1992). Communication: Cross-Cultural Applications of
the Physicians Art. *Canadian Family Physician, 38*, 1159-65.

Monet J. (1992). A Multicultural Canada, Then and Now. *Com-
pass, 9*(6), 21-23.

Ontario Ministry of Health. *Let's Work Together*. Policy Paper.
Ministry of Health, 1991.

South Australian Health Commission. (1988). *Migrant Health
Unit*: Adelaide: The Commission.

Spector R.E. (1985). *Cultural Diversity in Health and Illness*. Nor-
folk: Appleton-Century-Cross Press.

Statistics Canada. (1992). *Ethnic Tongue Data 1991 census of the
Population*. Ottawa: catalogues No. 93-313 and 93-315.

ONTARIO MINISTRY OF HEALTH
MULTICULTURAL HEALTH GUIDELINES

1. Identification of the Community

Health care organizations serving the community should recognize the diversity within the community and its component cultural/racial populations. There are differences within and among cultural/racial populations, including specific disadvantaged groups, which must be acknowledged if appropriate services are to be developed.

Considerations

* Have all populations within the community, including disadvantaged groups, been appropriately identified?
* What are the basic demographics of the target communities and their populations (i.e., demographics including age, sex, socio-economic status, education, as well as cultural/racial composition of the community as a whole)?
* What is the migration/immigration history and patterns relevant to the community?
* Have there been specific health issues that stem from an ethnocultural basis identified within the community?

Example

Health care organization programs and services that acknowledge and identify the percentage of new immigrants and populations within a catchment area, the cultural/racial composition of the community, and any specific health issues related to ethnocultural background.

2. Policy Statement/Commitment

Health care service organizations should establish an intention to serve the entire community in a statement of objectives, or in a policy or position statement. Any program or service intended to address specific cultural/racial needs should also identify its purpose.

Considerations

* Do the policies of the organization/agency planning the service establish a responsibility to provide equitable and accessible programs or services to all cultural/racial populations of the community in its catchment or service area?

- Is there a policy statement of accessibility or equity of care included in the by-laws and mission statement?
- What mechanisms are proposed to encourage community participation in all stages of the planning, delivery, and evaluation of the program or service?

Example

Health care service organizations that include in the planning process a policy statement governing the organization and its program and services, to meet the needs of all community populations within the entire organizational operation, and within any proposed programs/services, as an embodiment of its policy.

3. Participation and Representation of the Community

Health care service organizations should establish participation and representation from the various community populations they serve at the earliest stages of developing programs and services, and through the implementation process.

The representation may be individuals identified by the community to represent or express its concerns. Members of the organization's Board or Council, or the membership of the organization/agency, may emanate from and reflect the diversity of the community.

It must also be recognized that there are some groups within populations that may be especially disadvantaged and that will require specific attention to ensure that participation in the planning process (e.g., immigrant and racial minority women, seniors, etc.).

Considerations

- Which groups or individuals identified the need for the service/program?
- Which groups or individuals are involved in the planning?
- At what stage of the planning have the community representatives been involved?
- What is the sponsoring organization or agencies' relationship or involvement with the communities being served?
- Has there been an effort to identify specific disadvantaged groups and to include them in the planning process?

Example

Health care service organizations that solicit the support of community groups or representatives in planning stages, or community groups that work with health organizations or institutions to develop needed services.

4. Community Support

Health care service organizations should elicit the support of the community through appropriate approaches. If programs and services are to be effective in meeting needs, they should be supported by the community. Expressed support through such methods as a community consultation process should be solicited prior to the commencement of programs or services.

Considerations

• What form of community support has been solicited and given (e.g., financial donations, fundraising, formal recognition/liaison, volunteer efforts)?

Examples

Letters of support for proposed programs or services from individuals or from organizations having ethnocultural or multicultural representation. Provisions for ongoing involvement, such as a community consultation process, also help maintain community support.

5. Ongoing Community Liaison

Once established, programs/services should include some formal vehicle within the organizational structure for communities' ongoing representation and participation in decision making.

Considerations

• Is there a commitment from senior management and staff to appropriate ongoing community participation?
• How is ongoing community participation provided for and encouraged in the decision-making process?
• What is the nature of the financial controls? Has there been appropriate resource allocation to support effective community participation, and multicultural policy and program initiatives?
• What are the parameters of community participation in the decision-making process?

- Is there a communication strategy proposed internally to promote better understanding of community involvement and to assist the implementation of changes?

Example

Health care programs and services that establish Community Advisory Committees, to monitor ongoing operations and participate within a defined process with agreed upon parameters.

6. Necessary Cultural and Linguistic Components

Health programs and services should be sensitive and responsive to differences in cultural values, norms and practices, as well as to different linguistic needs. To serve communities equitably, programs and services must respond to the cultural norms, values, practices and linguistic diversity of the community.

Considerations

- Which languages will be provided for, and how?
- How will programs or services reflect cultural norms and values and needs of the community?
- How will client information be collected to identify linguistic/cultural/ethnic variables?

Examples

Programs or services that have identified a translation policy, or that will provide for translation/cultural interpretation, and are sensitive to religious or dietary differences within the community.

7. Staffing Practice and Training

The principles of equity should be reflected in all employment practices of all programs and services of health care service organizations. This would include recruitment, hiring, performance appraisal, promotion and the provision of a harassment-free work environment. In addition, staff should be afforded opportunities for training and development to improve their knowledge and responsiveness to cultural and racial sensitivity.

Considerations

- How does the program or service provide for the hiring of a cultural/racially representative staff at all levels of the organization?

- What specific continuing education/in-service training programs will be made available for the cross-cultural education of the health care providers?
- Are cross-cultural or race relations skills part of the assessment and evaluation criteria of the performance appraisal process?
- How will the organization establish accountability for equity measures, and will there be a penalty for nonperformance?

Example

Health care programs or services that utilize the skills of staff representative of cultural/racial groups at both management and staff levels, and that provide specific cross-cultural training and education opportunities for all staff.

8. Co-ordination Across Organization Programs and Services

Ongoing interaction and co-ordination with programs and services should be established with other systems, programs and services. In an environment where many cultural community needs are being met across a variety of areas, co-operation and co-ordination with other programs and services minimizes duplication to effort and fragmentation of services. Furthermore, such co-ordination can allow for improved longer-term/strategic planning across areas, as well as provide the flexibility to meet changing needs in the community as shifts in demographics and/or changes in health needs emerge.

Considerations

- What will the program or service contribute to the existing service network?
- What interactions, liaisons or integration with other service areas will be needed for the functioning of the program or service?
- Is there a system of referral for ancillary or related programs and services in place?
- Will there be cross-over or sharing with other organizations/agencies?

Example

Programs and services serving cultural/racial needs that establish interactions/linkages with the array of existing services, such as home-support services, public health services, multicultural service agencies, etc.

9. Evaluation

Evaluation should be an integral part of any program or service. To assess the degree of effectiveness of a program or service for cultural/racial sensitivity, responsiveness and accessibility, community involvement in the evaluation process must be a significant component.

Considerations

- Has the community been invited to participate in defining the measures of success, developing the tools for evaluation, and the preparation of the final report?
- Is there a mechanism in place to ensure the ongoing monitoring and evaluation of the program to reflect the needs of current populations or community?
- Will the community have easy access to evaluation information?

Example

A health care service organization that uses, for example, a Community Advisory Committee that could participate in the overall design and analysis of the evaluation process for the program or service. Use of such a group could ensure that all communities have an opportunity not only to voice their comments, but also to be informed of the results of the evaluation and the changes that will be made.

PROPOSAL REVIEW CRITERIA FOR CULTURAL/ RACIAL SENSITIVITY AND AWARENESS IN HEALTH CARE PROGRAMS AND SERVICES

Purpose of the Proposal Review Criteria

A set of criteria has been developed to rate the cultural and racial sensitivity of health care program/service proposals. These criteria can assist Ministry staff in assessing and reviewing proposals in terms of their cultural and racial sensitivity and responsiveness.

Identification of the Community

1. To what extent are demographics identified in the proposal; i.e., age, sex, socio-economic status, education level, cultural/racial composition, first language preference, length of residence, etc.?
A) Extensive data are available (full demographic information).
B) Moderate data are available (adequate but not extensive information).
C) Minimal data are available (less than adequate information).
X) Data not provided.

Policy Statement/Commitment

2. Does the policy of the health care service organization proposing the program/service acknowledge its responsibility to provide equitable and accessible service to all cultural/racial communities in the service area?
A) The policy is stated clearly and is known by others.
B) There is an intention to develop policy.
X) Policy is not addressed in the proposal.

Community Participation

3. Have the proposers of the program/service established mechanisms that include community participation in the (i) planning, (ii) delivery, and (iii) evaluation of the program/service?
A) The community participates in all three components.
B) The community participates in 2 components.
C) The community participates in 1 component.
X) The community does not participate.

4. In planning the proposal, were community groups involved in (i) identifying the need, (ii) developing plans, and (iii) proposing the service?
A) Community groups were fully involved in all 3 components.
B) Community groups were involved in 2 components.
C) Community groups were involved in 1 component.
X) Community groups were not involved.
Identify the community groups involved in each component.

Community Representation

5. To what extent does the composition of the board and the executive of the program/service reflect the cultural/racial composition of the community?

A) Full representation as an established mechanism for community participation.

B) Partial representation, with some means of obtaining community input.

C) Some degree of representation, but no systematic means for obtaining community input.

X) No provision for representation or participation.

Cultural and Linguistic Components

6. What provisions have been made to provide the program/service in languages other than English/French for both translation and cultural interpretation?

A) Program/service proposes to use the resources of in-house staff, fee-for service, or available materials/resources to meet languages translation/interpretation needs.

B) Many considerations are given to program resources and language translation availability.

C) Few considerations are given to program resources and language use.

X) No provision for language translation or cultural interpretation given.

Staffing Practice

7. To what extent is the cultural/racial composition of the community served reflected within the organization management and at all staffing levels?

A) Fully, at all levels of staffing.

B) Moderately well, within most levels of staffing.

C) Minimal cultural/racial staffing.

X) Staffing issues not addressed.

8. Are cross-cultural skills and racial diversity acknowledged as important factors when selecting and developing staff and management personnel?

A) These are considered necessary in the selection and development processes.

B) These are desired in the selection and development processes.

C) These are minimally considered in the selection and development processes.

X) Not acknowledged.

Co-ordination Across Organization Programs and Services

9. How does the proposed program/service link and co-ordinate with similar programs/services of other organizations?
A) Interactions, liaisons and service integration are established, and co-ordinated initiatives are fostered.
B) Some interactions, liaisons and service integration have been considered.
C) Minimal external interaction has been developed. The service plans to operate independently.
X) Possible linkages to other program/services are not addressed.

10. How receptive are other health care service organizations to the proposed service/link and plan for co-ordination?
A) Other agencies fully support, and plan to link with and co-ordinate services.
B) Other agencies are somewhat supportive and intend to later link with the proposed service for co-ordination.
C) Other agencies are not resistant but do not see the need to link or co-ordinate with the proposed service.
X) Co-ordination is not addressed.

Evaluation

11. To what extent will community groups participate in defining evaluation criteria and assessing that the service provides what is needed?
A) Full participation and consultation in evaluation process, with ongoing involvement and full access to data.
B) Moderate participation and consultation in evaluation process, upon request, with less than full access to data.
C) Minimal involvement, with the expectation that information would need to be sought.
X) Community group involvement was not addressed.

- 3 -

Transcultural, Cross-Cultural and Multicultural Health Perspectives in Focus

Lynette Mensah

Values, beliefs and perceptions about health are culturally determined; the relationship between culture, health and illness has long been recognized to be culturally shaped. In this chapter we shall consider and put into focus the three perspectives of transcultural, cross-cultural and multicultural health. These terms are often used independently and sometimes interchangeably when discussing culture, health and health care. From each vantage one can propose culturally sensitive care. Each describes a number of similar sentiments about the provision of such care. But what precisely is meant by these varying descriptions of care, health and culture? Are they the same? Do each of these concepts speak to different aspects or components of the same phenomena? The precise meaning of these three concepts has often been perplexing to health professionals and the large community alike. In this chapter I endeavour to bring a measure of clarity and coherence to the three concepts. My purposes are to delineate and examine the context of each with reference to the meaning of culture and ethnicity within the health field, and to challenge health professionals to see a new paradigm for health and culture.

CULTURE

It is important at the outset to situate oneself by examining several views which describe culture and ethnicity. Culture is a term which has various definitions in the literature, each reflecting different theoretical concepts. Logan and Semmes (1986) note that culture is a pervasive phenomenon: it colours one's attitudes, values and beliefs about the world and affects one's interactions with the world. Leininger (1977) defines culture as the common collectivity of beliefs, values and shared understandings and patterns of behaviour of a designated group of people. Logan and Semmes (1986) note that in its simplest form, culture is a distinctive way of life that characterizes a given community; it is the shared practices, beliefs, values and customs that are passed down from generation to generation. Each person is born into a family unique in its cultural characteristics which shape behaviourial development. From one's lived experiences as a member of a cultural community it is evident that there are rules that govern behaviour. These are learned through verbal and non-verbal interaction within the family and community. Cultural rules are normatively implied from the behaviours within the group; people sanction what is acceptable and what is not. It follows, therefore, that should the rules be broken, this can cause feelings of discomfort.

Spelman believes that whereas culture refers to learned patterns of behaviour, culture is also a way of life that encompasses the ideals of a given group, their folklore, science, religion, philosophy, the ethos of a people as well as the norms which govern morality, interpersonal relationships, the family and social institutions. Also included are the verbal and non-verbal behaviour and such material habits as dress codes and food habits. Ogburn and Nemkoff (1950) identify additional components of culture, such as the communication system and artistic expression, religious and magical beliefs, basic human patterns such as competition, conflict and cooperation, societal controls and the customs and laws which provide us with an understanding of the universality of culture. Yet culture is not stagnant, but rather it is dynamic, adaptive and within limits permits individual freedom of self-expression, thus allowing for social change to accrue.

Gardner and McMann (1976) see culture as a process through which is articulated the meaning found in our experiences; it is what we come to think of as the meaning of life. Culture therefore provides a prescription for daily living and decision making.

Furthermore, it is through cultural conditioning that people learn to think well of themselves and of the values and beliefs that give substance, stability and meaning to their lives. For some cultural groups, many aspects of culture may be so highly valued by its members that these are considered to be right and not open to questioning. It is undoubtedly a truism that the schema of culture affects how one perceives health and illness and when and from whom one seeks health care. In many cultures, folk healers or other individuals are consulted for advice and treatment of illness.

The question of ethnicity is an important link in the cultural chain and requires exploration. The concept of ethnicity is complex; however, the primary characteristics include common geographic origin, language and religion. But, it is much more than these: ethnicity colours the way a person or group perceive and experience life and emotions as well as health and illness. Ethnicity also describes a sense of community transmitted over generations by families.

Fienstein (1982) describes that aspect of ethnicity as peoplehood, a sense of commonality or community derived from networks of family relations which have over a number of generations been the carriers of common experiences. In short, ethnicity in this sense means the culture of a people and it includes the values, attitudes, perceptions, needs, and the modes of expression of identity and behaviour, whether or not we are conscious of our ethnic identity.

Ethnic identification may often be seen as an internal sense of distinctiveness and/or an external perception of distinctiveness. Ethnic affiliation with a value system and with those people who shape that system provides members with a comfortable sense of security, belonging and understanding. As Henderson and Primeaux (1981) note, ethnicity is an interactive process through which individuals share their lives with like others; they feel a sense of identity and common fate. Masi (1992) says that an ethnic group is seen as sharing a common ancestry of history and has distinctive patterns of family life, language, values and social norms. It is not surprising therefore, that ethnic groups vary in the way they view illness and health and how healing takes place. For example the orientation of Western medicine, which is predominantly of Anglo-Saxon origin, is to treat a diseased organ. In contrast, a Native American orientation is to view illness and disease as a lack of harmony with nature. Their approach to health care is to treat the whole person and to include the active participation of the family, the neighbours, and the community.

Even though culture and ethnicity are often used interchangeably within the realm of health care, Lynam (1991) cautions us to be aware of this folly. She points out that one's cultural roots can have a basis that is not solely determined by ethnicity. Similarly, sharing the same ethnic background does not necessarily mean sharing the same culture. We also need to be clear that ethnicity differs from race, in that racial background refers to a person's specific physical and structural characteristics such as skin pigmentation, stature and facial features. These characteristics are transmitted genetically. On the other hand, ethnic identity is a function of socialization.

The marriage of culture and ethnicity to the analysis of the context of health and health care has given birth to the transcultural, cross-cultural and multicultural paradigms of health and health care as determined by the social context in which one lives. As Kleinman (1978) notes, as medical systems are part of social and cultural systems. Furthermore, culture and ethnicity play an integral role in the interactions between the recipient of care and the providers of care.

In the beginning of this chapter I noted that confusion sometimes exists in the language used in describing the relationship of health and culture because there is ambiguity and misunderstanding about the three concepts (transcultural, cross-cultural and multicultural). What emerges from a review of the health literature is that there is a general agreement on the underlying goal of all the concepts. That goal is the provision of culturally sensitive care. However, there is less agreement about what each concept truly represents. The following analysis will assist or challenge health professionals to examine the meaning of each concept.

TRANSCULTURAL CARE

Transcultural health care—what is its nature, purpose and goal? What does it mean? According to the proponents of the transcultural concept, the focus is based upon a comparative study and analysis of different cultures with respect to their caring behaviour, health and illness values, beliefs and patterns of behaviour. The term "transcultural" focuses on human care, and the health and environmental contexts (Leininger, 1978). The essence of the concept is that helpers have a knowledge and understanding of (or the skills to understand) the beliefs, values, lifeways and practices of cultural groups so that helpers can provide care to all. From a transcultural perspective, the knowl-edge base is drawn largely from anthropology, the humanities and other social sciences. The focus is upon the care-giver. The transcultural approach enables the provider of care to recognize and understand the values, beliefs and health practices of di-verse cultures and to provide care in a culturally sensitive and appropriate manner, which includes acceptance, addressing concerns, identifying universal traits, understanding and knowl-edge of the group's cultural values and one's analysis of their own role and behaviour. Transcultural is the language often used in health care and more specifically within the nursing discipline.

CROSS-CULTURAL CARE

The nature of cross-cultural care is based on the assumption that the client and the professional helpers are of different cultural backgrounds. For example, the helper may be a majority group person drawn from the dominant culture, while the client comes from a minority. This approach recognizes the utilization of ethnographic information in the planning, delivery and evalu-ation of services for minority and ethnic groups clients. The cross-cultural approach reflects a primary focus of applying anthropological concepts and research findings to the disci-pline. In essence, the cross-cultural approach to health care seeks the provision of culturally sensitive care by those who are responsible for the operations and functioning of health services in cultural communities. Cross-cultural language is often used in health care and more specifically within the discipline of social work. The focus is upon the care.

MULTICULTURAL CARE

The multicultural health concept recognizes a major weak-ness and gaps in the two preceding perspectives. The multicultural health perspective further explicates and devel-ops the construct of health and cultures as it relates to the Canadian experience. This view is shaped by our environment, including the organizational and societal processes. This ap-proach in Canada is directly related to the nature or reality of Canadian society and to the Multicultural Policy of 1971.

Multicultural health is defined as health care which is both culturally appropriate and culturally sensitive. Masi (1990) says this definition includes concepts of ethnic and race relations; it does not refer to health care focused on a particular cultural community; it seeks to provide a structured and integrated approach to health care. The goal is broad as culturally appropriate sensitive health care includes cultural and racial sensitivity and awareness in health care programs and services, both at the institutional and community level. In other words, **systems change** is critical to address in order to be responsive and effective. The focus is upon the total health system. The multicultural health ethic incorporates racially and culturally sensitive, responsive and acceptable care for all populations within the community. It takes into consideration the linguistic, racial and ethnic factors as they relate to health and health care. Concomitantly, the multicultural health approach does not fragment services; rather it makes them more effective and applicable to a broader range of groups. Not only are concerns for cultural, ethnic and racial needs paramount in this approach but the overriding principle is equity in terms of access for all persons regardless of their racial or cultural background. These services should exist within a universal access system.

The multicultural health concept brings a broad and comprehensive approach to the arena of health and culture; it supports the underlying elements of care being provided in a culturally sensitive and appropriate context as espoused by the transcultural and cross-cultural perspectives, but it also brings to the forefront critical underlying or systemic issues such as equity with reference to access and participation to institutions, programs and systems in health care.

Multicultural health philosophy does not refer to health care focused only on a particular cultural community. That does not provide a structured and integrated approach to health care; it is by far more inclusive.

Throughout this text reference is made to the fact that today in Canada we are increasingly aware of the varied cultural and racial groups who comprise the demography of Canada. This is a pluralistic society which is officially recognized through the adoption of our multicultural policy and subsequent legislation. This entrenchment of multiculturalism within Canadian society brings to the fore the need to multiculturalize all systems, including the health care system. The multicultural health concept recognizes the importance of ethnic, racial, religious and cultural factors in facilitating or impeding health care of individuals and families. It helps us to focus upon the discrepancies between the community's needs and the health care agendas of organizations, institutions and professionals in responding to the pluralistic realities that exist in Canada today. A challenge is before us and is being proposed to the same institutions, professionals and cultural communities in the Canadian context. There is a need to recognize the limitations of the perspectives of transcultural and cross-cultural health care which embody a limited view of the relationship of health and culture. We can adopt the more comprehensive and inclusive multicultural health perspective. This vision of health care is uniquely Canadian. The objective is to promote equity in health care especially with reference to systems change.

More changes are needed. For example, change is needed in education in the way we prepare our future health care providers, and curricula change is needed so that multicultural health issues are appropriately and formally addressed. These changes should be integrated in the system and not treated as an afterthought, or addendum. The key principle here is a reorganization or modification of current health policies, programs and services to take into account the linguistic, racial, ethnic and cultural features of Canadian society. There is opportunity now to be proactive. We have a clear vision of the changing demography, and if we are committed to provide the best in health care, much can be done within the confines of our current expenditures on health to institute corrective action. Health professionals and the health care system can change and keep pace with and plan change to serve the diverse communities of Canada. Change requires altering old coping patterns and ways of doing things which are no longer effective. The thrust should be to confront old and new needs, demands and problems.

For practising health professionals, it is timely to take pluralism or diversity into account, to re-examine the important role culture plays in how people view and make decisions about their health. We all need periodically to re-examine our own cultural and professional biases, and to be cognisant of the current diversity in the communities we serve.

At the institutional level, as communities, agencies and organizations seek to better address the health needs of our pluralistic society, change needs to be based on an increase in cultural awareness. This could be the starting point for engendering equity. Successful structured system changes will mean change in the way we communicate with programs, and in how services are planned and developed.

The perspective of multiculturalism identifies a responsibility on the part of those who are given the mandate to develop health goals and policy to be alert and not to ignore the nature of the community. This will require the inclusion of input of cultural and ethnic groups early in the process; full participation at the inception of issues and policies is critical if health care is to be effective and efficient.

The concept of multicultural health has been in the forefront in Canada in recent years, and even though considerable work has been accomplished in this direction, there needs to be further work to implement the concept. The multicultural health perspective as delineated challenges care providers and the health systems to ensure all health care allows full access. This is what multicultural health is truly about.

REFERENCES

Anderson, J. (1986). Ethnicity and illness experience: Ideological structures and the health care delivery system. *Social Science and Medicine, 22*(11).

Feinstein, O. (1982). Why Ethnicity. In J.M. Anderson, O. Feinstein and I.A. Smith (Eds.) *Ethnic America:* A book of readings. Michigan: To Educate the People Consortium.

Goodenough, W.H. (1966). *Cooperation in Change.* New York. Russell Sage Foundation.

Henderson, G. & Primeaux, M. (1981). *Transcultural health care.* Menlo Park, CA: Addison Wesley.

Kleinman, A. (1978). International health care planning from an ethnomedical perspective: Critique and recommendations for change. *Medical Anthropology.* 2.

Krech, D., Crutchfield, R.S. Ballachey, E.L. (1962). *Individuals and Society.* New York. McGraw Hill.

Leninger, M. (1978). *Transcultural Nursing: Concepts, theories and practices.* New York. John Wiley and Sons.

Leninger, M. (1977). Transcultural nursing: A promising sub field of study for nurses. In Reinhardt, A. & Quinn, M. (Eds.) *Current Practice in Family Centred Nursing.* St. Louis. CV Mosby.

Lipson, J.G., Meleis, A. (1985). Culturally appropriate care: The case of immigrants. *Clinical Nursing, 7*(3).

Logan, B. & Semmes, C. (1986). Culture and Ethnicity. In B. Logan & C. Dawkin (Eds.) *Family Centred nursing in the community.* Menlo Park. CA.: Addison Wesley.

Lynam, J. (1991). Taking Culture into account: A challenging prospect for cardiovascular nursing. *Canadian Journal of Cardiovascular Nursing*, Vol. 2., No. 3.

Masi, R. (1992). Communication: Cross-Cultural Applications of the Physicians Art. *Canadian Family Physician, 38,* 1159-65.

Spelman, S. (1981). High risk considerations throughout the life span. In C.O. Helvie (Eds.) *Community health nursing theory and process.* Philadelphia. Harper & Row.

Section 2

Policies and Theory

Introduction

As Canadians we have generally accepted the following concepts: that health services should be universal; that the ethnic, racial and cultural background of the clients or communities are important; and that equity and equality of care are of value. How these principles translate into policy governing health care, services and programs has not yet been well defined. The acknowledgement of racial and cultural components as part of all health interventions is sometimes poorly understood.

There have been many approaches or initiatives undertaken in the field of multicultural health. Some have been very successful; others have not fared so well. Sometimes the reason for the failure is the lack of system support for the initiatives, or a poor understanding of how the endeavours fit within the context of the broader health care system. If theory, education, care, programs and services related to multicultural health are to be successful in the long term, they must be supported by policy which integrates these issues within a more global framework, and by administrative as well as human and financial resources.

In this section we have featured authors who have made contributions toward the recognition of general multicultural health policy within the health programs and services, and in some chapters there is specific application of those policies within the operational structure.

- 4 -

The Montreal Children's Hospital: A Hospital Response To Cultural Diversity

Heather Clarke

Most Canadian hospitals were founded at a time when the majority of the country's population was of European origin. Today, the population is increasingly diverse, a fact that is reflected in the growing cultural and linguistic diversity of hospital clientele and staff. As a result, the institutions now face many special challenges. Front-line professionals may encounter difficulties overcoming the cultural and linguistic barriers that arise between themselves and their patients. Managers may find that traditional management styles and techniques do not necessarily represent an effective method of working with or motivating a multicultural workforce. Administrators may become aware that hospital policies and practices need to be re-examined in the context of the evolving hospital community. All parties are constrained by budgets that permit few new expenditures.

The difficulties that result from such factors can have a major impact upon hospitals, and may at first appear to be insurmountable. However, it is both necessary and possible for institutions to respond. The present chapter is designed to share some of the experiences and enthusiasm that has been generated at The Montreal Children's Hospital as it has attempted to meet the needs of its culturally diverse staff and clientele. The chapter reviews past developments and future plans, and outlines some of the lessons learned by the hospital since it initiated its Multiculturalism Programme.

MULTICULTURALISM PROGRAMME
THE MONTREAL CHILDREN'S HOSPITAL

1. History

The Montreal Children's Hospital is a 214-bed tertiary-care paediatric hospital affiliated with McGill University. It provides more than 185,000 consultations per year and receives up to 450 patients in emergency daily, making it one of the busiest paediatric hospitals in North America. An estimated one-third of the patients speak French as their first language, one-third speak English and the remainder use other languages in the home. The more than 2,000 staff members come from over 45 ethnic groups and speak more than 50 languages and dialects.

Interest in multiculturalism at The Montreal Children's Hospital began when front-line staff members expressed the need to know more about the different cultures of their patients. In March 1984, the Clinical Staff Advisory Council, a body comprised of all of the paramedical professionals in the hospital, established a work group on multiculturalism whose task it was to determine the staff needs and how they could best be met. They began by inviting a few speakers from key cultural communities to address the staff. Within a year, the work group had evolved into a standing committee on multiculturalism that was composed of five physicians, five paramedical professionals and a representative of the hospital administration. In 1986, a grant was received from the Secretary of State to establish a hospital-wide Multiculturalism Programme that was to serve as a pilot project in the Canadian hospital sector. This Programme became an integrated part of the Hospital in 1991 and is funded from the institution's global budget.

2. Objectives

The main objectives of the Multiculturalism Programme are as follows:
- to encourage the understanding of and respect for cultural values, beliefs and practices throughout the hospital community;
- to develop resources and educational programs that will assist the hospital in meeting the needs of its culturally diverse community;

- to enhance the liaison between the hospital and the cultural communities both by promoting use by the hospital of community resources and by encouraging community participation in the hospital; and
- to promote cross-cultural sensitivity in other health and social service institutions.

The services that are offered include cross-cultural staff development opportunities such as workshops, seminars and colloquia; coordination of interpretation services within the hospital; information, consultation and referral services; the organization of, and participation in activities with a cultural community focus; and the operation of a multimedia lending library that specializes in cross-cultural issues in health care and intercultural education.

Over the years the importance of multiculturalism within the hospital has grown. The original committee, which at first monitored the growth of the Programme, later worked to facilitate communication between the Programme and the hospital staff. With the appointment of departmental representatives to act as liaison people, this committee was disbanded and replaced by the Multiculturalism Steering Committee, which reports to the Executive Director. The hospital's Mission Statement now declares that the institution is committed to "understand, respect and reflect the cultural and linguistic diversity of the community it serves".

Meanwhile, the Quebec government has been trying to adapt health and social services to meet the needs of the changing population. In May 1989, the Ministère de la Santé et des Services sociaux du Québec (MSSSQ) announced its aims and action plan entitled "Accessibility of Services to the Cultural Communities". This was followed in March 1990, by a similar plan at the regional level, which identified 40 institutions in the Metropolitan Montreal region that would, in turn, develop institutional plans. In May 1991, the Board of Directors adopted The Montreal Children's Hospital's plan to enhance accessibility of services to the various cultural communities. This plan was subsequently approved at the regional level by the Conseil de la santé et des services sociaux de la région de Montréal Métropolitain (CSSSRMM), the body coordinating health and social services in the Montreal area, and finally it was submitted to the MSSSQ for its approval. Such a lengthy process might at first seem excessively bureaucratic; it is, however, evidence of the Ministry's commitment to the realisation of its objectives.

Here are the highlights of the hospital's plan:

- to maintain the services of the Multiculturalism Programme in a cost-effective manner;
- to develop human resource initiatives that will attract candidates from the different cultural communities and will ensure that hiring, promotion policies and performance evaluations are free from discrimination;
- to adapt patient and cafeteria menus so that they reflect culturally diverse dietary preferences;
- to increase collaboration between the hospital and the cultural communities so as to stimulate the creation of partnership initiatives;
- to elaborate institutional communications policies that reflect and respect the cultural diversity at the hospital;
- to increase the amount of written information available to the clientele in different languages;
- to foster closer collaboration between the hospital and the universities and colleges in order to ensure that students benefit from their experience in a multicultural setting; and
- to improve the structure of existing cross-cultural staff development activities and develop an educational program that facilitates sequential learning.

As can be seen, cross-cultural sensitivity is a concern that is not limited to the Multiculturalism Programme alone but is becoming an integral part of the institution. The following is an account of some experiences setting up the Programme at The Montreal Children's Hospital that may be of benefit to other institutions that wish to embark on a similar process.

ESTABLISHING THE MULTICULTURALISM PROGRAMME

First Steps

Each institution is unique and has its own special needs and concerns. At The Montreal Children's Hospital, as in many hospitals, individuals at different levels throughout the institution felt that they were not equipped to meet the challenges posed by the growing cultural diversity of staff and clientele. As already noted, at The Montreal Children's Hospital, the concern was first voiced at a meeting of the Clinical Staff Advisory Council (CSAC). Without really planning it, the speech therapist who spoke at that meeting had selected the ideal forum. CSAC had the credibility and the network needed in order to generate hospital-wide support. Once the issue had been raised, CSAC established a multiculturalism work group, which canvassed direct patient-care personnel to determine their needs and then invited speakers from ten communities to address staff concerns. However, it also saw that the increasing cultural diversity of staff and clientele would have a major effect on the institution. It thus raised the issue again in another important forum, during the hospital's strategic planning process. Again the subject was well received. This time the result was the establishment of a new standing committee on multiculturalism composed of members of CSAC, the Council of Physicians, Dentists, and Pharmacists and the hospital administration.

Setting Goals

In the enthusiasm of embarking upon a new project, it is natural to want to move quickly. Since the person that was hired in 1986 to develop The Montreal Children's Hospital Multiculturalism Programme came from outside the institution, the process there began slowly. The coordinator had to begin by learning about the hospital and its clientele. However, even when the individuals or groups spearheading the initiative are familiar with the hospital, it is important to allow time to conduct a needs assessment, a crucial first step in order to identify realistic and appropriate goals for the Programme. This requires an examination of the context in which the initiative is to take place: the internal context (the institution itself) and the external context (the social and political environment in which it is located). One can begin by asking several questions:

For the internal context:
- Is multiculturalism a priority?
- How diverse is the staff?
- How diverse is the clientele?
- What languages are spoken by the staff and clientele?
- What cultural or racial groups are present?
- Are there tensions between groups?
- How is the institution structured?
- What efforts are already being made to make services accessible and appropriate?
- What attempts are made to respond to the diversity of staff and clientele at the management and administrative levels?
- What goals and needs related to cultural diversity have already been expressed?

- What financial and human resources are available?
- Who is in favour of the initiative?
- Who is against it?

For the external context:

- What is the cultural, racial and linguistic composition of the surrounding area?
- Are there tensions between groups?
- Are there other similar programs or initiatives elsewhere?
- What are the community resources that might be utilized?
- What are the municipal, provincial and federal government priorities and policies?

By studying the context, it is possible to determine the degree of change required and the factors that operate for or against the achievement of this change. At The Montreal Children's Hospital, there were several positive and negative forces that had to be considered. (Table 1)

The information obtained was subsequently taken into consideration in planning the Programme. Although the initiators had not set out to conduct a formal force field analysis, they have since learned that this is, in effect, what they had done. As a result, they suggest that this can be an excellent planning tool. A force field analysis consists of five steps:

1. Determination of what needs to be changed.
2. Identification of negative and positive forces that may influence change.
3. Prioritization of forces.
4. Decision regarding which forces are to be influenced.
5. Creation of an action plan.

3.   Creating a Plan

In designing a plan at The Montreal Children's Hospital, it was decided that an effort should be made to maximize the positive forces. The first step was to utilize the knowledge and the influence of the Multiculturalism Committee. Committee members took every opportunity to speak about the Programme and personally introduced the new coordinator to key individuals throughout the institution. The Programme had been assigned an office in an isolated corner of the hospital. The Committee was instrumental in having the office moved to a high-traffic area where it would be accessible to all staff.

Table1
The Montreal Children's Hospital, 1986

Positive Forces	Negative Forces
Favourable political climate	Lack of financial commitment on the part of the hospital
Culturally diverse staff and clientele	Absence of paid time for staff to attend sessions
Approval of the Executive Director	Scepticism on the part of some who saw no need for the program
Support of political bodies within the institution	Fears that the program might lead to stereotyping
Active Multiculturalism Committee with links to many departments	
Multidisciplinary interest	
Hospital Mission Statement recognizing diversity of clientele	
Family-centred approach to care	
Pride in institution's reputation as an innovator and teaching hospital	
Initiative looked upon favourably by the community and other institutions	
Financial support of the Secretary of State	

Secondly, the Programme had to develop credibility and establish the importance of the issues it was to address. This was done first by identifying respected individuals throughout the hospital who took the culture of the patients into consideration when working with them and then by drawing attention to such efforts. Two additional benefits of this tactic were, first, that it legitimized and encouraged the work of these staff members and second, it demystified the idea of cross-cultural care for other staff.

Meanwhile, action also had to be taken to counter the four negative forces mentioned earlier. First, the lack of sources of provincial funding for institutional initiatives in cross-cultural and race relations in the health sector promised to be a long-term problem as Secretary of State support was only granted on a temporary basis. The Quebec government saw funding for the needs of the cultural communities as a responsibility of the Ministère des Communautés culturelles et de l'immigration du Québec (MCCIQ). Thus, the Programme had to demonstrate not only that it was important to the hospital but that its work should legitimately be funded by the MSSSQ. The problem was resolved by submitting a development project to the MSSSQ. The argument was made that the ministry could maximize the benefits of the pilot initiative at The Montreal Children's Hospital by helping the Programme build upon and share its experience with others. The result was a commitment for three years' funding.

The second obstacle was that staff members were given little time for education or development activities of any kind. This meant that the activities of the Programme would have to compete for attention with other educational opportunities both inside and outside the institution. In order to ensure that activities would be well attended, the hospital staff were canvassed to determine their needs, and Programme activities were then tailored accordingly.

A third negative force was scepticism on the part of some members of the institution concerning the importance of cultural issues. The Programme took a non-confrontational approach to this problem, trying to entice people to become interested and to demonstrate the benefits to be gained by considering cultural issues. To counter the belief that there was no real commitment to multiculturalism and that the Programme would consist mainly of "song and dance", events focused on displays of folklore were completely avoided for the first two years.

Fourth, the fear that the Programme would lead to stereotyping was allayed by stressing not only differences but also similarities. A concerned effort was made to point out that people of different origins may have much in common and that, at the same time, there is great diversity within each cultural and ethnic group.

ACTIVITIES OF THE MULTICULTURALISM PROGRAMME

Staff Education and Development

The Programme had four main spheres of activity: staff development, interpretation, community liaison and documentation. The Multiculturalism Committee and the coordinator of the Programme decided that staff education and development were the first priority. This is still a major part of the Programme. In the 1990 - 91 fiscal year, educational activities within the hospital accounted for more than 1,470 participant hours. There are plans to build upon the activities that are already being offered and where possible, to create new opportunities that will allow for progressive learning. Given the educational role of the hospital, an increasing effort will be made to collaborate with college and university professors in order to create mechanisms and structures that will allow students to draw maximum benefit from their placements in a multicultural setting.

Any education and development activities must be geared to suit the needs of the particular institution and the population that is targeted. At The Montreal Children's Hospital, it was important to determine and choose speakers and workshop leaders who were appropriate for the sessions being offered. It was also necessary to plan sessions that used a variety of different types of format, educational methods and resources. Based upon the hospital's experience, the following six categories of activity were found to be particularly effective:

1.   Orientation Sessions

A presentation on multiculturalism was included during the orientation programs for new employees that were offered within the hospital. This introduced new staff to the cultural diversity that was present and to the impact that this might have on their work within the institution. These sessions also served to make new employees aware of the resources available through the Multiculturalism Programme and to recruit interpreters. Such presentations are effective since they require a minimum of resources and reach a captive audience.

2.   Presentations in existing educational programs

With a limited budget, existing educational programs such as the many regularly scheduled rounds in the hospital could provide a ready-made forum for the presentation of cultural issues. The fact that these issues were addressed in such a respected context also lent them added credibility.

3.   Intercultural seminars

Short presentations or seminars were used to raise awareness of cultural issues, as well as to provide a forum for discussion. The present intercultural seminars that are held at the hospital grew out of the first series organized in 1984. They are still offered as lunchtime sessions that are available to all staff and are videotaped for the Multiculturalism Programme library. However they differ in several ways from the initial presentations. In 1984, the Work Group tried to find "community representatives" to give cultural portraits of specific groups. This presented two problems. First, few people felt prepared to be the spokesperson for their entire community. Second, the extensive list of questions that presenters were asked to address in a one-hour session led them to speak in generalities. This, and the fact that speakers were introduced as being "representatives" of their cultural groups, tended to lead to sterotyping on the part of the participants who failed to see the diversity within the speaker's culture. Today, before each session, participants are reminded of the fact that great variations exist within any group and are told that speakers will be sharing their own particular experience and knowledge. Over the years, an increasing amount of attention and time has been allocated to the proper selection and briefing of presenters and to the focusing of topics. The seminars now take the form of panels, discussions or formal talks by health care professionals, academics, cultural community workers or clients.

4.   Mini-workshops and workshop series

Given the limited time available for staff development, it was found necessary to offer some short workshops that were one to three hours in length. They addressed such issues as cross-cultural communication, working through interpreters and cross-cultural interviewing. Where necessary, multiple sessions were also developed to deal with different aspects of a single topic, such as the series Culture and Patient Care. This allowed for in-depth learning over a period of several weeks.

5.   Major workshops

Major workshops were also offered that varied in length from one to several days and were tailored to meet the needs and learning styles of particular groups. Such workshops went beyond the point of simply providing information, they also helped participants to recognize their own culture and that of their professions and to understand the impact that these cultures had upon their work. The experience revealed that it is unlikely that any one cross-cultural facilitator will be appropriate for all groups of staff members (managers, nurses, doctors, housekeeping personnel, etc.). It also showed that workshop leaders had to be well briefed about the institution and the needs of the participants in order to be able to offer sessions that were effective.

6.   Departmental sessions and series

Particular departments or clinics sometimes had specific needs that could best be addressed within the departmental context. In recent years, the Programme has been offering more individual sessions and workshops at the departmental level to respond to the particular needs of the staff engaged in nursing, human resources and housekeeping, among others. It is predicted that as expertise increases within the various target groups, the Multiculturalism Programme will gradually become less active and will play an advisory role. In fact, a number of physicians and other professionals are already incorporating cultural considerations into their own teaching, both inside and outside the institution.

Interpretation

Even when resources are very limited, a great deal can still be accomplished in the area of interpretation. At The Montreal Children's Hospital, the number of interpreter requests is considerable. In 1992-93 fiscal year, the Multiculturalism Programme was able to arrange 873 interpretations for a total of 36 languages and dialects. Since 1986, consultations with staff, other institutions, interpreters and community groups have led to improvements in the structure and functioning of the hospital's interpretation service. Interpretations are now coordinated by the Multiculturalism Programme which has access to more than 150 staff members who, when necessary, leave their place of work to interpret, as well as to selected individuals and organizations in the cultural communities. When requests are received, interpreters are selected in accordance with the linguistic and cultural knowledge required for each case. Two sets of guidelines have been developed, one for interpreters and the other for staff using their services. Departments are encouraged to post the procedure for obtaining interpreters beside the telephone. These changes and the cross-cultural interpretation training offered by the Programme have greatly improved the service. Meanwhile, the Régie régionale du Montréal-Centre, formerly the CSSSRMM, is developing a regional interpreters' bank. The Montreal Children's Hospital is not only participating in the pilot phase, it is also acting in an advisory capacity to the regional board throughout the process.

Multiculturalism Library

It is likely that those responsible for any multicultural initiative will begin early in the project to collect materials that might be of use to others within the institution. This is the moment to develop a filing or cataloguing system that will continue to be workable as the collection grows. The Multiculturalism Library at The Montreal Children's Hospital is a sub-library of the hospital's Medical Library. It includes both printed and audio-visual materials on different cultures and on cross-cultural health care. Almost all of its holdings are catalogued by the main library. The only exception is the articles in the vertical file that are cross-referenced in a card file in the sub-library. However, there is a problem in employing the main library cataloguing system in that the categories generally used for culture and cultural issues are limited. Thus, it proved necessary to add more detailed themes to the sub-library card files. Meanwhile, cataloguing items through the main library can make the collection available, not only to staff, volunteers and students working within the institution, but to others via the interlibrary loan system.

Community Liaison

The community can be a valuable resource. Cultural community organizations provide services that complement those of the hospital. They can also be a source of speakers, interpreters, resource people and referrals to professionals who are able to communicate in the language of the clientele. However, community groups are notoriously underfunded and their generosity must not be abused. In return, a hospital can help community groups to advertise their events and their services. At The Montreal Children's Hospital, special tours are given to immigrants; space is provided for distribution of community newspapers, and organizations are invited to access the resources of the Multiculturalism Library and to attend cross-cultural seminars and workshops.

In serving a multilingual clientele, it is sometimes essential to provide materials in languages other than English and French. A staff survey conducted in 1990 showed that, although some such materials existed in the hospital, they were still limited in number and the quality of the translations was not always appropriate. There are now plans to establish a special committee to review existing materials and to make recommendations regarding revisions and acquisitions. An important source of information about the resources that are available will be the resource listing that was first drawn up by the Affiliation of Multicultural Societies and Services of British Columbia, and later revised and expanded by the Multicultural Health Coalition of Ontario.

Another important aspect of community relations is ensuring that the members of the cultural communities find themselves reflected in the institution. Thanks to the collaboration of schools and community groups, there are approximately 12 children's art displays each year in the main registration area of the hospital. Visitors to the hospital are welcomed in 46 languages by means of a mural inside the entrance. They also see the racial diversity of the staff and clientele reflected in images throughout the institution. Communication policies soon to be developed will ensure that not only the environment but the materials distributed to parents, the items sent to the media and the internal audiovisual presentations reflect, as much as possible, the diversity of the hospital community.

There are other policies and practices that need to be scrutinized. They are the ones that go beyond image and govern the daily life of the institution. The Montreal Children's Hospital has committed itself to examine its hiring policies, promotional practices and performance evaluations to ensure that they are free from systemic discrimination and that they do not contain discriminatory elements that might be prejudicial to members of certain cultural or racial groups.

NETWORKING

No hospital should work in isolation. A great deal can be learned from other hospitals. It is impossible to note all of the initiatives that are now being taken in Canadian hospitals but it is important to mention a few. In Vancouver, the Mount Saint Joseph Hospital is taking a "top down" approach aided by committee attached to the board. The Winnipeg Children's Hospital has established a training program for its native medical interpreters. In Toronto, Doctors Hospital has developed close ties with the surrounding multi-ethnic communities; the Hospital for Sick Children has a well-developed interpretation service; Mount Sinai Hospital is known for its Chinese outreach program and Central Hospital prides itself on its multicultural care. In Montreal, several hospitals are working to approve accessibility of their services including Hôpital Sainte-Justine which like The Children's is a paediatric institution.

In the development of the Programme at The Montreal Children's Hospital, it also proved useful to examine work conducted outside the hospital sector. Among the cross-cultural initiatives that were particularly relevant were those of the Children's Aid Society of Metropolitan Toronto, the United Way of Greater Toronto and the Ottawa and Vancouver police forces. Meanwhile, since the process of multiculturalizing an institution is one of effecting organizational change, many of the same challenges and obstacles that were faced by other institutions, such as Quebec's Ministère des communications which was introducing office automation, were encountered.

Since its inception, the Programme has found it necessary to keep abreast of the rapid changes in the field of cultures and health. This it does via participation and collaboration in various conferences and other activities. Networking is also made possible by membership of Programme, or its staff, in a number of organizations and committees devoted to cultural issues. This has brought the Programme to collaborate closely with organizations such as the Canadian Council on Multicultural Health and its provincial affiliate (Conseil de la santé multiculturelle - filiale du Québec), l'Alliance des communautés culturelles pour l'égalité dans la santé et des services sociaux, the Center for Research Action on Race Relations and, at the provincial government level, with the MSSSQ. As a result, The Montreal Children's Hospital has come to be seen as a leading advocate in the cross-cultural field.

CONCLUSION

Over the years the Hospital has come to understand that not only does adaptation to cultural diversity take a great deal of time, it necessitates embarking on a process of institutional change that affects not only service delivery but institutional policies, procedures and practices. Among other things it involves the development of cross-cultural education and development for staff at all levels, the elaboration of appropriate interpretation services, the gathering and sharing of resources, the development liaison between the institution and its community, networking with other institutions and acting as an advocate for multicultural change.

Any interested in establishing a program similar to that in Montreal will be pleased to know that a manual is being prepared based upon the experience at The Montreal Children's Hospital. Enquiries can be directed to:

Multiculturalism Programme
The Montreal Children's Hospital
2300 Tupper Street, Room C-108
Montreal, Quebec
H3H 1P3

SUGGESTED READING

Canadian Council on Multicultural Health. (1992). *Health Care for Canadian Pluralism: Towards Equity in Health.* Toronto: Canadian Council on Multicultural Health.

Québec. Gouvernement. (1989). *Accessibilité des services aux communautés culturelles: orientations et plan d'action 1989-1990.* Québec; Bureau des services aux communautés culturelles, Ministère de la Santé et des Services sociaux du Québec. Québec: Gouvernement du Québec.

— —. (1986). *Guide d'implantation de la bureautique.* Québec; Direction de la coordination interministérielle. Direction des communications. Ministère des communications. Gouvernement du Québec.

Multicultural Health Coalition. (1992). *Multicultural Health Resource List.* Toronto: Multicultural Health Coalition.

Thomas, Barb. (1987). *Multiculturalism at Work.* Toronto: YMCA of Metropolitan Toronto.

United Way of Greater Toronto. (1988). *Multiculturalism Works: A Guide to Organizational Change.* Toronto: United Way of Greater Toronto.

— —. (1991). *Action Access Diversity! a guide to multicultural/anti-racist organizational change for social service agencies.* Toronto: United Way of Greater Toronto.

- 5 -

A Changing City: The Response of the City of Toronto Department of Public Health

Maria Lee
Maria Herrera

The City of Toronto Department of Public Health has adopted the Mandala of Health as the model to be followed for developing public health programs in the city (Figure 1). This model is based on the concept that a person's health is significantly affected by many complex interactions between the individual and his or her particular family, community and culture.

The Mandala also emphasizes the importance of understanding the demographic characteristics of the city's population. Toronto is, and will remain, a major reception area for new Canadians. Over the years many different ethno-racial groups have made the city their home. For example, a large number of Vietnamese refugees arrived in Toronto during the early 1980s; many Tamil refugees came to the city after the massacre in Sri Lanka in 1983; Somalian refugees have been among the more recent arrivals. In basing its health policies on the Mandala, therefore, the Department of Health has had to recognize such population shifts and to respond to the growing racial and cultural diversity within the city.

Commitment to a multicultural health policy was first articulated by the Department of Health in 1978, when it published a report that recognized the importance of culturally and linguistically appropriate programs, and of citizen participation in public health programs (Toronto, 1978). In 1988 it adopted the

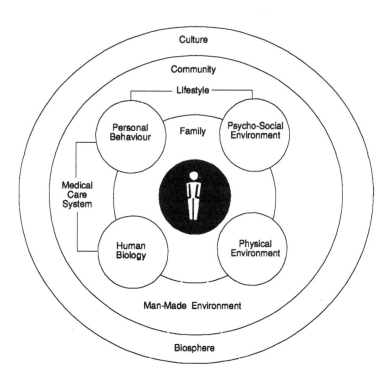

Figure 1: The Mandala of Public Health

policy outlined in *Healthy Toronto 2000—A Strategy for a Healthier City* (Toronto, 1988). In this publication multiculturalism is identified as one of three priority areas for the department: "In view of the cultural diversity of Toronto, our efforts must be culturally appropriate and directed to those communities with the greatest inequalities...Each of the Department's programs will reflect the Department's three priority concerns...to reduce inequalities in health...to meet diverse cultural needs...to empower individuals and communities."

COMMITMENT OF DEPARTMENT OF PUBLIC HEALTH, CITY OF TORONTO

A Multicultural Task Force on Access to Services was formed in May 1988 with a mandate to examine how the Department of Health policies and procedures impacted on the accessibility of public health services to all ethnocultural and racial communities of Toronto. The Task Force was made up of senior management personnel from all the disciplines represented within the Department and reported directly to the Department Management Team. The Task Force presented the *Report on Multicultural Access to Public Health Services* in March 1990. This report outlined the multicultural values of the department and the objectives of its multicultural policy. It also made recommendations for actions to address outstanding issues with respect to multicultural access. The report was approved by the Board of Health, which is a standing committee of City Council and is responsible for setting policies for the Department of Public Health.

The Department's initiatives would not have been successful without the strong support of the Toronto City Council. In January 1987, City Council approved a multicultural policy and an implementation strategy in its report *Multicultural Access to City Services*. This report endorsed a review of policies and procedures that present barriers to the cultural communities. The city's Multicultural Access Program was subsequently put in place and became a source of support and a resource for the Department's own multicultural programs.

AREAS OF ACTION

The areas of action to improve access to public health were clearly articulated in the *Report on Multicultural Access to Public Health Services*. This report becomes the blueprint for many multicultural initiatives in the Department. It was stated that the mission of the City of Toronto Department of Public Health is "to enable all people in the City of Toronto to be as healthy as they can be." In order to ensure that the Department's programs are accessible and relevant to persons of all races and cultures, the following multicultural values were defined:

1. All City of Toronto residents have the right of equal access to health care services, regardless of ethnic origin or linguistic skills.
2. It is the responsibility of the Department to provide culturally and linguistically appropriate public health services.
3. Department staff and management structure should strive to reflect the city's ethnic composition through equal opportunity initiatives.

4. The Department is committed to working with community groups to address issues of poverty, unemployment, discrimination and racism, which affect the lives of many people and are barriers to access to health.

Moreover, the Department has made a commitment to achieve the following: develop a capacity to communicate with the many cultures in Toronto using languages and materials that are culturally sensitive and at the appropriate literacy level; provide services that are culturally appropriate, and have a workforce that is flexible and reflects the ethno-racial diversity of people in the city; collect data and conduct research in issues related to culture, race and health in order to identify gaps in health programs. It should develop appropriate promotional programs and aim to foster an environment in which the department and/or community groups can assist each other in developing culturally appropriate health care.

The Department has identified certain areas where action is desirable, but there are impediments that need to be removed before the goals of the department can be met. The following is an outline of the major initiatives.

Recruitment and Hiring

There are several barriers to having a workforce that reflects the cultural and racial diversity of people in Toronto. Sometimes it is hard to match the needs of the various cultural groups with staff of particular language skills because there is a lack of skilled personnel in that community. The terms of the existing collective agreements and union contracts may also inhibit hiring new professionals. Foreign-trained professionals who might be well qualified for such positions often have difficulty acquiring the necessary Canadian credentials. To overcome these barriers, the Department has planned to work with the city's management services in the following areas:

1. to complete a job inventory to identify present and future vacancies that are not restricted by licence requirements, as well as positions that would be enhanced by language and cultural skills;
2. to re-evaluate job interview methods to ensure that there are no cultural biases;
3. to develop an aggressive outreach program in the various cultural and racial communities (advertisements for jobs would be placed in multicultural media);

4. to provide scholarships and loans to unlicensed profession-
    als to obtain further education and receive Canadian creden-
    tials; and
5. to advocate for increased flexibility in hiring people for
    contract positions.

Staff Training and Orientation

The Department provides three levels of training for all its
staff. First level; promotes general awareness of multicultural
health issues. Second level; develops work-specific/culture-
specific training; and third level; provides in-depth training on
racism, human rights and on how to manage a multicultural
work force.

Succession Planning and Equal Opportunity

The Department is planning to update its succession and
career-pathing reports and help supervisors acquire the skills
that are necessary to counsel staff in career-pathing and development. As well, the Department will develop a plan to hire
people who are from diverse cultural and racial backgrounds
within the licensed disciplines of public health nursing, inspec-
tion, medicine and dentistry. The plan will also include jobs not
restricted by licence requirements.

Data Analysis and Database Development

There are several challenges in the area of database development and analysis. First, there is a dearth of health data on
ethno-racial communities. Second, there is a need for the Department to develop a policy in this area, since such data when
acquired will have to be analysed by persons who appreciate the
sensitivity of statistics related culture and race.

Health Promotion

The health promotion strategies identified by the Department
and the Board of Health that are integral to the Department
programs include health advocacy, community development,
health education, media promotion and community relations.
Policy papers have been written on both health advocacy and
community development and strategies to implement the recommendations will be developed by multidisciplinary work
groups.

For health education, the Department has developed a protocol to ensure that printed health education materials are relevant both as to literacy and culture. The protocol involves focus
group testing with various sectors of the communities to ensure
health messages have been appropriately translated.

On the subject of media promotion, the Department aims to establish stronger links with the media, an important source of information to ethno-racial communities, and so that the Department and the media can work together in disseminating health awareness and information.

In the area of community relations, the department has participated in community events such as Caribana and the Kensington Festival. Participation not only increases the Department's profile with the communities, but also enhances the communities' receptivity to health messages.

Use of Foreign-Trained Professionals and Paraprofessionals

There is a need for flexibility and creativity in personnel policies in order to access the knowledge and expertise of foreign-trained professionals. As already mentioned, the Department will work with Management Services and the union to develop a policy that would make this possible.

Representation on Community Health Boards and the Board of Health

The community health boards provide the links between the community, the Board of Health and the Department of Health. At present, there is an inadequate representation from members of ethno-racial communities on these committees. The Corporation of the City of Toronto encourages adequate representation on these boards as well as on all the other committees of the corporation.

Networking at the Municipal, Provincial, National and International Levels

The Department will continue to network with all levels of government and with other countries to enhance opportunities to learn from the experiences of others. It is also important for the Department to articulate its policy regarding international visitors and international health projects.

New Immigrant and Refugee Policy

There is a need for all levels of government agencies to have a coordinated approach in assisting new immigrants and refugees. At present, the relevant municipal departments, provincial ministries and federal departments do not have a coordinated approach to provide support to the new Canadians. The Department of Health will develop a strategy so that it receives from Immigration and Health and Welfare Canada notification of the arrivals of immigrants and refugees, especially of groups that are at high risk. The Department will also work with other city departments to develop protocols to ensure effectiveness and efficacy of the programs.

Interpretive Services

The Department has acquired the services of a non-profit community organization to provide staff with cultural interpreting services. As well, the department will work with the City Clerk's Department to make better use of the language skills of the staff. A screening mechanism for language ability will be developed and a protocol will be put in place.

RESOURCES REQUIRED

A coordinated approach and effective planning is necessary to ensure accessibility and appropriateness of all health programs for the City of Toronto. Various resources both at the corporation and the Department levels are needed to ensure effective delivery of such programs:

- Cultural interpreters should be used for health education classes, community consultations and Board of Health meetings
- Members of the ethno-racial communities who review and proofread translated forms and materials must be recognized and compensated
- Advertising space should be purchased in multicultural media to provide information on health issues
- All staff should be given training on issues related to race, culture and health. Audio-visual training materials, fact sheets and training manuals should be produced to assist in the training and orientation programs
- Multicultural resources should be acquired such as audio-visual teaching materials, books and tapes
- Multilingual health education materials should be produced
- A multicultural health database should be established
- The staff and resource needs for each Health Area should be assessed

- Scholarships or interest-free loans should be provided to enable foreign-trained professionals to return to school and obtain Canadian licences and credentials.

SUMMARY

The City of Toronto Department of Public Health has made considerable progress in addressing the needs of the ethno-racial communities in Toronto. It is attempting to implement a coordinated and planned approach to multicultural health strategies that will not only enhance the Department's past initiatives but will ensure incorporation of multicultural considerations in all the Department's existing programs and services. The Department recognizes that all these efforts take time and need appropriate resources; that strategies are multi-sectoral, multi-faceted and multidisciplinary; that there should be commitment from management, staff and the community; and that there should be a strong political will to accomplish the designated goals.

Only in this way will truly accessible and relevant public health programs be achieved.

REFERENCES

Toronto, City of. Board of Health. (1978). *Public Health in the 1980s*. May. Toronto: Board of Health.

— —. (1988). *Healthy Toronto 2000--A Strategy for a Healthier City*. September. Toronto: Board of Health.

— —. (1990). *Report on Multicultural Access to Public Health Services*. Toronto: Board of Health.

— —. Department of Health. (1984). *Career Pathing and Succession Planning in the Department of Public Health*. December. Toronto: Board of Health.

— —. (1986). *Equal Opportunity Action Progress Report*. December. Toronto: Board of Health.

— —. (1991). *Putting Words to Work: A "How-to" Guide for Staff*. Toronto: Board of Health.

- 6 -

First Nations Peoples in Urban Settings: Health Issues

Chandrakant P. Shah
Gloria Dubeski

This chapter is dedicated to the Late Dr. Gloria Dubeski who committed her life to humanity by engaging in international work in underdeveloped areas of the world.

The obstetrician and a medical student were seeing patients in a downtown medical office. One of these patients was a Native woman with heavy vaginal bleeding. An examination led to a provisional diagnosis of gonococcal endometritis; a hemoglobin level done in the office yielded a shockingly low value of less than 5 g/dl (normal range 12 to 14 g/dl). The medical student could not understand why the patient had not come in sooner, nor how she could sit so quietly without complaining in the waiting room. The diagnosis of a sexually transmitted disease, however, did fit in with the student's impression of Natives, even though she had not treated Natives before. The obstetrician, seemingly a kind and professional practitioner, then instructed the patient to take a bus the six miles or so to the hospital where she would be admitted. It was obvious the woman was unfamiliar with the city, and had no knowledge of the city buses. The student felt ashamed, thinking that a non-Native patient would have travelled immediately by ambulance, but did not say anything.

As health care workers, most of us have dealt with Native patients in our training or practice. Thus, we can think back to our own experiences, as has one of the authors (Dubeski) in the above example, to examine our attitudes toward Native patients. We can ask ourselves how much we actually know about their circumstances, and how much we have sought to learn. This author was able to recognize that her reactions at the time were based on a negative stereotyped image of Natives, which were not only uninformed, but discriminatory. For many of us, it has taken the events of Meech Lake, the Oka crisis, Aboriginal land claims and recent constitutional negotiations to focus our interest on Native concerns; yet we still fail to take any active steps to educate ourselves about people of the First Nations.

In order to provide health care services that are culturally sensitive to the urban Native population, providers need to have an understanding of issues that are relevant to this group. These include the fundamental differences between the aboriginal people and other ethnic groups; their cultural diversity as well as their common cultural features; the Aboriginal concept of health; the basic demographics of the First Nations peoples, especially those in urban areas; their overall health status; the problems (both general and health-specific) that Natives face in urban areas, and the services that are now available or are still required. Since none of these topics can be fully dealt with within a chapter such as this, it can only be hoped that the reader's awareness in these areas will be increased and that his/her interest will be stimulated enough to learn more.

HISTORICAL PERSPECTIVE

Native Canadians are not simply members of yet another ethnic group in Canada's multicultural mosaic. They are descendants of the founding races of North America who arrived on the continent thousands of years ago. They are thus not immigrants themselves, nor the descendants of recent immigrants, as are all other Canadians. Their particular history during the last few hundred years makes them distinct. It is not one of new worlds explored and conquered, nor one of refuge from persecution and poverty, as was true for many immigrant groups, but rather one of invasion and loss. Since the time of first contact with Europeans, the indigenous peoples have experienced decimation of their populations, relegation to reserves and loss of their culture and identity through policies of assimilation, discrimination and disregard for their civil rights (Canada, House of Commons, Standing Committee, 1990; Miller, 1989).

NATIVES IN CANADA

A common misconception is that Natives in Canada form a homogeneous cultural population. This is not the case; within the major groupings of status and non-status Indians, Inuit and Métis there is much cultural and linguistic diversity of which non-Natives may be unaware. Eleven major Aboriginal language families can be found in Canada and some of these themselves include many distinct languages. The three largest families are Algonkian (which includes Cree, Ojibwa and Micmac, among others), Athapaskan and Eskimoan (including Inuktitut) (McMillan, 1988). There are many cultural subgroups within or crossing over these linguistic boundaries. The Inuit people, who will not be addressed specifically within the context of this chapter, have their own distinct history and culture. The Métis are descendants of the mixed-blood unions between European men, primarily the French fur traders, and Aboriginal women. They make up a sizable proportion of the current day Native population, especially in urban areas.

The terms status and non-status Indians were arbitrarily created by the passage of the Indian Act in 1869. For those persons whom the government has registered as "Indians," the Department of Indian and Northern Affairs has accepted certain responsibilities under the Indian Act (Frideres, 1988). Non-status Indians are people of Aboriginal ancestry who, for any of a number of ad hoc reasons, are not registered as "Indians" by the federal government, and are thus not considered eligible for the government services provided to status Indians. Many Indians lost their "status" on receiving an education; status women lost theirs by marrying non-status Indians, Métis persons are not considered "status." The Native Council of Canada represents the interests of non-status Indians and Metis, and argues that they should have status as well (Canada, House of Commons, Standing Committee, 1990). In the interim, the federal and provincial governments often disagree on their relative jurisdictions. A 1985 amendment to the Indian Act (Bill C-31) permitted the restoration of status to those who had lost it. This meant that status Indian women who had lost their status by marrying non-status Native men, regained it for themselves and their children (Miller, 1989).

TRADITIONAL NATIVE CONCEPTS OF HEALTH

Because of the wide traditional cultural diversity in the Native population as well as the varying effects of cultural suppression and assimilation experienced by members of this population, it is impossible to consider one Native concept of health. Certain features can however be discussed that apply to most traditional cultures.

Aboriginal health beliefs were holistic in nature and formed part of an integrated belief system, in which the individual person was in harmony with his/her community and with nature. Health did not relate only to the physical characteristics of the person, but to the social, psychological and spiritual aspects as well. Health depended on a balance of all its elements; if one was neglected, the others might suffer. Thus, the traditional emphasis was on prevention rather than on treatment, and on a balance which was to be maintained, not only within the person, but between that individual and the surrounding natural world. This view of health is only now coming to be accepted by the modern health care establishment in contrast to the previously held view of health as being the absence of disease.

In Malloch's description of healing traditions in the Anishnawbe people (1989), Woman was the earth, the nurturer; she had great natural healing powers which she practised in a preventive manner in the home. She may also have been a herbalist for her community. Man, however, had to develop his powers and relationship with the earth through instruction, ceremonies, fasting and the sweat lodge. The knowledge he developed had to be used for the benefit of the community. In order to fulfil their role in creation, men were usually chosen to be the medicine people, although women with gifts for healing were certainly recognized.

In the past, traditional healers were of various types, including shamans, herbalists and group medicine societies. For example, in Ojibway society, four basic groups of health practitioners existed; the Midewiwin or Grand Medicine Society, the Wabeno, the Jessakid and the Mashkikiwinini, or herbalists (Young, 1988). The Midewiwin's primary function was the curing of illness, but it also had great religious significance. Periods of instruction and initiation rites took members successively through the various levels in the hierarchy (McMillan, 1988). Whatever the practices of a particular medicine man were, his intent was to maintain and restore the balance between the body, mind and spirit of an individual.

Ceremonies and treatments varied among clans. One example was the Shaking Tent ceremony of the Ojibway shamans. In this, the shaman would sing and drum within a small lodge to call spirit helpers to assist in a cure. Their arrival would be accompanied by a shaking of the tent, and voices heard within (McMillan, 1988). Every tribe observed its own rituals for the use of medicinal herbs. Because medicines from the natural world were considered sacred, they had to be collected and treated with care and respect to honor the spirit of the medicine (Malloch, 1989). Medicine bundles were common to many cultures, and contained instruments, sacred objects and herbs, passed down from healer to healer.

Knowledge of herbal properties was well developed, and many Aboriginal remedies were taken up by the Europeans. Their derivatives may be found in the pharmaceuticals we use today. One example is a tea made from the bark of willow or poplar trees, which was used to treat headaches and other pains. The active ingredient, salicin, is very similar to today's indispensable and ubiquitous compound, acetylsalicylic acid (Weatherford, 1988). Jacques Cartier used a Huron tonic made from the bark and needles of an evergreen to effectively treat his men for scurvy. Two hundred years later, James Lind read of Cartier's experience and "discovered" a cure for the disease (Weatherford, 1988).

OTHER TRADITIONAL CONCEPTS

While generalizations to all members of an ethnocultural group should be avoided, especially to such a heterogeneous one as the Native population, an awareness of common traditional Native concepts that differ from the dominant North American pattern is fundamental for health professionals working in a cross-cultural setting.

Time

Rigid schedules and clock-watching historically were not of importance to Natives, who were used to seasonal work, which, when applicable, had to be completed regardless of the amount of time it took. At other times, schedules were irrelevant. Similarly, an emphasis was given to the present, rather than to the future, in contrast to Western society, which values insurance plans and accumulations of interest. The means of livelihood in traditional Native societies, such as hunting, trapping and fishing, made patience a necessity again, a quality out of keeping with the tense rapid pace of the non-Native lifestyle (Kirkness, 1973).

Family

Native families were traditionally extended, and not necessarily defined by close blood ties. The family was of utmost importance, and not only the extended family, but also the community were involved in the upbringing of children (Toronto, Department of Public Health, 1989). This has sometimes been misinterpreted by non-Native person who have often presumed a condition of neglect, when a birth parent has left children in the care of other family members; such children have been inappropriately removed from their homes and communities.

Children

Child-bearing has always been a natural and healthy part of life in Native communities. Large families and young maternal age at first pregnancy have not been generally considered undesirable, particularly in the light of a supportive extended family and community. Native children were usually exposed to a model of learning that permitted them to observe until tasks were mastered, and to apply inductive reasoning and problem solving.

The Elderly

Aged persons were traditionally very respected in Native societies, and played an important role in community life and government. Their experience was valued, and they were well cared for by their families (Kirkness, 1973).

Religion

In the past, religion for Natives was not a discrete compartmentalized entity, but was present in all activities, including medicine. Beliefs were animistic, that is, all elements in nature were endowed with spirits, including minerals, plants and all animals. Man had no special place in creation, but had to honour and live in harmony with its other members. This was very much an ecological approach, and the importance of harmony and continuity is reflected in the use of symbols involving circles, such as the Circle of Life, and all of the forces and colours of nature (the four winds, the elemental colors, etc.)(Toronto Department of Public Health, 1989).

Other Values

There are many other principles that distinguish traditional Native culture from the modern North American belief system, only some of which are briefly mentioned here. Cooperation, tolerance and sharing were desirable and necessary traits in Native communities. These values contrast with the European culture now dominant in North American, which could well be described as competitive and materialistic. Non-interference was another Native principle: Natives would not tell each other what to do as this would be considered ill-mannered. The open expression of anger was frowned upon (Brant & Brant, 1983).

MODERN VALUES AND CONCEPTS

Today, native societies are in transition. The above concepts are traditional ones, and may not apply to many Aboriginal people today. Many, however, are still applicable and should be considered by health care providers who work with this population.

Native healing practices suffered greatly from cultural suppression by the Europeans and from the ravages of imported diseases. Under these pressures, the numbers of skilled healers dwindled, and their knowledge often died with them. Today, Natives generally understand and accept current scientific concepts such as the germ theory of disease, but, as well, accord importance to the role of environmental, spiritual and non-physical factors that form part of their broader holistic view of health (Toronto, City of, Department of Public Health, 1989). Traditional remedies and healers may often be used in conjunction with Western medical treatments.

The extended family structure has broken down and it is common to see, both on reserves and in cities, disrupted families and solitary elderly who are deprived of the caring and support of their relatives. Because large families and teenage pregnancy are still more common in Native populations, young and/or single mothers find themselves particularly disadvantaged by the erosion of the family unit.

However, traditional family values are often still evident in Native practices. Members of the extended family may be involved in caring for a particular family member, and many relations may visit a Native patient in hospital. They should not be discouraged. Family members can be incorporated into the care of patients, and provide resources and assistance to facilitate early discharge and recovery.

Health care providers should be aware that Native persons from a traditional background may not always adhere to the Western practice of punctuality for appointments. The current North American practice of volunteering and requesting personal information during client-service provider interactions is not compatible with Native tradition. An apparent reluctance to provide information thus should not be interpreted as lack of concern or hostility. Moreover, rather than appear to disagree, a Native person may indicate understanding of and assent with a professional's advice, when this may not be the case.

FACTORS CONTRIBUTING TO CHANGE

Many factors have contributed to the breakdown of the traditional family unit and loss of cultural values. One of the most devastating has been the residential school system, which operated from the late nineteenth century until the 1960s. In this system, the federal government gave the Protestant and Catholic churches control over the education of Natives on reserves across Canada. It was hoped that the missionaries could "civilize" the Indians by making them Christians, a process which often entailed the removal of Native children from their families to residential schools, where they were forbidden to speak their language or observe their own religious and cultural practices. Despite the good intentions of some of the proponents of this system, the overall effects were catastrophic. Entire generations lost their cultural identity, their self-esteem and their language. In addition, the physical, psychological and even sexual abuses that occurred in these schools continue to affect their victims today, long after the schools have ceased operation (York, 1990).

Another practice which contributed to the destruction of the Native family was the removal of Native children from their families by well-meaning child welfare agencies, and their subsequent adoption with non-Native families in Canada and the United States. This affected thousands of children during the 1960s and 1970s, whose birth parents were considered inadequate to provide for their needs. "For the country as a whole, aboriginal children were being taken from their families almost five times more frequently than non-native children. By 1980, about 15,000 native children were under the control of child welfare agencies across Canada, and three-quarters of all adopted Indian children were placed in non-native homes," (ibid., 206). Native efforts finally resulted in inquiries into this practice and a recognition of the "cultural genocide" that had resulted from it. In Manitoba, where the practice was most widespread, a policy was developed in 1984 to seek placement for Native children in Native families first, if removal is actually warranted; and across Canada, Native-controlled child welfare agencies have been established. As with the residential schools, however, the effects of the misguided zeal of non-Native workers are still being felt by today's young Native adults and their families.

These are only a few examples of practices which have contributed to the historic marginalization of the First Nations people. As a result, Natives find themselves disadvantaged in social, political and economic terms. They are (without even considering biological and organizational factors) also disadvantaged because of the resulting effects of these factors on their health. The Report of the Standing Committee on Aboriginal Affairs, *Unfinished Business: An Agenda for all Canadians in the 1990s*, states that: "This decade is an especially appropriate time for Canada to address the unacceptable socio-economic status of aboriginal people and the many outstanding issues respecting their political and legal rights. Canada has an obligation to achieve some substantial progress on aboriginal affairs matters as part of the global struggle to ensure a universal respect for human rights and self-determination." (Canada, House of Commons Standing Committee, 1990, 29) This unenviable history has resulted in a health profile that is, in many ways, particular to the Native population in its characteristics and severity, and also in the measures required to address the existing problems and barriers to health.

It should also be emphasized that improved health for Natives cannot be achieved solely by access to and use of health sector services. A comprehensive view of health must be taken and a framework used such as the Health Field concept proposed by Marc Lalonde (1974). This concept states that the health of an individual is the product of the interaction of four elements: human biology, environment, lifestyle and, finally,

health care organization. Native health cannot be assessed without proper consideration of all of these elements. For example,
the environment element includes not only physical parameters
(for example, housing, food and water), but also social and
economic conditions. When fundamental environmental determinants such as housing and income are grossly inadequate,
efforts to improve health based solely on medical services will
be ineffective. Another concept, which is complementary to
Lalonde's framework, is that of health as "a resource which
gives people the ability to manage and even to change their
surroundings...a basic and dynamic force in our daily lives,
influenced by our circumstances, our beliefs, our culture and
our social, economic and physical environments," (Epp, 1986, 3)
This view of health, espoused by the Minister of National Health
and Welfare, again emphasizes the wide perspective that must
be taken in examining the health of an individual or community.
Therefore, the discussion that follows is not limited to biology
and health care organization, but tries to encompass many of the
broader issues that have an important impact on Native health
today. Only when the wider context is considered can the
deplorable gaps and barriers to adequate health in the Native
population be fully recognized, and appropriate commitments
made to address this inequity.

THE CURRENT NATIVE SITUATION

Demographics

Norris (1990) provides a review of the demographics of Aboriginal people in Canada, using recent Canadian census data.
The proportion of Natives in the total Canadian population has
been increasing since the 1930s. In the 1981 Census, 2.0% of the
total population was composed of Indians, Métis and Inuit,
compared to 1.4% in 1941. In the 1986 Census, the first year in
which either single or multiple origin could be reported, 2.8% or
the population (or 711, 725 persons) reported single or multiple
Aboriginal origins, and 1.5% reported single Aboriginal origin.
The term "single" here refers to persons reporting only Native
ancestry, and "multiple" refers to persons with mixed Aboriginal and non-Aboriginal origins. The population according to
Aboriginal group was 531, 445 Indian, 128, 640 Métis, and 33,465
Inuit. In 1986, 68% of the status Indian population of 387, 829
persons lived on reserves (Canada, House of Commons, Stand-

ing Committee, 1990). Because of the amendments to the Indian Act in 1985, the number of status Indians has been increasing since that time. It is estimated that by the end of 1991, 92,000 registrants and their children will be added to the status Register (Canada, Indian and Northern Affairs Canada, 1989).

The Territories, followed by the Western provinces, have the highest proportions of Native persons in their populations; while Ontario is the province with the largest Native population, in terms of absolute numbers. Two-thirds of all North American Indians (status and non-status) are concentrated in Ontario and British Columbia, two-thirds of Métis are in the Prairies and the majority of Inuit are in the Territories (Norris, 1990).

Urban/Rural Population

Data from the 1986 Census reveal that 38.4% of persons with single Aboriginal origin live in urban areas (59.3% of Métis, 35.8% of Indians, and 17.4% of Inuit), compared to 72.4% of Native persons with multiple (or mixed) origin, and 76.4% of the total Canadian population. As in the non-Native Canadian population, women outnumber men in urban areas. However, this differential is more marked in the Native population (ibid.).

The Canadian Native population has a younger age structure and is aging less rapidly than the total population (Figure 1). The mean age for the Canadian population is 34 years, as compared to 23 years for Natives. Young adults (aged 20-34) make up a larger proportion of the urban Native population (one-third) than the rural Native population (one-quarter).

While Native fertility has been declining, particularly in the last two decades, birth rates are still twice as high as in the non-Native population. Native birth rates are still highest on reserves.

Migration

Overall, Natives are more mobile than non-Natives. Those living outside of their Native communities change residences more than the general population; those Natives in their original communities move less than the general population. More Natives from reserves are moving to large cities but, as well, an increasing number of migrants to reserves are coming from metropolitan areas. Women are more mobile than men, particularly when migrating from reserves.

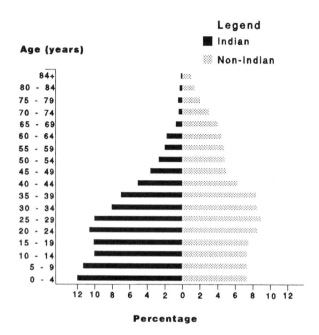

Figure 1: A Comparison of the Age Composition of the Canadian Indian and Non-Indian Populations, 1986.

(Source: Statistics Canada, 1987)

The largest off-reserve populations, numerically speaking, are found in British Columbia and Ontario, while proportions of off-reserve Indians are highest in the larger Western cities of Winnipeg, Regina and Vancouver, and are also high in many smaller urban centres in the West. Ontario and Quebec off-reserve Native populations are largest in Montreal and Toronto, but are more concentrated (by proportion of the population) in smaller northern centres. Off-reserve populations in the Atlantic provinces are more dispersed (Canada, Indian and Northern Affairs Canada, 1980). Exact data on the numbers of Natives in urban centres are difficult to obtain, owing to lack of participation in the Census, and difficulties in ethnocultural identification.

Natives move to urban centres for several reasons, but economic necessity is the major one (Stanbury, 1975; Maidman, 1983). Family problems or illness, and educational needs are also common underlying reasons. The largest proportion of moves made by Natives are made alone (40%), followed by moves accompanied by spouse and/or children (24%) (Maidman, 1983).

Young adults of working age are most likely to move off-reserve. Educational levels in urban Natives tend to be higher than those in rural Native populations; although, overall, educational levels in Natives are lower than in the total Canadian population. This situation is gradually changing, however: younger Natives tend to be better educated than their elders (Canada, Statistics Canada, 1984).

Problems Faced in Urban Centres

A number of studies have examined the problems that Natives face in urban centres. These are identified as mainly social and economic in nature and they have a major impact on health. Natives in cities, when compared to non-Natives, have higher rates of unemployment, lower incomes and worse living conditions. Shah (1988) summarized the major self-identified problems of urban Natives as unemployment, inadequate housing, limited education, alcohol abuse, lack of cultural awareness and discrimination. Much higher rates of unemployment in Natives can be related, in part, to lack of training, physical disability, family responsibilities and discrimination (Stanbury, 1975). However, the pervasive effect of "welfare colonialism," that is, the ongoing dependency relationship arising out of government policies, should also be recognized. Incomes of urban Natives, while higher than those of rural Natives, are still significantly lower than those of non-Natives living in cities (House of Commons Standing Committee on Aboriginal Affairs, 1990), reflecting the low status jobs that Natives tend to have. One of the most serious problems facing the urban Native is the lack of good affordable housing. Not only is housing more difficult to find for Native people, but that which is available is often of poor quality and substandard with regard to plumbing, size, appearance, insulation, wiring, location and other factors (Maidman, 1983; Saskatchewan Senior Citizens' Provincial Council, 1988). In addition to the traditional problems stemming from poverty, Native families moving to urban areas are faced with the diffi-

culties of a different, insensitive culture and racial discrimination. All of these conditions contribute to an unhealthy environment and lifestyles, impair social and psychological function
and predispose individuals to physical illness.

HEALTH STATUS OF NATIVE PEOPLE

Available information on the health status of Natives in
Canada relates for the most part, to on-reserve or status Indian
populations. The life expectancy of status Indians has always
been much lower than that of Canadians in general. While the
gap is decreasing, the most recent estimates indicate that a male
status Indian has 8.4 years less life expectancy than a non-Native
male, and a female 7.3 years less than her non-Native counter-
part (Health and Welfare Canada, 1988). While infant mortality
rates have declined in registered Indians, in 1985 the Indian rate
was still twice as high as the Canadian average (Canada, Indian
and Northern Health Services, 1988). The shocking differential
in life expectancy between Natives and non-Natives reflects not
only socio-economic conditions, lifestyle behaviours, geographical isolation (and thus lack of access to services), and cultural
barriers, but also the impact of our "Indian" policies, which have
created conditions of dependency and loss of cultural identity.

Leading causes of death for the registered Indian population
for 1980 to 1984 were injury and poisoning (33.6%), diseases of
the circulatory system (23.3%), neoplasms (9.5%) and diseases of
the respiratory system (8.7%) (Figure 2). For the total Canadian
population, the four leading causes were: diseases of the circulatory system (44.5%), neoplasms (25.8%), injury and poisoning
(8.0%) and diseases of the respiratory system (7.3%) (Canada,
Indian and Northern Health Services, 1988).

Age-specific death rates for Indians are much higher than the
general Canadian population rates, and are only surpassed by
the latter after the age of 80. Cause-specific mortality rates are
significantly higher in the Native population (both sexes) for
infectious and parasitic diseases, diabetes mellitus, alcoholic
psychosis and alcoholism, pneumonia, kidney disease, acci-
dents and violence. In addition, Native women have a higher
mortality rate for cervical cancer and diseases of the circulatory
system than non-Native women (Mao, et al., 1986). Suicide rates
continue to be much higher in Indian populations. For the period

1980 - 84, the highest age-specific suicide rate for Indians was in the 20 to 24-year age group, and was five times greater than the Canadian rate (Canada, Indian and Northern Health Services, 1988).

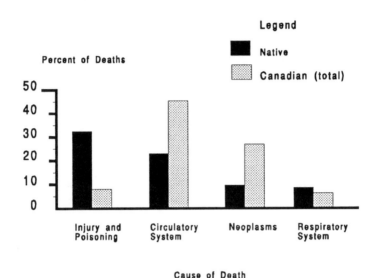

Figure 2: Major Causes of Death, 1980-84, Native and Canadian Populations.

(Source: Indian and Northern Health Services, 1988, p. 13-14)

Morbidity

Other important health problems, in addition to the above causes of mortality, include anemia, respiratory diseases, arthropathies, hearing and vision impairment and dental problems. Tuberculosis rates are declining but are still much higher in Indian populations than among non-Natives. Mental health disorders, often related to alcohol or substance abuse, are prevalent. Anxiety, depression and family violence are considered major problems in many communities (ibid.). Native Canadians have a higher proportion of disabled and handicapped persons than other Canadians (Shah, unpublished data). Obesity, poor nutrition, smoking and hypertension are common and are important risk factors for disease.

Specific Health Problems in Urban Areas

To some extent, generalizations can be made that the health status of Natives in urban areas is similar to that documented for registered Indians on reserves, but with added problems linked to their urban circumstances.

The stresses of adaptation and acculturation have been used to explain alcohol abuse in urban areas (Brody, 1971); and alcohol abuse increases the incidence of many health problems, including cirrhosis, pneumonia, fetal alcohol syndrome, malnutrition and child neglect. Substance abuse of various types is an ongoing problem in the urban Native population, particularly in the transient and indigent population. Certain emotional disorders such as depression, anxiety, substance abuse and self-destructive behaviour can be related to the economic deprivation and social disorganization that Natives face in urban areas. As well, significant stress is caused by conflict between traditional Native values and those of the dominant North American culture.

Elderly Natives in the city are at higher risk of health problems for a number of reasons. Their educational level is lower than that of younger Natives, and they tend to have low incomes and substandard housing. They often live alone, cut off from the supports of family members at a time when they have increased need for assistance, particularly given the high prevalence of chronic disorders and disabilities in this group. Many have migrated to the city from reserves late in life when adaptation to a new and hostile environment is even more difficult (Saskatchewan Senior Citizens' Provincial Council, 1988).

Native women living in the city may experience the multiple risk factors of poverty, single-parenting and discrimination. Native women, in general, are frequently victims of family violence. The Ontario Native Women's Association conducted a study on Aboriginal Family Violence (1989) that revealed that, while 1 in 10 Canadian women experience a form of abuse, 8 out of 10 Aboriginal women have been, or can expect to be, abused or assaulted. Their children are also at risk for abuse, and appropriate services for both mother and child are not often available.

Barriers to Health Care

Organization of Health Care Services

Health care service delivery is a major difference. On a reserve, health and medical services are usually provided through the Medical Services Branch of National Health and Welfare and the Department of Indian Affairs and Northern Development (DIAND). Drug and other benefits are included. In the city, however, Natives must use the provincial health care system, with which they are not often familiar. Status Indians are still eligible for drug benefits and coverage of their provincial premiums, if other programs (such as Welfare) are not applicable. For all Native newcomers to the city, whether eligible for benefits or not, the provincial and municipal systems are foreign and confusing. This creates major difficulties in access. This situation is exacerbated by the fact that the federal and provincial governments continue to disagree regarding their relative jurisdictions in delivery of services. Farkas and Shah (1986) conducted a survey of public health departments in Canada to determine the extent of programming provided to urban Natives. They found that most departments had no data on the health status and needs of this group, and little or no programming for Natives. In part, they felt that this could be attributed to confusion between levels of government as to their responsibilities toward urban Natives.

Communication

Natives may have communication difficulties with health care providers, not only with respect to language but also cultural communication patterns. One major problem, even when services are accessed, is the lack of medical records and patient history information, especially when chronic problems exist. Also, in addition to a shortage of health care providers with cultural awareness and sensitivity towards Native circumstances, there is still a genuine dearth of trained Native health care professionals.

Pattern of Utilization of Health Services

Native persons tend to use health care services as a last resort, after seeking assistance from family and friends. There may be denial of their condition or minimization of the problem when they do present for treatment. Walk-in clinics and hospital emergency rooms are often used, particularly so by the transient population. Inappropriate use of health services may also lead to increased hospitalization rates (Shah and Farkas, 1985). Compliance with treatment may be low because of a lack of understanding of or confidence in the treatment or practitioner, cultural inappropriateness, lack of money to buy medications and unstable living conditions (Toronto, Department of Public Health, 1989).

Lack of Cultural Awareness in Health Care Providers

Most non-Native health professionals are unaware of Native concepts and values, not only with regard to health and illness, but also other values, as previously described, which affect their behaviour as patients or seekers of service. A patient who shows up late for an appointment, volunteers little information and is seemingly reluctant to answer or ask questions my be construed as being deliberately difficult and obstructive. This patient may not have attended the physician for routine matters, including immunization, because he/she did not feel ill. Also, in conjunction with the treatment prescribed by the Western practitioner, the patient may be using medicines provided by a native healer. The provider may not have any knowledge of the social, economic and political realities of Natives, and thus be unable to understand the particular circumstances of his/her patient. This gap in understanding may prove frustrating to both parties, and lead to a lack of trust, misdiagnosis, noncompliance and failure to return for needed follow-up and/or referral. It should also be noted that ignorance about the wider problems of the urban Native on the part of the health care provider means that the provider may not place the same priority on the patient's medical problems, and may fail to link the patient with services of other agencies, which may be more urgently required.

MEETING NEEDS OF URBAN NATIVES

Current Initiatives

In recent years, many Aboriginal initiatives in the health care sector have been developed to address Native problems appropriately. These changes are occurring in various settings such as hospitals, community health centres, community agencies, mental health programs and educational institutions. Some examples are given below.

1. Hospitals

Native interpreters are now being used at hospitals in cities such as Winnipeg, Regina and Montreal. These persons are required to be not only translators, but culture brokers, advocates and liaison workers. The Toronto East General and Orthopedic Hospital has a mental health outreach program for Natives.

2. Community-Based Services

Community Health Centres, which provide a range of culturally sensitive services for Natives, are now being established (for example, Anishnawbe Health Toronto). In many cities across Canada, friendship centres supply interpreters, fill a liaison role and assist Natives from reserves who have come for medical treatment. They may also provide some health programs or substance abuse services (for example, Alcoholics Anonymous). In recent years, there has been a revival of interest in traditional medicine, and applications of the Aboriginal model of health, which incorporate these methods, have been successfully used in mental health and substance-abuse programming in hospitals and urban care centres (Baker, 1988).

The federal government funds substance-abuse treatment and rehabilitation programs such as Pedahbun Lodge in Toronto, Crowfoot Sunrise Lodge in Calgary and others in Lethbridge, Edmonton and Winnipeg. Provinces may also contribute to these programs (Shah, 1988).

3. Public Health Agencies

City health departments have been slow to examine the health status of or provide services for urban Natives (Farkas & Shah, 1986). Calgary and Toronto have conducted needs assessments of Natives in those cities (Obonsawin Irwin Consulting Inc., 1984; Toronto, Department of Public Health, 1989; Calgary Social Services Department, 1984). Edmonton's Board of Health established an Urban Native Health Working Group in 1986 to improve services to Natives living in Edmonton. In 1988, it hosted a national workshop on the needs of urban Natives. Some of its initiatives have included the use of Native Community Health Representatives in Native areas, cross-cultural training of non-Native health care providers, development of resources for Natives and liaison with other agencies providing services to

Natives. The efforts of these other bodies, for example, the Urban Native Child Welfare Interagency Committee and the Alberta Social Services Child Welfare Services, should also be recognized for their impact on Native health.

4. Educational Institutions

Finally, some universities and colleges are beginning to address the problems of a lack of trained Native health care professionals, and the lack of cultural awareness and sensitivity of non-Native providers. For example, at the University of Toronto, the Indian Health Careers Program was established to recruit Aboriginal students into health science programs, promote access to these programs, provide support services to Aboriginal students and to provide cultural workshops on Native health issues and traditional practices (Indian Health Careers Program, 1989). A similar program had already been established at the University of Manitoba. An annual visiting lectureship provided by Native experts to sensitize non-Native professionals on Native health issues was first held in 1990 at the University of Toronto.

RECOMMENDATIONS

Edmonton's Urban Native Health Working Group set out an action plan to deal with identified issues in that city's urban Native population. Recommendations given by that group are applicable to most cities. They include:

- clarifying jurisdictional boundaries;
- giving information to Natives regarding available services;
- promoting increased sensitivity of non-Native providers;
- employing more Natives in the health care system;
- developing Native referral centres for facilitation, advocacy and interpretation; and
- supporting programs provided by Natives for Natives (Paton, 1988).

However, health problems of urban Natives cannot be met solely by improving access to culturally appropriate services. While gaps in these areas continue to be large, others remain such as gaps in housing, employment, education, justice, access to community agencies and resources, and cultural awareness in general. These are priorities for urban Natives themselves (Maidman, 1983). Health per se is not always high on this list, but one can recognize that the identified issues are indeed determinants of health. The recent proposed amendments (1992) to Constitutional Act, 1982 to incorporate the inherent rights to self-government for all Aboriginal peoples, including non-status Indians and Métis could have brought about the long overdue desired changes. Unfortunately, it did not happen. There is a pressing need to resolve jurisdictional disputes between all levels of government to address outstanding Native concerns.

REFERENCES

Baker, F.W. (1988). Summary. In T. Paton (Chair), *Inner City Health: The Needs of Urban Natives, Proceedings of the Ninth Symposium on the Prevention of Handicapping Conditions* (65-67). Edmonton, Alta.

Brant, C.C., & Brant, J.A., (Eds). (1983). *The Native Family: Traditions and Adaptations. The Transcribed and Edited Proceedings of the 1983 Meeting of the Canadian Psychiatric Association Section on Native Mental Health.* Ottawa.

Brody, H. (1971). *Indians on Skid Row.* Ottawa: Department of Indian and Northern Affairs.

Calgary Social Services Department. (1984). *Native Needs Assessment.* Calgary, Alberta: The Department.

Canada. Health and Welfare Canada. (1988). *Health Indicators Derived from Vital Statistics for Status Indians and Canadian Populations 1978-1986.* Ottawa: Minister of National Health and Welfare.

— —. Indian and Northern Affairs Canada. (1980). *Indian Conditions: A Survey.* Ottawa: Minister of Indian Affairs and Northern Development.

— —. (1989). *Basic Departmental Data: 1989.* Ottawa: Minister of Supply and Services Canada.

— —. Indian and Northern Health Services, Medical Services Branch. (1988). *Health Status of Canadian Indians and Inuit: Update 1987.* Ottawa: Health and Welfare Canada.

— —. Parliament. House of Commons. Standing Committee on Aboriginal Affairs. (1990). *Unfinished Business: An Agenda for All Canadians in the 1990s.* Second Report of the Standing Committee on Aboriginal Affairs. Ottawa: Queen's Printer.

— —. Statistics Canada. (1984). *Canada's Native People.* Ottawa: Minister of Supply and Services.

— —. Statistics Canada. (1987). *Census Canada 1986.* Ottawa: Statistics Canada.

Epp, J. (1986). *Achieving Health for All: A Framework for Health Promotion.* Ottawa: Minister of National Health and Welfare.

Farkas, C.S., & Shah, C.P. (1986). Public Health Departments and Native Health Care in Urban Centres. *Canadian Journal of Public Health, 77,* 274-76.

Frideres, J.S., (1988). *Native Peoples in Canada: Contemporary Conflicts, 2d ed.* Scarborough, Ont.: Prentice-Hall Canada.

Indian Health Careers Program. (1989). The Indian Health Careers Program: Preparing Our Youth to Serve First Nations. *Canadian Woman Studies, 10*(2,3), 125-26.

Johnston, P. (1983). *Native Children and the Child Welfare System.* Toronto: Canadian Council on Social Development in Association with James Lorimer & Co.

Kirkness, V.J. (1973). Education of Indians and Metis. In D.B. Sealey & V.J. Kirkness (Eds.), *Indians Without Tipis: A Resource Book by Indians and Metis* (137-71). Winnipeg: William Clare (Manitoba).

Lalonde, M. (1974). *A New Perspective on the Health of Canadians.* Ottawa: Minister of Supply and Services.

Maidman, F. (1983). *Native People in Urban Settings: Problems, Needs and Services. A Report of the Ontario Task Force on Native People in the Urban Setting, 1981.* Toronto.

Malloch, L. (1989). Indian Medicine, Indian Health: Study Between Red and White Medicine. *Canadian Woman Studies, 10*(23), 105 - 12.

Mao, Y., Morrison, H., Semenciw, R., & Wigle, D. (1986). Mortality on Canadian Indian Reserves 1977-1982. *Canadian Journal of Public Health, 77* (July/August), 263-68.

McMillan, A.D. (1988). *Native Peoples and Cultures of Canada.* Toronto: Douglas and McIntyre.

Miller, J.R. (1989). *Skyscrapers Hide the Heavens: a History of Indian-White Relations in Canada* Rev. ed. Toronto: University of Toronto Press.

Norris, M.J. (1990). The Demography of Aboriginal People in Canada. In S.S. Halli, F. Trovato and L. Driedger (Eds.), *Ethnic Demography: Canadian Immigrant, Racial and Cultural Variations.* Ottawa: Carleton University Press.

Obonsawan Irwin Consulting Inc. (1984). *Report on the Health Status of Native People in Toronto.* Downsview, Ontario.

Ontario Native Women's Association. (1989). *Breaking Free: A Proposal for Change to Aboriginal Family Violence.* Thunder Bay, Ontario.

Paton, T. (1988). Urban Native Health Working Group. In T. Paton (Chair), *Inner City Health: The Needs of Urban Natives, Proceedings of the Ninth Symposium on the Prevention of Handicapping Conditions.* (72-77). Edmonton, Alta.

Primeaux, M., and Henderson, G. (1981). American Indian Patient Care. In M. Primeaux and G. Henderson (Eds.), *Transcultural Health Care* (239-54). Menlo Park, California: Addison-Wesley Publishing.

Saskatchewan Senior Citizens' Provincial Council. (1988). *A Study of the Unmet Needs of Off-Reserve Indian and Metis Elderly in Saskatchewan.* Regina, Sask.: The Council.

Shah, C.P. (1988). A National Overview of the Health of Native People Living in Canadian Cities. In T. Paton (Chair), *Inner City Health: The Needs of Urban Natives, Proceedings of the Ninth Symposium on the Prevention of Handicapping Conditions* (2 - 45). Edmonton, Alta.

Shah, C.P., & Farkas, C.S. (1985). The Health of Indians in Canadian Cities: a Challenge to the Health Care System. *Canadian Medical Association Journal, 133,* 1 Nov., 859-63.

Stanbury, W.T. (1975). *Success and Failure: Indians in Urban Society.* Vancouver, B.C.: University of British Columbia Press.

Toronto, City of. Department of Public Health, Health Promotion and Advocacy Section. (1989). *The Native Canadian Community in Toronto.* Toronto: City of Toronto Department of Public Health.

United States Congress. Office of Technology Assessment. (1986). *Indian Health Care: Summary.* Washington, D.C.: Office of Technology Assessment.

Weatherford, J. (1988). *Indian Givers: How the Indians of the Americas Transformed the Work,* New York: Fawcett Columbine.

York, G. (1990). *The Dispossessed: Life and Death in Native Canada.* London: Vintage (U.K.).

Young, T.K. (1988). *Health Care and Cultural Change: The Indian Experience in the Central Subartic.* Toronto: University of Toronto Press.

The Universal Right to Health: An Ideological Discourse

Audrey L. Kobayashi
Mark W. Rosenberg

There is an international rhetoric surrounding the issue of the right to health. Contradictions between the principle and the provision of universal health care can be found in developing as well as developed countries, tied not only to economic conditions but to ideological systems. The right to health is expressed within a larger discourse on the nature of human rights. Examples from several countries illustrate the importance of understanding the nature of this discourse within historically specific contexts. Achieving universal health requires going beyond consideration of economic and policy constraints to address the process by which cultural definitions of health and human rights are constructed.

In 1978, delegations from 134 governments attended the World Health Organization (WHO) conference at Alma-Ata. It resulted in the Declaration of Alma-Ata (World Health Organization, 1978). This and the subsequent *Health for All by the Year 2000* declaration (World Health Organization, 1979) are representative of the international rhetoric of the right to health. An examination of the principles evinced in these documents and others compared to the delivery of health care in developing as well as developed countries demonstrates profound contradictions between rhetoric and reality. The purposes of this paper are to argue that these contradictions needed to be tied not only to economic conditions, but to ideological systems within their historically specific contexts and to place the right to health within a larger discourse on the nature of human rights.

To accomplish these goals, we develop our thesis in three parts. First, we review the Alma-Ata and Health for All declarations to demonstrate the international rhetoric of the right to health. Second, we review evidence from various studies of the delivery of health care in developing and developed countries to illustrate the contradictions between the rhetoric of the right to health and the reality. We focus on access issues at the regional, rural versus urban, inter-urban and intra-urban scales and on the lack of specific services for women, children, the elderly and racial groups in order to show that the contradictions need to be tied not only to economic conditions but to ideological systems within their historically specific contexts. Third, we make the case for placing the right to health into the larger discourse of human rights. We conclude by arguing that the achievement of universal health requires going beyond consideration of economic and policy constraints to address the process by which cultural definitions of health and human rights are constructed.

THE INTERNATIONAL RHETORIC OF THE RIGHT TO HEALTH

Several themes can be identified in the international rhetoric of the right to health. In the Alma-Ata Declaration (World Health Organization, 1978), these include: health as a **fundamental** human right (Resolution I); inequality in health status as a **common** concern to **all** countries (Resolution II); the **right** and **duty** of people to contribute to the planning and implementation of their health care (Resolutions IV and VI); government **responsibility** for the health of the people (Resolution V); health as a component of the **spirit** of social justice (Resolution V); primary health care as **essential** and **universally accessible** (Resolution VI); health as **peace** (Resolutions III, VI, and X); and the **equation** of economic and social development with health (Resolutions I, II, III, VI and X) (emphasis added).

Similar themes are repeated in various "Health for All", WHO and WHO regional group documents. In the Pan American Health Organization's, "Health for All by the Year 2000 Strategies," (1980, 179) primary care must be applicable to "the entire population" and organized "to guarantee economic, cultural, geographic and functional accessibility" (ibid., 180) (universal access). "It is emphasized that the community must participate in analysing its own needs and developing possible solutions (ibid., 181) (right and duty). In another section (ibid., 182), the involvement of the health sector in regional and national development is discussed (equation of economic and social development with health). Inter-country cooperation strategies and Technical Cooperation Among Developing Countries (TCDC) are also discussed (ibid., 183-84) (common concern to all countries).

In addition to endorsing a general rhetoric of the right to health, governments also endorse goals for specific populations (Pan American Health Organization, 1980). Argentina, Bolivia, Brazil, Chile, Colombia, Costa Rica, Cuba, Ecuador, El Salvador, Guatemala, Guyana, Honduras, Jamaica, Mexico, Nicaragua, Panama, Paraguay, Peru, Uruguay and Venezuela all endorsed the goal of emphasizing health care for deprived urban and rural groups, and within them high-risk families, including mothers and children under five years of age. Some countries also included workers, the elderly and school children and adolescents as priority groups for health improvements.

Such endorsements are made by developed countries as well (Pan American Health Organization, 1980). The Canadian government's position equates health, social well-being and income security with living socially and economically productive lives. Strategic objectives are supposed to achieve **adequate** access to **appropriate** health care services and social services are to be provided for those who are disadvantaged. "Health equity is linked to social equity."

In the United States strategy to achieve "Health for All by the Year 2000," access to services for all Americans is one of three elements emphasized. Within this general element of their strategy, the United States government identifies specific high-risk and vulnerable groups (the mentally impaired, migrants, women, children, adolescents and Native peoples) and recognizes that no person should be unable to afford needed health services (universal access). Explicit recognition is also given to the private sector in the refinement of objectives, the identification of problems, measurable goals, objectives and program planning.

ACCESS TO HEALTH CARE: RHETORIC AND REALITY

In contrast to the international rhetoric of the right to health, in this section we examine case studies from various developing and developed countries to illustrate the reality of access to health care. Emphasis is placed on inter-regional, inter-urban and intra-urban differences in access to health. Focus is also given to the differential treatment of women, the elderly, the young and racial groups. These studies also serve to demonstrate the importance of seeing the differences between rhetoric and reality within their specific ideological and historical contexts.

Differences between Rhetoric and Reality in Developing Countries

The apartheid health care system of the Republic of South Africa provides a stark illustration of the linkages between "gross violations" of human rights and access to health. Turshen's (1986) study of the Ciskei bantustan shows that infant mortality rates and malnutrition are extreme. Rural rates are even worse than urban rates within the bantustan. The high rates of morbidity and mortality of children and adults in the Ciskei are directly linked to the South African government's manipulation of the organization of the labour process. Whereas 81 percent of the white population is covered by medical aid schemes, only 1 percent of the black population is covered in South Africa (ibid., 890). In the Ciskei and other bantustans, the health care system is urban-based but the population is essentially rural-based. Compounding this mismatch between the delivery system and the lifestyle of the population is the absolute lack of health care resources.

Andersson and Marks (1989) make the connection between ideology and health care explicit in their analysis of the allocation of health resources in southern Africa. Their analysis shows that prior to independence of southern African countries and in the case of the Republic of South Africa where apartheid continues, much higher rates of morbidity and mortality existed for people living in rural areas and for the black population whereas the allocation of health care resources heavily favoured urban areas and the white population. The explanation for this cannot be ascribed to objective need or technical breakdown, but can be found in class domination and class alliances (Andersson & Marks, 1989). Andersson and Marks (ibid., 520-22) point to the particular mental and physical problems faced by women generated by the intersection of patriarchial forms of gender relations and the organization of production in southern African countries. The third element of their analysis is to treat "race" and "tribe" as social and ideological constructs to show how these designations are used to gain or deny access to health care (ibid., 522-23). A fourth element of their argument is to show how in post-independence southern Africa health care has been used in the process of reform or as part of the broader apparatus of social control. The final element of Andersson and Marks' paper is to remind the reader that although variations in the health care systems of southern African countries do exist, attempts at improving access to health care are constrained by the geopolitics of a global economy.

Raikes (1989) links women's health in East Africa to their growing roles in production and social reproduction of the household. She argues (ibid., 448) that maternal and child health services (MCH) have remained "centred on women's reproductive role with little attention being paid to their wider health needs." Lack of access to safe and hygienic MCH services leads to infertility, death from illegal or failed abortions and unsanitary child delivery. With the increases in the number of women in production roles in rural and urban areas, malnourishment, disability and physical and mental abuse are growing health problems not addressed by most MCHs. In urban areas, sexually transmitted diseases, especially among women forced into prostitution, are another of example of the need for broader definitions of services than those already in use.

In Nigeria the right to medical care is guaranteed. Alubo (1987) shows, however, that the difference between rhetoric and reality is that status, power and privilege determine who gets medical services and the type of medical service. Through an analysis of various development plans, Alubo shows that the rhetoric of development recognizes that while most of the population is rural, most of the medical services are found in urban areas. Although this has been the case for years, the reality is that each successive régime has failed to address the issue. This combined with a system of special facilities and services for the privileged and élites of Nigerian society insures that the differences between rhetoric and reality remain great.

The difference between the rhetoric of the right to health and the reality are not confined, however, to the developing countries of Africa. For example, Simonelli (1987) links the process of modernization and access to health care in Baviacora, a rural municipio of the state of Sonora, Mexico. In focusing on infant mortality, she shows that the introduction of the artifacts of modernization led to impressive declines in morbidity and mortality for infants between 1955 and 1984, but that these same forces have led to increases in deaths due to trauma, chronic conditions and endemic diseases since this time. With the economic crises of the 1980s, Simonelli argues that the state is no longer able to support the infrastructure of modernization, even though the population has adjusted its lifestyle to a health care system based on modern technology. A rural population can no longer purchase the health care services created, pharmaceutical products on which it is based are in short supply, and the price of basic foods has increased, compromising nutritional requirements.

Differences between Rhetoric and Reality in Developed Countries

In developed countries, the differences between rhetoric and reality over the right to health are most clearly illustrated within the contradictions of the "privatisation" debate and access to abortion services. If it is the young and the rural populations who make up the majority of the total populations who suffer in developing countries; it is the elderly and the rural populations who are smaller parts of the total populations who suffer in developed countries. If it is the black majority who suffer in South Africa, it is visible minorities who suffer in developed countries. In both geographies of the world, it is women who share a common suffering.

Perhaps, the most stark illustration of the differences between rhetoric and reality in a developed country is the number of people in the United States who have no health insurance whatsoever. In 1985, the number of people who fell into this category was 31.3 million or 13.3 percent of the total population (United States, 1988, 92). Although the differences in the percentage of males and females without any health insurance coverage are minimal (14.6 for males and 12.0 for females), the differences by racial group are substantial (ibid.). Among the white population, 12.4 percent had no health insurance coverage whatsoever. Among the black population, no health insurance coverage jumps to 19.3 percent of the population, and among people of Hispanic origin, 27.0 percent had no health insurance whatsoever (ibid.).

In a study of the privatization of hospital services in New York City, McLafferty (1988) shows how "high need groups, including the elderly, the poor, and ethnic minorities" are the losers in the process of hospital closures and restructuring. In her case study, she shows that the reorganization plan of two voluntary hospitals was going to mean the loss of obstetric and paediatric services in an area with some of the highest infant mortality and low birth weight baby rates in New York City (New York City Department of Health 1984 as cited in McLafferty, 1988, 145).

Rosenberg (1988) has shown how abortion services in Canada discriminate among women regionally and by city size. He also shows how socio-cultural and political-economic factors affect access to abortion services, legal and illegal. Since 1988, the Supreme Court of Canada has ruled that the laws governing abortion are unconstitutional in Canada. Instead of accepting this ruling, the federal government has introduced a new abortion law that continues to place women and physicians in legal jeopardy over the right to health.

THE RIGHT TO HEALTH AND HUMAN RIGHTS

The examples cited above show that substantive rights are insufficiently matched in practice, and that in most of the world women and visible minorities suffer double disadvantage, caused by general limitations to medical access as well as specific limitations of subordinate social groups. This double disadvantage applies across the spectrum of rights recognized within the International Covenant on Economic, Social and Cultural Rights (Davies, 1988).

The acknowledgement of human rights in principle has not brought about a realization of rights in practice, policy and legislation, for many reasons. There is a series of impediments to the full implementation of programs that includes an array of simply practical problems, including technological, economic and infrastructural underdevelopment that impede progress towards universal solutions; problems of a legal nature that range from political legislative obstacles to the difficulties of interpreting declarations of rights; consequent problems of co-ordinating international and national legislation and jurisdiction; the dilemmas that attend the provision of rights on an individual and a collective basis, especially in situations complicated by questions of national self-determination; and limitations upon enforcement or remedy mechanisms for achieving human rights.

A second order of problems occurs at an ideological level, in achieving consensus on the nature of rights to be guaranteed. The United Nations documents give priority to civil and political rights, which are relatively clearly specified, over economic, social and cultural rights, of which the right to health is one. The latter rights are more flexibly defined, and their implementation is to be accomplished progressively rather than immediately, according to available resources as determined by individual member states (Weissbrodt, 1988, 8). An obligation to recognize a right is not in itself, however, a guarantee of affirmative action; the right to health is not the right to be healthy. The flexibility of definitions of health, and the emphasis upon local resources, therefore, can be used with equal ease as an excuse for non-action or as a device for grassroots empowerment. Furthermore, the right to health presupposes a definition of health which is historically contingent, and which occurs within a shifting cultural context. The ideological nature of this definition, and its link to relations of power that define fundamental social conditions, make representations of health highly partial and subject, therefore, to differential access. This recognition propels our argument into an extremely complex realm of moral, philosophical and legal controversy.

Within the more limited scope of this essay, however, our concern now turns to the issue of how access to health care is compromised as a result of the extension of the notion of natural right to the notion of natural difference, where difference, based on inherent aspects of "race" and sex, becomes the basis for the social construction of inequality. The natural rights discourse is, we argue, contradictory in its definition of rights, and so becomes an impediment to the very social changes it propounds.

The notion of the right to health in international terms is part of the post-World War II "world revolution" in human rights (Humphrey, 1977), whereby the 19th-century concept of state sovereignty gave way to a recognition of universal and fundamental human rights that transcend state boundaries (Weissbradt, 1988). The WHO is a product of this natural rights philosophy, based on the twin principles of the fundamental right of the individual to "the enjoyment of the highest attainable standard of health" and the fundamental obligation of all states for "the provision of adequate health and social measures" in a spirit of cooperation with other member states.

All of the international conventions on equality rights derive from the principle of natural rights, expressed in Article 1 of the Universal Declaration of Human Rights, that "All human beings are born free and equal in dignity and rights" and therefore (Article 2) entitled to rights and freedoms "without distinction of any kind, such as race, colour, sex, language, religion, political or other opinion, national or social origin, property, birth or other status." Within the logic of this claim for primordial equality, it follows that if equality is naturally given, it is the unnatural, a state of inequality, that is socially constructed. It is, therefore, the obligation of human beings, through the auspices of their state organizations, to maintain the balance of nature by dismantling the social barriers to equality.

It could be argued, however, that the idealization of equality that occurs in natural rights theories is of little help in the provision of equality rights in common life. Furthermore, the transcendental notion of rights established in the United Nations discourse provides no inherent justification beyond the rights themselves, and leaves the specification of rights open to a wide range of interpretation. As Lowey (1987) points out, such a view is a static one, and has limited scope for social change. It leads to a notion of justice as formal, external, immutable, unrelated to "human needs and human experiences" (ibid., 787). The achievement of rights will be severely limited, then, until it is more widely recognized that both equality and inequality are socially constructed. Individuals are not born equal, but are born into socially constructed situations of inequality. Rights, then, are neither natural nor inherent, but constructed as a form of social relationship.

What Loewy and others who envision rights provision within a pragmatist philosophy of community negotiation fail to recognize, however, is that construction of rights and meanings occurs according to the terms of power by which social relations are structured. Power is no simple process, but is fractured along the complex lines of social, political and economic formation, and given strength in the intersection of cultural beliefs and practices. This principle is becoming well established in feminist scholarship, where not only is the construction of gender seen increasingly as one of power (for reviews see Connell 1987; Tong 1989), the social construction of the "body" as expression of gendered identity is carried over to expression of the "body politic" in which the full terms of power are expanded to encompass the individual and the state.

This relationship has obvious medical application, developed, for example, by Lock (1988), who reports a "disjunction between belief and body" that results in a reconstruction of menopausal symptoms to conform not to subjective experience but to a state rhetoric that supports the "oft-repeated mythology about the nuclear family, modernization, and the loss of traditional values that many middle-aged women, together with the majority of Japanese appear to accept as reality" (ibid., 55). Thus "medicalization" of national life takes into account the complex of interest—the state, health care professionals, men and women—that converge within the nexus of power by which the complex strategy of national development emerges. Our concern for health, then, takes a critical turn, pivoting from a position that propounds the inherent right to health, to one that uncovers the social means by which relations of power that subordinate gendered and racialized members of society also make them more vulnerable to the inadequacies of health care and other public service provisions.

We have labelled this process a "discourse" because it involves the production of meaning within an ideological framework, that is, of the meaning of "health," of "gender," of "race." Such production of meaning structures social relations, in which a "hierarchy of acceptability" to use Miles' (1989, 51) terminology, emerges to represent hegemonic priorities, which "shift constantly, reflecting the changing dynamics of gender, race/ethnic and class relations over time" (Ng, 1989, 10), as well as the shifting ways in which such definitions project nationalist agenda toward an international screen.

The work of Michel Foucault exposes the terms of such an agenda in his historical analysis of the links between cultural definitions of "illness" (1973) and "sexuality" (1978). His analysis of discourse takes shape in two ways. First, as Jackson (1989, 167) has shown, it "allows the reader to move between individual statements and the social relations of power through which those statements are articulated and given meaning, moving back and forth from 'text' to 'context'." This analytical project provides a methodology to link "text" and "context" in order to uncover the ambiguities, tensions and contradictions between individual experience and social structure or between what we have called, somewhat loosely, "rhetoric" and "reality."

Such analytical distinctions, however, are only that. A second feature of analysis of discourse is that it is more than a probing or deconstruction of formal language; it is the cultural process itself by which meaning and power are negotiated. Again, as Jackson notes (Jackson, 1989, 167): "For Foucault, relations of power are never external to a discourse; rather, they are immanent in it and operate through it."

Using the case studies presented above as examples, the forms of social relationship most strongly connected to the inaccessibility of health care are patriarchy and racism, rooted in cultural constructions of "gender" and "race," two terms that define fundamental characteristics and categories of human beings, and that provide a basis for an ideology of difference and a justification of systemic inequality sustained through cultural practice. These notions are invoked through a discourse that defines human places, and through which health is racialized and gendered. They need to be linked to the international rhetoric on human rights, or contextualized, in order to uncover the ways in which the gap between recognition of right and provision of right is culturally constructed.

Thus the health effects of such practices as criminalization of abortion, genital mutilation, stigmatization of sexual preference and medical apartheid are normatively condoned or supported and given moral justification in ways that do not conflict with the state's commitment to international striving for human rights. The stigma of AIDS is bound to the stigma of sexual preference and to "race," high levels of infant and maternal mortality are de-emphasized in proportion to the devaluing of women's place within society, and male professionalism supercedes traditional methods of health care, such as midwifery, that are usually the domain of women.

To understand how such situations of inequality come about in what seems to be defiance of accepted standards of equality, it is necessary to penetrate the discourse through which value systems that sustain inequality come about. For however oppressive they may be, value systems work because the are valuable, and are given cultural legitimacy. This means that it is not sufficient to recognize, for example, the equality of men and women in gaining access to the medical professions; we need also to challenge the process by which the professional standards set by men retain a higher status while the practices traditionally performed by women continue to be debased. Similarly, it is not sufficient to provide equal access to all "races"; it is necessary to challenge the cultural notion of "race" itself, and the ideology of difference by which human beings have become categorized on the basis of skin colour (European Parliament, 1985; Said, 1985). Nor is it sufficient to accept the right to health on principle; the gap between the right to health and access to health can only be bridged through an interrogation of the means by which health itself is culturally constructed.

CONCLUSIONS

Despite the strength of rhetorical claims for Health for All as a universal commitment, discrepancies between policy objectives and the actual provision of health care continue in both developed and developing areas of the world. While the problems in provision of health care need to be understood in light of economic, political and technological impediments, it is also necessary to understand the specific cultural contexts in which ideologies of difference are used to construct and to justify inequality.

To make this claim is not to reject the goal of Health for All, or to denigrate the progress that has been made in international cooperation to achieve high standards and universal access. It is to suggest that the challenge to provide new ways of thinking about health will be met in part through a critical understanding of the extent to which concepts of health are thoroughly contextual, and replicate the relations of power, sustained by cultural norms, through which inequality is effected. It is to challenge the discourse of human rights in which contemporary notions of health care have developed, in order to uncover the means by which practices such as patriarchy and racism lead to unequal access to "equality."

REFERENCES

Alubo, S.O. (1987). Power and privileges in medical care: an analysis of medical services in post-colonial Nigeria. *Social Science and Medicine, 24*(5), 453-62.

Andersson, N., & Marks, S. (1989). The state, class and the allocation of health resources Southern Africa. *Social Science and Medicine, 28*(5), 515-30.

Connell, R.W. (1987). *Gender and Power*. Cambridge: Polity Press.

Davies, P. (Ed.) (1988). *Human Rights*. London and New York: Routledge.

European Parliament. Committee of Inquiry into the Rise of Fascism and Racism in Europe (1985). *Report on the Findings of the Committee.* Luxembourg: European Parliament.

Foucault, M. (1973). *The Birth of the Clinic.* London: Tavistock.

— —. (1978). *The History of Sexuality Volume I: An Introduction.* (Hurley, R., Trans.) New York: Vintage.

Humphrey, J. (1977). The world revolution and human rights. In A. Gotlieb (Ed.), *Human Rights, Federalism and Minorities.* (147-79). Toronto: Canadian Institute of International Affairs.

Jackson, P. (1989). *Maps of Meaning: An Introduction to Cultural Geography.* London: Unwin Hyman.

Lock, M. (1988). New Japanese mythologies: faltering discipline and the ailing housewife. *American Ethnologist, 15*(1), 43-61.

Loewy, F.H. (1987). Communities, obligations and health care. *Social Science and Medicine, 25*(7), 783-91.

McLafferty, S.L. (1988). The politics of privatization: state and local politics and the restructuring of hospitals in New York. In J.L. Scarpaci (Ed.), *Health Services Privatization in Industrial Societies.* New Brunswick, N.J.: Rutgers University Press (130-51).

Miles, R. (1989). Migration discourse, British sociology and the 'race relations' paradigm. *Migration, 6,* 29-54.

Ng, R. (1989). Sexism, racism, nationalism. In J. Vorst et al. (Eds.), *Race, Class, Gender: Bonds and Barriers.* Society for Socialist Studies, Between the Lines 5.

Pan American Health Organization (1980). *Health for All by the Year 2000. Strategies.* Washington, D.C.

Raikes, A. (1989). Women's health in East Africa. *Social Science and Medicine, 28*(5), 447-59.

Rosenberg, M.W. (1988). Linking the geographical, the medical and the political in analysing health care delivery systems. *Social Science and Medicine. 26*(1), 179-86.

Said, E. (1985). An ideology of difference. In H.L. Gates, Jr. (Ed.), *'Race,' Writing and Difference.* Chicago and London: University of Chicago Press.

Simonelli, J.M. (1987). Defective modernization and health in Mexico. *Social Science and Medicine, 24*(5), 453-62.

Tong, R. (1989). *Feminist Thought: A Comprehensive Introduction.* London: Unwin Hyman.

Turshen, M. (1986). Health and human rights in a South African Bantustan. *Social Science and Medicine, 22*(9), 887-92.

United States, Bureau of the Census. (1988). *Statistical Abstract of the United States. 108th Edition*. Washington, D.C.: U.S. Department of Commerce.

Weissbrodt, D. (1988). Human rights: an historical perspective. In P. Davies (Ed.), *Human Rights*. 1-20. London: Routledge.

World Health Organization. (1978). *Alma-Alta 1978: Primary Health Care*. Health for All Series No. 1. Geneva: WHO.

— —. (1979). *Formulating Strategies for Health for All by the Year 2000*. Health for All Series No. 2. Geneva: WHO.

Section 3

Professional Practices and Education

Introduction

If persons providing care are to have the requisite knowledge, skills, and dispositions, they must first acquire them. Some will bring cultural knowledge to the health care field but not know how to apply it. But even then the practitioner who has the knowledge and the skills to apply the knowledge may be deterred by a professional ethos which demands scientific technological care or which deculturates the potential practitioner.

Recruitment of candidates in the health professions has often been left to the vicissitudes of the educational system. There are increasing demands for equity. How such demands will be implemented remains to be seen. When we need them, we open the doors; when we have an adequate number we move to close the door. But no matter how wide open the door, we must still confront educational questions that involve professional as well as ethical standards.

However, whether the health professionals are simply inducted here or are totally educated in Canada, there are implications for the society and for the health professionals who function in a pluralastic society. What should society require? Health professionals who can function transculturally? But who is culturally sensitive? Should cultural health care be left to the ethnocultural practitioner? Should a nurse or a medical doctor practise without a knowledge and understanding of cultural behaviours? Increasingly health professional programs and those who plan them are becoming more willing to include cultural knowledge, skills and dispositions in education.

Why has there been resistance responding to these questions? In some instances, the resistance has been based on outright prejudice or ethnocentrism. In others it has been based upon what some would call a misguided belief that medicine or nursing care is scientific and technological in its orientation; that the folk ways and beliefs must be set aside. On some occasions the resistance has been systemic, or has resulted from the unwillingness of the professional leadership to change. Even some so-called innovative reports on seniors, AIDS or health planning have neglected to incorporate cultural factors. Resistance has many faces.

The articles on education focus upon what might be done to incorporate cultural considerations. There are also suggestions as to how health education facilities might teach leaders, everyday practitioners and the health educators to effect change and to deal with resistance to change.

What is the community base for the education of health professionals? What should candidates be **taught** about the interrelationship between themselves, their professions and the community? What involvement should the community have in the kind of education professionals receive? The degree of detachment of some programs to the cultural realities of the communities and to the potential patients or clients is sometimes exceedingly high despite the fact that educational theory and practice tell us that experientially based education is one of the best methods of learning and teaching.

- 8 -

Multicultural Health Care: An Introductory Course

Hope Toumishey

Daily life occurs within a cultural context in which each person's values and beliefs shape, modify and sanction their decisions about how to live. It follows therefore, that personal definitions of health and illness are culturally determined and are acted upon within the boundaries of social acceptance. The delivery of professional health care, if it is to be culturally appropriate, sensitive and responsive, can be assured only if health practitioners understand the importance of cultural behavioural conditioning for both their clients and themselves. Such conditioning can facilitate helpful communication and joint decision-making during therapeutic interactions.

Education to raise awareness of cultural factors in health occurs through the literature, seminars, workshops, conferences, courses and research. While these efforts are significant, there are still many educators who are unaware of such resources or who remain unconvinced of the need to gain this specialized knowledge. Those who do recognize the importance of this matter favour the incorporation of multicultural health care as a major component in accredited health educational curricula.

There are various opinions on how students in the health professions should be taught about the influence of cultural factors on health-seeking behaviour. Those who advocate that this theme should be completely integrated throughout the entire curriculum argue that only such an approach will ensure that clients consistently receive culturally sensitive and appropriate health care. However, this approach also requires that all faculty be very knowledgeable about culture and health, and be competent in demonstrating how to incorporate the cultural nature of clients in practice. Since this is not yet the case, the usual practice has been to offer introductory courses that will provide students with a basic foundation of knowledge on multicultural health. The student is then expected to assume personal responsibility for continuing to gain the additional knowledge and skill required to incorporate cultural factors in clinical practice.

Guidelines for incorporating cultural factors in curricula for health disciplines are limited. Most educators have relied informally on the work of others while drawing heavily on their own understanding of the essential cultural concepts that are relevant to their respective disciplines. A consensus does seem to be a slowly emerging, however, on what interdisciplinary knowledge should be considered fundamental to the study of multicultural health. In the main, these cultural concepts are primarily identified in the medical anthropology and nursing literature and increasingly from medicine and social work. Suggested content for introductory multicultural health courses for these disciplines are provided by Branch (1976); Kay (1978); Leininger (1978); Koss (1979); Rubel (1979); Byerly and Brink (1979); Henderson and Primeaux (1981); Chrisman (1982); Berlin and Fowkes (1983); Spector (1985); Hayes (1986); Toumishey and Pocius (1986); Lipson (1988) and Christenson (1989).

It should be noted that, for any study on cultural factors, basic knowledge about anthropological concepts is important. Therefore, it is advisable that students complete introductory courses in anthropology and medical anthropology prior to entering any course on multicultural health. What students learn specifically from anthropologists includes relevant information about cultural orientations and lifeways, as well as methods of observing and systematically recording this behaviour. This knowledge, when combined with normal methods of clinical observation, dramatically increases their understanding of health and illness behaviour within diverse cultural contexts.

The application of this knowledge in professional practice, however, requires that students also receive additional direction on how to incorporate cultural factors when providing health care. As Lipson states: "teaching of straight anthropology is not sufficient for teaching nurses (also applicable to other health disciplines) to use cultural perspectives in practice, teaching and research....An approach which includes knowledge (content), a focus on attitudes and self-awareness, and an opportunity to apply cognitive and affective learning in a practice situation, provides superb graduates who are well prepared to do excellent work as well as help other nurses consider cultural variables in nursing care" (1988, 5). The following outline and discussion of an introductory course on multicultural health provides this specific direction.

THE INTRODUCTORY COURSE IN MULTICULTURAL HEALTH CARE

The overall purpose of this course is to help students begin to acquire knowledge and understanding of cultural and racial diversity so that they will successfully incorporate awareness of such factors in their professional practice.

In order to achieve this, careful consideration must first be given to what specific objectives can be feasibly met in the course, given the available resources and time constraints. Since the range of cultural context is too extensive to cover in detail in any course, a number of general concepts are introduced that are intended to stimulate the students' interest in the subject, and to provide them with enough basic information and beginning skills that they will be able to implement this knowledge in their professional practice in a safe and culturally sensitive manner.

In this chapter, the discussion of these concepts is modelled on a conceptual framework entitled "Multicultural health: basic concepts for an introductory course for health practitioners" (see Figure 1). The discussion will be limited to a few major points considered basic to each of the concepts, and to selected authors who provide valuable related information and analysis. The precise manner in which these concepts are addressed in any learning situation is, however, the prerogative of faculty.

In Figure 1, the conceptual framework is divided into three sections. Section 1 includes three major components that are common to all cultures, the understanding of which are essential for the development of a trusting relationship between clients and their care-givers. These components are **culture and cultures, values and beliefs, and intercultural communication.** Section 2 focuses on health related factors that determine the conduct of the application of the above three general concepts in professional practice. These factors are **health-seeking behaviour and health care options.** Section 3 focuses on cultural factors that influence the conduct of **therapeutic interactions,**

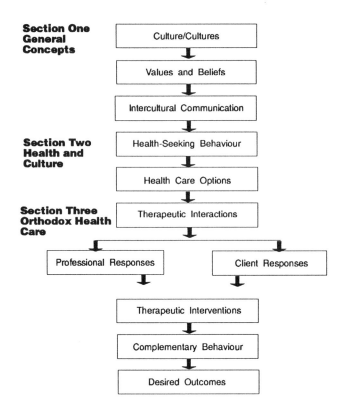

Section One
General
Concepts

Culture/Cultures

Values and Beliefs

Intercultural Communication

Section Two
Health and
Culture

Health-Seeking Behaviour

Health Care Options

Section Three
Orthodox Health
Care

Therapeutic Interactions

Professional Responses   Client Responses

Therapeutic Interventions

Complementary Behaviour

Desired Outcomes

Figure 1 - Multicultural health: a basic conceptual framework for a multidisciplinary introductory course.

and decision-making for therapeutic interventions that are appropriate to the cultural nature of clients and that are administered by health practitioners who function within the dominant orthodox health care delivery system.

Section One: General Concepts

Culture and Cultures

Developing a basic understanding of multicultural health requires that students have no doubt that culture is the dominant factor that determines health values, beliefs and behaviour, the etiology of disease and illness and the interpretation of these phenomena. Similarly, they need to understand that the organization of curing and caring activities takes place within a cultural context. Health care as a cultural activity cannot be seen as merely the efficacious application of prescribed techniques. Certainly technical procedures are essential when required, but sensitive holistic health care goes beyond these skills and extends out to the community and culture of the client. Should these factors be overlooked, then caring becomes at best "an exercise in the imposition of an ethnocentric authoritative allocation of professional (i.e. middle class) values, where the client is defined as a passive recipient of what is professionally designated as appropriate efficacious treatment. To ignore the client's cultural background with all its ramifications is to deny the existential and possibly the ontological dimensions of humaneness" (Morley, Toumishey & Pocius, 1982, 1).

In the study of culture and cultures and their relevance for health, these are three major factors to be considered. First, such study forces health practitioners to recognize that they, to, are rooted in their own culture and that they bring their "personal cultural beliefs" to each interaction with their clients. Having this awareness will lead them to expect that there may be some difficulty in communicating empathy, congruence, respect and acceptance when they interact with clients who adhere to a culture different from their own. Also, practitioners who do not deliberately examine their own cultural orientation may be prone to imposing on clients certain cherished and "habitual" interventions, which may not necessarily be the best method in helping clients reach their desired state of wellness.

The second factor is learning that person and group cultural orientations are all subject to change. This is especially true where people are in transition from one cultural orientation to another. The adjustment behaviour of such people was termed by Oberg in 1954 as culture shock. It can be precipitated by choice, through immigration, or defection, or by force, through becoming refugees; on through moving from one community or family to another; or through temporary or permanent admission to new systems and institutions such as hospitals and nursing homes. Brink and Sauders (1989) have reformulated Oberg's original premises like a concept model that can be adapted by health professionals in the context of health settings. They postulate that if normal life changes are stressful and require physical and behavioural adjustments, how much more of a "shock" are dramatic life changes such as those that occur when a person faces illness and/or death. This shock is compounded when it is experienced in an unfamiliar cultural setting.

The third factor is the recognition that health care cannot be appropriately planned without attention to the cultural environment(s) within which people have to make adjustments to change. For example, although Canada is one of the most polyethnic societies in the world and is a country whose ethnic diversity is officially recognized by both the federal and provincial governments, many Canadian-born people or immigrants still encounter overt cultural, ethnic and racial prejudice. Since such attitudes can contribute to loss of self-esteem and cultural identity, health practitioners must determine their own attitudes and possible biases towards clients from cultures which are different from their own. This will ensure that they are not inadvertently interfering with the rights of these clients to access to equitable and culturally sensitive comprehensive health care. The examination of ethnic pluralism in Canada, as described by Dreiger (1989) and the study of the Canadian Charter of Rights and Freedoms proclaimed in 1982 and the Multiculturalism Act of 1988 are invaluable as a means of gaining some understanding of the dominant social and political realities of living in a pluralistic country.

Values and Beliefs

An open mind is essential when attempting to recognize the relativity of one's own culture compared to others. To understand any culture, one must try to understand its symbolic world. This symbolic world is ordered by value systems inherent in all cultures which are formulated and sanctioned through what Blumer (1969) calls symbolic interactionism. He states that symbolic interactionism rests on three premises: that human beings act toward things on the basis of the meanings that the things have for them; that the meanings of things arise from the social interaction that one has with one's fellows; and that one handles and modifies these meanings through an interpretative process that is used by the individual when dealing with the things he or she encounters.

In any interaction between a client and a professional therapist, the meaning of health and illness as it relates to the circumstances that have brought the participants together is thus rooted in the values which each of them hold; these values are expressed symbolically in a manner that may or may not be fully understood. Therefore, the therapist must not only make the effort to gain as much insight as possible about the value orientations of the client in order to provide culturally appropriate care, but must also know upon which personal and professional values he or she will make decisions for the well-being of the client. This clarification process increases awareness of value priorities, and of the degree of consistency between the values held, and the related personal and professional attitudes and behaviour of each of the participants.

The examination of values as the fundamental determinants of human behaviour requires a search for similarities of values among the participants. It is only after this understanding is reached that value differences can be intelligently explored. This search for similarities can be guided by the hypotheses of Kluckhohn and Mowrer (1944), who identified four major determinants of personality which they term as universal, communal, roles and idiosyncratic as well as four levels of expression of personality which they call biological, physical and environmental, social and cultural. Building on their work, Kluckhohn in 1953, and Kuckhorn and Strodbeck in 1961, provided a conceptual system that allows for a systematic ordering of value orientations within the framework of five common-universal-problems, each of which has three possible solutions. These problems are: 1) innate human nature which can range from evil to good; 2) the relationship between humans and nature where people are either subjugated by nature, in nature, or have control over nature; 3) time orientation in the past, the present or future; 4) valued personality type; and 5) types of relationships which may be lineal, collateral or individualistic. Put in the form of a grid, this framework is useful for generally identifying value profiles for specific cultures. When using this process, care must be taken not to stereotype clients as no two persons in any one group will totally share and act upon their values in exactly the same manner. Such variation may be minor in nature but still significant in their manifestations.

Beliefs differ from values in that they are representations of the way people view their world. What they and others in their social group agree to be true, is true, if not necessarily logical. Beliefs are largely determined by what people are conditioned to believe, want to believe, and have to believe to meet certain basic needs and for continuing acceptance by others in their social group. According to Raths, Harmon and Simon (1978), the importance of a belief depends on how connected it is to other beliefs and what consequences it has on other beliefs. Beliefs learned from direct experience and shared by others are very connected and, therefore, very central.

In health, for example, beliefs related to the causation of an illness or injury takes on particular significance because they govern the actions that are taken to relieve discomfort associated with the illness or injury. Causation beliefs generally held by health professionals in orthodox health systems are related to germ theory, lifestyle behaviour and environmental toxicity. Clients, however, may hold quite different causation beliefs relating to their personal health problems. Murdock (1980) discusses the diversity of theories of causation around the world, which range from the theory that medicine is an applied science to the theory held by the majority of the world's population that medicine is applied religion. He classifies these theories into four major categories which he calls natural causation, supernatural causation, animistic causation and magical causation. These classifications are useful tools when conducting health histories since clients will act according to what they believe is the cause of their illness, which may not necessarily coincide with the diagnosis of a professional practitioner. The relevance of studying causation beliefs is also supported by Morley who states: "One must seriously ask oneself whether superstition and myth, in the derogatory or non-specific connotations of these words, are not due to our judging a given people from our conceptual standpoint rather than theirs...When the trouble was taken to find their concepts, then it became evident that everything made sense and that their behaviour and cultural norms followed as naturally and consistently from their particular categories of natural experience as ours do from our own" (1978, 1).

Most important, professional health practitioners must recognize that it is not sufficient to base ethical considerations only on the values that they personally hold. This is particularly relevant in that, as Williams points out, "the present North American monolithic view of human nature and culture can lead to the bioethical considerations which are inadequate when caring for multicultural clientele" (1990, 3). Williams also noted that in the discussions, at the conference on "Transcultural Dimensions of Medical Ethics" in Washington, DC (April 26-27, 1990), speakers consistently demonstrated that the emphasis of the bioethical approach in medical decision making is actually a minority position within the global community. Such misinterpretations of the diverse cultural values of clients can lead to value conflicts that inevitably will reduce their right to culturally sensitive, equitable quality health care. The conduct of a concurrent ethical analysis, with the cultural aspects present in any given therapeutic interaction in mind, will contribute to resolving the dilemmas associated with such conflict.

Intercultural Communication

The importance of developing skill in intercultural communication through the use of language and other symbols during interchanges in a therapeutic interaction can be facilitated through an examination of intercultural communication theory, and through critical analysis of the communication dynamics present during such interactions. Attempts to achieve consensus about subject-matter among people of various cultures is further complicated when the participants speak different languages since they are usually unaware of the implications of their own respective speech habits. As Fuglesang explains, "the notion of rationality or logical reasoning has in any culture the twist of that culture....When we indulge verbally in our logical faculties, we do not sense that the phenomenon of our language surrounds and controls us, the speakers, as an element outside our critical consciousness" (1982, 18).

Hall and Whyte (1989) provide further insight into how cultural affects communication in their discussion on how convention permits or demands the amount and type of physical contact and the intensity of emotion that accompanies the communication. They explain how culture determines the timing of interpersonal interactions, the place where it may occur, the spacial distance between participants and the acceptable tone of voice for the interaction. Communication difficulties are further compounded through a lack of understanding of the meanings of culture specific signs, symbols, gestures, emotional connotations, historical references, traditional responses and pointed silences. Hall and Whyte provide some general approaches to facilitate effective interactions among people of diverse cultures. These include the recognition that one's personal convictions are in no respect more "eternally" right than someone else's, and that conversational patterns exist and need to be accommodated in any interaction, be they personal or therapeutic.

Singer (1987) focuses primarily on perception and identity in intercultural communication. He expounds on the value of existing communication theories but has modified these theories to fit his perceptual focus. He proposes a number of premises, beginning with a definition of a perceptual group, which he defines as a number of individuals who perceive some aspect of the external world more or less similarly, but who do not communicate this similarity of perception among themselves. However, should this group communicate this similarity, they are transformed into an identity group. The more individuals continue to share their perceptions with others, the more likely will they be able to identify to differing degrees - and at different levels of consciousness - with other value systems. At this level, should direct conflict occur among simultaneously held group identities, an attempt will usually be made to find some third identity to accommodate, neutralize, rationalize and/or synthesize these conflicting systems. The application of these theories facilitates understanding of why difficulties may occur in intercultural therapeutic interactions where the client and the therapist do not share a cultural definition of the situation in which they are communicating.

Another confounding factor in intercultural communication is that Western-oriented therapists generally view problems brought by clients in terms of linear cause-effect relationships. However, the subjective realities of the non-Western socialized client will, in all probability, have been shaped by a different cultural conditioning for addressing problems and causal relationships. This inevitably leads to incongruence between the participants' respective interpretations of the situation and their expectations as to outcome. Overcoming this incongruence requires that participants in an intercultural interaction take responsibility for learning as much as possible about the cultural and social realities of each other before and during each such event.

The understanding of such communication barriers can be enhanced if the directions of Fuglesand and Brownlee (1978) are followed: in describing applied intercultural communication for educators and health workers in developing countries, they provide explicit information on which communication strategies are effective or preventive to intercultural understanding. They also give clear guidelines to communication process to facilitate constructive interchanges with those seeking health care. Careful selection of the major components of these theories for study, can help in formulating effective communication strategies appropriate for therapeutic interactions with clients from diverse cultures.

Section Two: Health and Culture

Health-seeking Behaviour

Health-seeking behaviour is generally governed by belief, tradition, experience, knowledge and the extent to which people have access to alternate options for health care services. The study of concepts such as culture, cultures, values, beliefs and intercultural communication assists in the process of gaining understanding of the reasons why people behave in certain ways and how this behaviour affects health, and responses to illness.

It is important to understand that the experience of illness is not necessarily identical to any biomedical interpretation of disease, but is rather an individual's perception of illness, which is constructed from belief and knowledge at the time and place in which it occurs. Because definitions of health and acceptable illness and health-seeking behaviour are essentially culturally determined, there are inevitable variations in the way people perceive and response to health-threatening situations, and in the choices that they make form the alternative sources of health-care services to which they have access.

Chrisman and Maretzki question "what links could be sought in the cultural environment in which individuals grew up to the nature of the adult world in which they matured, and how could these linkages be related to behavioural expressions and cultural labelling of behaviours" (1982, 3).

The search for such links in relation to health is assisted by Chrisman who suggests that the elements in the health-seeking process are symptom definition, illness-related shifts in role behaviour, lay consultation and referral, treatment actions and adherence (1977, 353). He explains that, while these elements may describe health-related actions that a sick person may exhibit, they are not necessarily sequential. This process is dynamic and strongly influenced by actions taken in the past and the present.

There are many other theories and discussions on health-seeking behaviour in the literature (for example, see Kleinman, Eisenberg and Good (1978); Good and Good (1981); and Romanucci-Ross, Moerman and Tancredi (1983). Their material is helpful in that it provides some explanation as to why there is great diversity in perceptions of illness and health-seeking behaviour.

Health Care Options

Given the number of available alternative options for health care, it is important to understand what is generally inherent within these options, and on what criteria personal choices among these options are based. To facilitate this understanding, the "Pathway to Health" model was developed by Toumishey (see Figure 2). This model shows five major steps along the pathway to health, from the moment of self-awareness of a health problem to its final outcome. Steps 2 to 5 relate specifically to the four major health care systems most commonly used when in need. These are self care, folk and popular care, unorthodox care and orthodox care.

Each of the five steps in this model are presented in a logical order in which health seeking probably occurs. The arrows point toward the direction (pathway) most likely to be followed in the option selection process. This order does not mean, however, that people will not revert to any of the other options when strategies that are initiated by self or others fail to provide the desired outcome.

Also identified in this model are the two choices that people have when deciding to accept or reject therapies associated with each of the five steps to health. These are denial of significance of the presenting symptom(s), which negates the need to act or validation of the significance of the symptom(s) as health-threatening, which requires immediate action by self alone or by reference to others for help.

Step One: Self-awareness

The conscious awareness of a potential or real health problem for oneself starts the process for option selection for the relief of the presenting symptoms. Whereas in some instances people may attempt to deny that they have a problem, most seek first to validate whether there is a need to act immediately for comfort and restoration of health, or whether they can safely delay such action for a while.

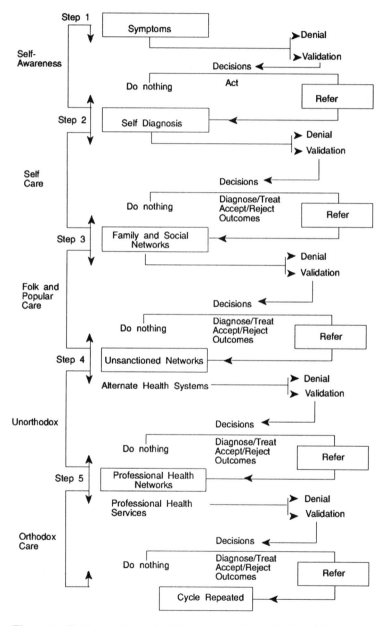

Figure 2 - Pathway for selecting care options for health

Step Two: Self Care

Where there is some or no history of the presenting symptom(s), self diagnosis of the cause of the complaint is usually made first in the hope that the situation is of minor concern and temporary in nature. If so considered, tested home, folk, and/or over-the-counter remedies previously considered as effective for similar symptoms may be tried.

Step Three: Folk and Popular Care

When self-care efforts fail to provide the desired symptom relief, help is commonly solicited from others, usually within family and social networks. Those who are considered to have knowledge and experience and are trusted as "healers" are approached for advice, direct interventions and support throughout the entire period of discomfort. These resource people generally suggest either folk and/or popular remedies.

Additional alternate approaches may be to request a pharmacist to recommend non-prescription remedies or to seek and act on health information available in the popular literature. For some conditions, this information may be appropriate, but the fact that many people resort to these measures, even when contraindicated, is an indication of the strength of their desire to remain in personal control of decision making for their health, and thus to try any method that promises immediate or early relief and/or cure of the disrupting health condition.

Step Four: Unorthodox Care

When the above options fail to provide the desired relief, unorthodox therapies may be considered, if they are seen to offer fast and effective solutions to acute or chronic illnesses or injuries. Unorthodox therapies are those which are provided by particular practitioners who may use specific healing strategies that are not officially sanctioned within the orthodox professional health care system or by government. These practitioners include homeopathists, naturopaths, shamans, faith or psychic healers, indigenous traditional healers and, in some instances, chiropractors.

In Canada, health practitioners who provide care in other major world-health systems such as Ayerveda, Unani, Humerol and African or Chinese medicine are also considered to be providers of unorthodox health care services. It is understandable that they are many in Canada's ethnocultural societies who put their faith in these culturally specific, time-tested and honoured approaches to health care. Such practitioners are often consulted while the patients are under the care of orthodox physicians.

Step Five: Orthodox Care

The majority of people in Canada are generally comfortable in seeking care from practitioners who function within orthodox professional health networks. The dominant orthodox health care system in Canada, as in most other developed countries, offers high calibre services to meet more health needs of people, yet are not always considered as a primary option for needed care. The selection of these services depends largely on personal perceptions of the seriousness of the presenting symptoms and discomfort; personal interpretations of the value of past experiences as clients in the system; present perceptions of the attitudes of physicians and other professional practitioners, and levels of trust in their competence and the availability of and equitable access to their services.

The examination of cultural factors that influence decision making by clients for seeking or rejecting the professional services offered by the orthodox health system provides practitioners within this system with the opportunity to become acutely sensitive to the human need for respect and support of personal health-related values and beliefs when ill. It also alerts them to the need for clients to act as participants in planning for their own health in a complementary way, rather than to accept solutions imposed on them by therapists passively, without consultation.

To facilitate understanding of why people choose from the options available in the above health systems, the "Constructs Comparisons" of major health systems was developed to show the basic elements within each of the major constructs held in common by these systems (see Table 1).

This comparison serves to demonstrate some of the similarities and differences of each of these systems, but are not complete or extensively elaborated upon. They are, however, sufficient to stimulate interest in examining these options in greater depth. Also, the variations in philosophical bases that determine the specific approaches and strategies used for health in each of these systems provide an opportunity for a comparison of evaluation with those found in the first three systems with those found in the orthodox health system, where practitioners are criticized for not taking sufficient account of the health values, beliefs and traditional practices of their clients.

Table 1
Construct Comparisons of Major Health Systems

Construct	Folk	Popular	Unorthodox	Orthodox
Values	Humanistic. Humans as part of nature.	Humanistic in part. Profit making.	Humanistic in part. Profit making.	Humanistic but mainly on scientific basis.
Beliefs	Total nature of person involved. Controlled by nature. Illness caused by magic, spiritual or natural means.	Self care with direct access to remedies by purchase. Partly control nature. Varied causation beliefs.	Usually one specific causation belief. Some biomedical base. Can manipulate nature in part. Cure at source.	Biomedical focus. Theories of causation: germs, stress and environmental. Strong belief in ability to control nature by science.
Meanings Explanations	Clear and known. Explanations: retribution, fate, mystical spirit agression and sorcery.	Often unclear. Many single explanations. Superficial knowledge. Some mystery.	Clear. Limited technology, research and drugs. Often one strong causation belief and one dominant therapy.	Varied. Focused on cause and effect. Mysterious in part due to sophistication.

Table 1 continued
Construct Comparisons of Major Health Systems

Construct	Folk	Popular	Unorthodox	Orthodox
Focus	Holistic caring. Family-centered. Prevention and curing.	Individual centered. Prevention and curing.	Holistic in part. Individual centered, mainly fragmented.	Holistic in part. Mainly individual centered. Fragmented control. Prevention and curing.
Settings	Community/home.	Anywhere.	Own offices.	Institutions, offices and homes.
Organization	Loose. Directed by events. Controlled within local areas and by local access to resources.	Commerical venue. Advertise to sell products. Over counter drugs controlled. Some freelance.	Varied. Some organized in professional associations. Legislative control limited.	Tends towards hierarchy and bureaucracy. Highly organized and controlled.

Table 1 continued
Construct Comparisons of Major Health Systems

Construct	Folk	Popular	Unorthodox	Orthodox
Motivation of Clients	Seek relief from familiar and significant persons. Limited or no access to options outside local area.	Readily available. Quick relief for self or others.	Direct access usually in urban areas. Limited intrusive and painful interventions.	Reasonable access. Trusted scientific base. Familiar with system. Rely on professionals when not able to self manage.
Expectations of Clients	Immediate relief. Accommodating and culturally sensitive. Familial and individual decisions.	Immediate relief. Mainly individual decisions.	Immediate or promise of relief. Mainly individual decisions.	Immediate or promise of relief. Individual and familial decisions.
Acceptance by Clients	Self generated. Many fatalistic. High faith in time-tested care.	Worthy of trial.	Faith in naturalistic and non-drastic intrusive interventions.	Faith in system becoming more demanding for explanations and involvement in planning care.

Table 1 continued
Construct Comparisons of Major Health Systems

Construct	Folk	Popular	Unorthodox	Orthodox
Practitioners	Familiar healers shared values and beliefs. High status. Education experiential. Some specialists. Profit making.	No defined role for healers.	Varied. Education formal/apprentic. Some specialists. Unidisciplinary. Profit-making. Limited legislative control.	Varied. Local and non-local. Diverse values. Formally educated. Many specialists. Use scientific research. Legislative control.
Therapies	Non-technical. Diagnostic. Direct client contact. Use natural products and rituals. May incorporate the supernatural. Short term.	Limited technology. Diagnostic. Natural and manufactured products. Limited client contact. Short term.	Varied complexity. Diagnostic. Direct client contact. Use of natural products and physical manipulations. Short and long term.	Complex. Diagnostic. Technical. Heavy drug use and surgery. Direct client contact. Short and long term.
Costs	Minimal. Shared by primary group. Fees usually in kind within limits of client.	Varied. Choice of individual. Depends on demand.	Varied. Depends on complexity of treatment.	Expensive due to complexity and extensiveness. Salaries and fees high. Clients may have insurance.

Section Three: Orthodox Health Care

Orthodox health care is provided through a process of therapeutic interactions between clients and professional practitioners during which interventions appropriate to the needs of the
clients are determined and accepted.

Therapeutic Interactions

All participants in therapeutic interactions bring with them
their cultural selves, which means that each will act primarily
upon what they value, believe and know with respect to the
clinical situation (see Figure 3). The basic personality development of people who share similar cultural and ethnic orientations
within particular sociocultural environments is, in part, formulated through early experiences. As a consequence of this sharing, they will have many elements of personality in common.
Likewise, those who do not share these early experiences will
have differing personality characteristics.

Individual personal characteristics are dependent on states of
physical and emotional growth, as well as on levels of integrated
human functioning in terms of sexual orientation, role status,
outlook, view of self, social responsibilities, levels of knowledge
and expectations for self. These characteristics all contribute to
the formulation of a personal perception of one's own health
status, and for a therapist, a perception of the overall status of
a client.

The past that personal characteristics play in a therapeutic
interaction is, therefore, crucial and will strongly influence the
conduct of the interchanges among the participants. A continuing awareness of this fact by all those involved is necessary to
ensure the development and maintenance of a positive and
trusting therapeutic relationship among them. It is this complementary behaviour, which also contributes to the making of
mutually acceptable professional and client judgments, within
the limits set by the structure of the orthodox health system, that
will hopefully lead to the desired outcome for all those involved.

During therapeutic interactions, professional practitioners
are morally and legally obligated to strive to meet the health
needs of their clients to the best of their ability. Clients, in turn,
are equally obligated to be sensitive to the cultural and professional background of their therapists in that, by seeking their
care, they give note that they support the established health
structures and services in which their therapists function. For

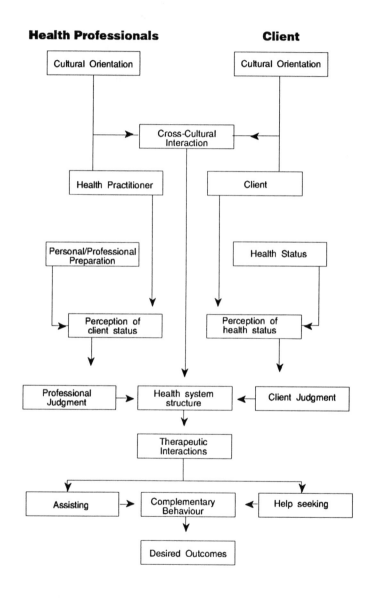

Figure 3 - Personal characteristics of participants in cross-cultural therapeutic interactions

many there is a "cultural congruency" in that they share the "cultural patterning" of the policy- and decision-makers within this health system. Difficulties may arise when this congruency does not exist. In these circumstances, it is the practitioners who takes first responsibility to accommodate to the realities of these clients and to reassure them that these differences are understood and recognized and will be taken into account.

Therapeutic Interventions

Therapeutic interventions are not solely the prerogative of professional practitioners. In most circumstances, while specific regimens are proposed and prescribed by them, the consent to adhere to the recommendations is governed by the will of the client. A consensus is, therefore, essential. Without it, the possibility exists that the desired outcome, from the client's point of view, could be in conflict with that of the practitioner.

To prevent this conflict, all planned interventions must incorporate those factors that influence the lifeways, and thus the health, of each individual client. These factors are discussed by Orque (1983) who proposes a Ethnic/Cultural System Framework in which she identifies the components of this system to be value orientations, language and communication processes, healing beliefs and practices, family and life processes, diet, religion, art and history. Kleinman (1978) expands on these components by giving recognition to the types of realities held in common by people. These are physical, biological, psychological, social and symbolical realities within a social world and a non-human physical environment. The application of these, and other models such as those by Leininger (1978), Spector (1985) and Waxler-Morrison, Anderson & Richardson (1990) provide the practitioner with direction for determining more exactly the health needs of clients that require professional intervention if the presenting problems are to be resolved.

Clients have a right and a responsibility to ensure that they participate in the determination of appropriate interventions on their behalf. Practitioners, on the other hand, have a responsibility to assist those clients who are hesitant to contribute to decision making. It is in this collaborative and complementary process that any interventions proposed will be seen to have a high probability of effectiveness for the well-being of the client. As well, the care that is delivered will be perceived to be sensitive and appropriate to the unique cultural and social circumstances of the client, thus facilitating his or her capacity to cope with the short- or long-term effects of the illness or injury.

CONCLUSIONS

This course has been offered for over ten years at one Canadian university. Students are asked to apply this knowledge in clinical practice, through two specific assignments. The first is designed to sensitize the student to the interplay of values, beliefs and communication styles among people who are participating in a particular unfamiliar cultural experience. Students are asked to analyse their personal responses to being a stranger in such an experience, which helps them begin to appreciate the responses that people are likely to exhibit when they are in an unfamiliar environment. (For specific information about the requirements for this assignment and the learning consequences for the student, see Toumishey (1989).

Second, students are required to conduct a cultural health assessment. It is designed to demonstrate the value of using systematic frameworks for observing, analyzing and explaining the health-seeking behaviour of an individual, and for determining sensitive interventions appropriate to the cultural nature of each individual client.

While the value of the content covered in this course has been evaluated by students as a positive learning experience, it can be extensively enriched by rigid attention to faculty and professional staff enforcement, and by follow-through in the consistent application of cultural health factors and related aspects in clinical practice—not just for students, but for all health care practitioners.

Finally, decisions on strategies for incorporating cultural factors in curricula for health disciplines are the prerogative of their educators. A major value of the interdisciplinary approach is that students in different disciplines have the opportunity to share their respective perspectives on their professional responsibilities to provide culturally appropriate and sensitive care; to gain insight into what they hold in common with practitioners in other disciplines in this respect; and to devise ways on how they can better work together to provide the comprehensive holistic health care their mutual clients require. The conceptual framework of this course is sufficiently general in scope to allow for modifications suitable to a unidisciplinary or multidisciplinary composition of students for whom it is intended.

REFERENCES

Berlin, E.A., & Fowkes, W.C. (1983). A teaching framework for cross-cultural health care. *The Western Journal of Medicine*, *130*(6), 934-38.

Blumer, H. (1969). *Symbolic interactionism: perspective and method*. Englewood Cliffs, NJ: Prentice-Hall.

Branch, M. (1976). Models for introducing cultural diversity in nursing curricula. *Journal of Nursing Education*, *15*(2), 7-B, 13.

Brink, P.J., & Saunders, J.M. (1989). Culture shock: theoretical and applied. In P.J. Brink (Ed.), *Transcultural nursing: a book of readings*. (2nd Edition) Englewood Cliffs, NJ: Prentice-Hall.

Brownlee, A.T. (1978). *Community, culture and care: a cross-cultural guide for health worker* (3-26). St. Louis: Mosby.

Byerly, E.L., & Brink, P.J. (1979). Model course V: cultural variation in nursing practice: A course for upper division undergraduate or graduate students in nursing. In *Teaching medical anthropology (1,* 55-66). Special Publication No. 1. Washington: Society for Medical Anthropology.

Chrisman, N.J. (1977). The health seeking process: an approach to the natural history of illness. *Culture, Medicine and Psychiatry 1*, 351-77.

——. (1982). Anthropology in Nursing: an exploitation in adaptation. In N.L. Chrisman & T.W. Maretzi. *Clinically applied anthropology: anthropologists in health science settings* (117-40). Boston: Reidel.

Chrisman, N.L., & Maretzi, T.L. (1982). *Clinically applied anthropology: anthropologists in health science settings*. Boston: Reidel.

Christensen, C. (1989). Stages in the development of cross-cultural awareness: A conceptual framework. *Counsellor, Educator and Supervisor*, *28*(4), 270-87.

Dreiger, L. (1989). *The ethnic factor: identity in diversity*. Toronto: McGraw-Hill Ryerson.

Fuglesang, A. (1982). *About understanding: ideas and observations on cross-cultural communication.* Upsalla: Dag Hammarskjold Foundation.

Good, B., Good, M. (1981). The meanings of symptoms: a cultural hermeneutic model for clinical practice. In L. Eisenberg and A. Kleinman (Eds.), *The relevance of social science for medicine.* Boston: Reidal.

Hall, E.F., & Whyte, W.F. (1976). Intercultural communication. In P.J. Brink (Ed.), *Transcultural nursing: A book of readings.* Englewood Cliffs, NJ: Prentice-Hall.

Henderson, G., & Primeaux, M. (1981). *Transcultural health care.* Menlo Park, CA: Addison-Wesley.

Hayes, J.R. (1986). Consultation-liaison psychiatry and clinical ethics: a model for consultation and teaching. *General Hospital Psychiatry, 8*(6), 415-18.

Kay, M. (1978). Clinical anthropology. In E.E. Bauwens, (Ed.), *The anthropology of health.* Saint Louis: Mosby.

Kleinman, A. (1978). Culture, cure and care: clinical lessons from anthropological and cross-cultural research. *Annals of internal medicine, 88*(2), 251-58.

Kleinman, A., Eisenberg, L., & Good, B. (1978). Culture, illness and care, *Annals of Internal Medicine, 88*(2), 251-58.

Kluckhohn, F.R. (1953). Dominant and variant value orientations. In C. Kluckhohn & H.A. Murray (Eds.), *Personality in nature, society and culture,* (2nd. Ed.). New York: Knopf.

Kluckhohn, C., & Mowrer, O.H. (1944). Culture and personality: a conceptual scheme. *American Anthropologist, 46,* 1-29.

Kluckhohn, F.R., & Strodtbeck, F.L. (1961). *Variations in value orientations.* Elmsford, N.Y.: Row & Peterson.

Koss, J.D. (1979). Ethnomedicine or comparative medical systems. In H.F. Todd, & J.L. Ruffini (Eds.), *Teaching Medical Anthropology* (29-40). Special Publication No. 1. Washington: Society for Medical Anthropology.

Leininger, M. (1978). *Transcultural nursing: concepts, theories and practices.* New York: Wiley.

— —. (1981). Transcultural nursing: its progress and its future. *Nursing and Health Care* (Sept.), 365-71.

Lipson, G.J. (1988). The cultural perspective in nursing education. *Practical Anthropology, 10*(2), 4-5.

Morley, P. (1978). Culture and the cognitive world of transitional medical beliefs: some preliminary considerations. In P. Morley & R. Wallis (Eds.), *Culture and curing.* Philadelphia: University of Pennsylvania Press.

Morley, P., Toumishey, L.H., & Pocius, G. (1982). Culture and caring: a report on the transcultural care course at Memorial University of Newfoundland, (Unpublished).

Murdock, G.P. (1980). *Theories of illness.* Pittsburgh: University of Pittsburgh Press.

Orque, M.S. (1983). Orque's ethnic/cultural system: a frameowrk for ethnic nursing care. In M.S. Orque, B. Bloch, & L.A. Monrroy. *Ethnic nursing care: A multicultural approach* (5-38). St. Louis: Mosby.

Raths, L.E., Harmon, M., & Simon, B. (1978). *Values and teaching: working with values in classrooms.* Columbus, OH: Merrill.

Rubel, A.J. (1979). Medical Anthropology: an introductory field for undergraduates. In H.F. Todd, & J.L. Ruffini. *Teaching medical anthropology,* (13-20). Special Publication No. 1. Washington: Society for Medical Anthropology.

Romanucci-Ross, L., Moerman, D.E. & Tancredi, L.R. (Eds.). (1983). *The anthropology of medicine.* South Hadley, Mass: Bergin and Garvey.

Singer, M.R. (1987). *Intercultural communication.* Englewood Cliffs, NJ: Prentice-Hall.

Spector, R. (1985). *Cultural diversity in health and illness.* (2nd Ed.). Norwalk, Conn.: Appleton Century Croft.

Touishey, L.H. (1989). Strangers among strangers: clients and health practitioners in health care settings. *Nurse Education Today, 9,* 363-67.

Toumishey, L.H., & Pocius, G. (1986). Transcultural health care: an introductory course for nurses and other helping professions. *Communiqué, 5*(2), 37-41.

Waxler-Morrison, N., Anderson, J., & Richardson, E. (1990). *Cross-cultural caring: a handbook for health professionals in Western Canada.* Vancouver: University of British Columbia Press.

Williams, J. (1990). Ethics in multicultural health. *Multicultural Health Bulletin, 6*(4), 2-4.

— —. (1990). Transcultural dimensions of medical ethics. Conference held in Washington DC, 26-7, April.

- 9 -

Education and Self Reflection: Teaching About Culture, Health and Illness

Margaret Lock

In order to develop the necessary skills with which to approach health care in a manner that gives due recognition to the significance of culture, it is first important to recognize that this entails a radically new way of thinking about and representing the body. It is not sufficient to regard culture simply as an extra variable to be taken into account when using a scientific, analytic approach to the body. Furthermore, students and clinicians need to be made aware that the analytic approach is one which is inherently contradictory to the idea that recognition of cultural variation is important. These fundamental points should be incorporated into every aspect of health care education beyond the teaching of the basic sciences. In this chapter, I will briefly consider certain assumptions inherent in a scientific approach to the body which impede a culturally sensitive approach to health care. I will then turn to the difficulties of defining concepts such as culture, race, and ethnicity, and will finally discuss the relationship of culture to the body in health and illness, and how the significance of this relationship may best be taught as part of health care education.

THE CULTURE OF ANALYTICAL MEDICINE

The dominant approach to education of health care professionals today is one in which the body is visualized as a conglomerate of various molecules and cells, systems, structures, and functions, elements which can best be understood in relative isolation from one another. Of course, this analytical approach has proved to be, and continues to be, an extremely powerful and indispensable method of dealing with the sick and ailing body. On the other hand, the dramatic successes of technologically based biomedicine often blind us to several interrelated assumptions which usually go hand in hand with this approach, but which need to be carefully examined when considering the relationship of culture to health and illness.

While it is generally recognized that beliefs and behaviours which form the basis for daily participation in any given culture have a profound effect on the epidemiology of disease, including, for example, diet, the avoidance of tabooed foods, the use of stimulants, indigenous ideas about hygiene and preventive medicine, it is usually assumed, both in the education of health care professionals and in clinical practice, that one can delve beneath the veneer of culture to the "truth", and arrive at a relatively stable transhistorical, transcultural, biological base. It is also assumed that the forms which various diseases take are for all intents and purposes, universal, and that, at least in theory, contemporary medical knowledge can be applied to all peoples throughout the world, with only superficial modifications. It follows that diagnosis and healing should be largely confined to observations and practices at the biological level (obviously some aspects of psychiatric and clinical psychology are exceptions) and that one must therefore try to "get inside" individual patients, and delve beneath their load of "cultural baggage." In other words, the "noise" of culture is thought to impede professionals who are attempting to provide good medical care for the diseased body.

In biomedicine the pathological effects of disease are assumed to produce physical changes in the structure and function of the human body which can be diagnosed as specific, named diseases. Furthermore, it is believed that, in the case of most illness, subjective physical sensations of distress can be directly correlated with the pathological process.

Diagnosis is the process of sorting out the signs and symptoms presented by an individual patient, and of then assigning them a name according to the recognized taxonomy of diseases. On the basis of a diagnosis, an appropriate therapeutic regimen is selected that will treat the pathology. The task of the health care professional is one of "decoding" patient complaints, of freeing up their statements from their cultural overload, and of converting observed evidence and subjective reporting into named diseases.

In order to produce well-trained practitioners, contemporary basic science and clinical education for health care professionals is concerned above all with teaching students about normal and pathological anatomy, physiology and biochemistry. The goal in this kind of approach is to develop systematization, uniformity, control, unequivocal categorization and reproducibility. Health care professionals must act, and act decisively: they need rational, clear guidelines from which to work, and they have to make vital decisions, often in great haste, about what must be done. An analytical approach to the body is indispensable in this task, and it is this type of knowledge that most health care education is designed to impart today.

On the other hand, as soon as one starts to talk about culture, the question of difference takes centre stage, and analytical precision is lost; so too is uniformity and reproducibility. Suddenly, all bodies are not the same; they speak different languages, attribute very different meanings to events, show variation in physical features, and have different ideas about what is health, what causes illness and what are cures for illness. Cultural variation is seemingly endless, and injects a frightening disorder into the systematized and controlled world of analytical health care.

The terms "multiculturalism" and "ethnically sensitive health care" are buzz words in Canada today, and numerous health care providers have voiced concern about resources that are inadequate to deal adequately with the more than 100 ethnic groups represented in the country. However, this concern frequently masks a tendency to think of cultural beliefs as just the frills and trimmings which get in the way of the real business of modern health care, namely the repair of sick bodies. A barely hidden desire to create a "shopping list" of cultural characteristics is sometimes discernible: Tamils do this, the Cree do that and Guatemalans do the other, in order to systematize and "tidy up" culture in the same way as are other epidemiological variables, such as smoking, age, gender or fertility rates. At the same time, the hope is to obtain better patient compliance by becoming sensitive to preconceived notions which patients bring to clinical encounters.

Paying attention to cultural difference can, therefore, be a thin disguise for obtaining compliance—for learning how, in effect, to coerce patients into doing what one thinks is best for them, while at the same time conserving an intact analytical approach to the body. Kaufert has called this trend the "boxification of culture" (1990).

THE CULTURE OF THE OTHER

Our failure to appreciate the salience and complexity of cultural variables in illness episodes was illustrated many years ago by the experience of Mark Zoborowski when he presented himself to the Veterans Hospital in New York in the 1960s to discuss a research project on cultural differences in response to pain. He was told that such a study would smack of racism, and that factors such as individual pain thresholds or temperament accounted for differing responses to pain and, moreover, that making ethnicity or culture into significant variables in health care would be unscientific (Zoborowsi, 1969). However, Zoborowski's study demonstrated that, despite their claims to the contrary, health care personnel did indeed treat patients with pain complaints differently depending on which cultural group the patient belonged to: some groups of patients were described as "taking their pain well," while others were viewed as "nuisances" or "alarmists." Zoborowski's study highlights a very important lesson, but one which is rarely emphasized in discussions of the relationship of culture to health, illness, and health care: while it is important to acknowledge the culture of the "Other," it is even more important to examine our own values and assumptions. One can enter into a cooperative relationship, that does not entail coercion and manipulation only when the cultures of analytical medicine and of health care providers are examined together with those of patients and their families. Self-reflection is more difficult than the recognition that others are strange and different, but is essential to ethnically sensitive health care. As one medical student from Trinidad put it: "It is as though some of us have culture, but the rest of you think you are beyond all that."

There is now a large body of knowledge that calls into question the assumption that modern health care is value-free (Lock & Gordon, 1988; Wright & Treacher, 1982; Weisz, 1990). Among other things, it has been shown that both the way in which health, illness and diseases are defined, and the meanings which are associated with illness episodes, not only by patients, but also by health care professionals, are culturally produced. There is cross-cultural professional variation, for example, in the recognition of signs and symptoms as significant or otherwise, and in the creation of diagnostic categories, which has a profound effect on the incidence, course, and outcomes of illness episodes (Corin, 1990; Good & Kleinman, 1985; Lock, 1986; Kleinman, 1986).

At a more general level, contemporary Canadian health care usually starts out from the assumption that the "normal" family is a nuclear one, that the fundamental social unit is an individual, that the preservation of individual rights are fundamental to good health care, and that the goal of therapy should be to reinstate the patient back into society as an autonomous individual. But, these assumptions do not appear "natural" in most cultures where the family, and not the individual, is taken as the basic social unit.

Practitioners of ethnically sensitive health care have to begin with an open mind, and must avoid the pitfalls, first, of dismissing cultural variables as superficial, and second, of assuming rigid categories, either biological or social, which are then taken as universal. The education of health care professionals should start out with a discussion of the way in which terms such as the individual, the family, the body, health, illness, death, life, depression, anxiety, and menopause, among many others, are not facts of nature that can be defined once and for all, but are concepts, the meaning of which shift throughout historical time and across cultures. If one is to give due weight to the point of view of patients and their families, then their understanding of these concepts must be elicited and respected. Furthermore, it must be pointed out that most of the key concepts which are freely used in the new literature on multiculturalism and health care, including those of culture, race, ethnicity, class, and gender, are also cultural constructs which are laden with multiple meanings and implicit values.

WHAT IS THIS THING CALLED CULTURE?

One comment overheard in the corridors of the national conference on Health Care and Multiculturalism in Toronto in 1989 was: "I'm really into culture right now." What could this person have meant? Symphonies at the O'Keefe Centre? Trips

such as those advertised in the New Yorker to Terra del Feugo
or New Guinea to see "exotic" cultures? Tissue culture? Petri
dishes of staphylococcus? Sugar-beet culture? Or was it Ukrainian folk dancers at the Winnipeg ethnic fair?

Williams (1976) has pointed out that "culture" is one of the
two or three most complicated words in the English language. It
was first used in European languages in a rather concrete fashion to convey the idea of a process, and in particular with the
tending of something, usually crops or animals. By the 16th
century this was extended by metaphor to mean not just crops,
but also human development, and especially the cultivation of
the human mind. A German philosopher named Herder, at the
end of the 18th century, first suggested that there are many
cultures throughout the world, and that by definition, all people
who have a shared way of life have a culture.

During the 18th and 19th centuries the word civility was often
used to distinguish educated people who were cultured and
enlightened from "uncivilized" peasants. Gradually this usage
was transformed into a notion which is still very much with us
today: that modern cities and their inhabitants are cultured,
whereas people who live outside cities are immersed in "rural
idiocy" (Williams, 1973).

Spencer's hypothesis of the evolution of societies, put for-
ward in the wake of Darwin's theory of the evolution of species,
gave a scientific foundation to the idea that some groups of
people are cultural while others remain "closer to nature" and
hence uncultured. It was assumed, of course, that European
civilization represented the pinnacle of evolutionary success,
the end of the long road from darkest Africa through numerous
primitive and barbaric groupings and groupings to the high
"white" culture of Europe and, eventually, North America.

The term culture retains all of these meetings according to the
context in which it is being used today. In our minds we tend to
set up oppositions between culture and nature (which needs
taming or cultivating); culture and the individual (whose basic
"biological nature" must be cultivated so that he or she can
function in social groups); culture and science (which is a
"factual" representation of the natural world, and is hence
ontologically different from cultural activities), and between
high culture (the civilization of cities, including the fine arts,
classical music and literature) and popular culture (with its folk
dances and costumes, ethnic foods and crafts).

Most of daily professional life today is thought of as rational and/or scientific, and hence separate from culture. We take "time out" to relax and indulge in cultural activities. However, in contrast, by drawing on the evolutionary meaning of culture, there is also a tendency to assume that "ethnic minorities," "immigrants" and "patients" for example, are on the whole irrational, unscientific and hence childlike or "primitive." Furthermore, a recognition of ethnicity is often associated with popular culture. These viewpoints are not completely groundless, because patients of all kinds are indeed less scientifically educated with respect to their bodies than are medical professionals, and some immigrants enjoy folk dancing more than classical ballet. Nevertheless, such viewpoints are prejudiced because negative value is usually attached to the lack of scientific knowledge with respect to the body, or what is assumed to be the "folksy" behaviour of the patient or immigrant.

We can now see that we have done a complete about-face over the past one hundred years with respect to the notion of culture. From claiming that only the educated élite are cultivated, we have moved to an unexamined assumption that only poorly educated peasants are completely immersed in culture, while the rest of us, have moved beyond culture into a rational, post- or supra-cultural world, which is grounded in science and hence is value-free. There is a real danger, then of jumping into a culturally sensitive approach to health education without first examining what we mean by culture and, even more important what our own values are with respect to the culture of the Other. How pluralistic are we really prepared to be? The history of cultural pluralism in Canada provides us with a grave warning. One other major concern is that the notion of culture is in danger of being seized on as a panacea, as the key which will open the door to a trouble free health care system, while once again the deeper more persistent problems which lie at the root of so much ill health, most particularly poverty, exploitation, and discrimination, remain unexamined.

ETHNICITY AND CITIZENSHIP

To function adequately as a human being it is essential to achieve a sense of individual identity and at the same time to participate in various social groups. This is achieved through socialization into a shared cultural heritage. Since much of the socialization process takes place using pre-verbal and non-verbal forms of communication, most of us cannot state clearly what we mean by belonging to a "culture," although we usually have an intuitive sense of its existence. Isolated, non-literature societies (of which virtually none remain today) often had no special name for themselves since they were the only people of any consequence in their known world. In complex societies, awareness of one's own culture is most often achieved through a recognition of difference. Once groups of people are thought of as "other," as being outside one's own culture and labelled as different, then a sense of ethnic affiliation has been created. Ethnic groups identify themselves and other peoples in one or more typical ways, usually through language, skin colour, by religion, a shared history and so on.

In the modern world, however, none of us are simply "ethnics"; our cultural identities are also created out of gender, class, occupational, and educational differences, as well as out of the individual social and familial milieux in which we are raised. Moreover, in countries such as Canada, we are also citizens with recognized rights. Such categories are not mutually exclusive: they are used indiscriminately, sometimes emphasizing gender difference, sometimes occupational affiliation, at other times, ethnicity or citizenry.

There is, furthermore, variation within any given ethnic group in terms of socio-economic and educational background and several languages and/or religions may involved. There is also the question of differences among first, second, and ensuing generations after immigration—when does one stop being an "ethnic"? As a moment's reflection indicates, no firm boundaries can be drawn between one ethnic group and another; over the centuries, migration, political coups, wars and intermarriage have ensured that ethnicity is an extremely fluid category which cannot be taken as a given or a constant. Recent research into ethnicity has shown that it is something that is reinvented and reinterpreted by individuals with each new generation and there is no such thing as a timeless, static concept of what it means to be, for example, a Mohawk or an Italian. Moreover, many of the geographical groupings which we now take as "natural" are the result of relatively recent political realignments, as events in Eastern Europe have clearly shown. Obviously, then, the concept of ethnicity cannot be used as if it is an epidemiological variable. It is, above all, a political category, and if it is to be useful at all, it must remain flexible and open.

In any given clinical encounter, then, both the care-giver and the patient should reflect on whether ethnicity is a useful category at all, and what meanings, including possible prejudicial ones, are being attributed to it.

RACE: A POLITICAL CONCEPT

The concept of race was first introduced into the biological literature by Buffon in 1749. Before this time there was apparently **relatively** little concern with human difference based on physical appearance. Three events contributed to the creation of race as a political concept: the formation of nation states, the subjection of the Native peoples of the Americas and the slave trade (Gould, 1979). It was only much later, at the end of the last century, that attempts were first made to formulate a scientific concept of race. This concept is grounded in the assumption that there are important and consistent discrete genetic differences between groups of people who are considered to form distinct human populations. A large body of research has demonstrated that this assumption is not correct, and the biological concept of race has been roundly refuted (see Cooper & David, 1986 for a good summary of this work). Nevertheless, this concept is still used in both epidemiological and public health research. Yet it is clear that the common public health categories of Black and Hispanic; for example, are, biologically speaking, absurd. Today in the United States many people are classified as Black whose ancestors would have been classified as whites; furthermore, all children of mixed marriages in which the father is Black are classified as Black. The term Hispanic is a very loose political/ethnic category which has no biological meaning at all. Despite these facts, some persist in using race as a concept, very often to make prejudiced and incorrect discriminations about behaviours which are ostensibly grounded in genetic difference. We slip all too easily from pseudo-science to value judgements. For example, sickle cell anemia which is thought of in North America to be a "Black" disease is widely distributed in the Middle East, around the Mediterranean, and in India and Africa, and it is absent in many parts of tropical Africa. However, because it is counted as a "Black" disease, there have been major political difficulties and prejudices in connection with screening programs (Duster, 1990; Weissman, 1990). The concept of race should, therefore, be discussed when teaching a **multicultural approach to** health care, and then discarded, first because it is not scientific, and second, because it is loaded with prejudice.

THE CANADIAN MOSAIC AND THE CONCEPT OF MULTICULTURALISM

The passage of the Multiculturalism Act into law in 1988 brought to a head a rising tide of concern over the need to make the Canadian health care system responsive to what is popularly known as the Canadian mosaic. The very notion of multiculturalism implies, of course, that immigrants and refugees are not expected to become assimilated (as is the case in the American melting-pot). In the Report of the Canadian Task Force on Mental Health Issues Facing Immigrants and Refugees, a careful distinction was made between assimilation and integration. Assimilation was defined as "a process of eliminating distinctive group characteristics which may be encouraged as a formal policy," (1988, 97) whereas integration was defined as "a process, clearly distinct from assimilation, by which groups and/or individuals become able to participate fully in the political, economic, social and cultural life of the country" (ibid., 98). The concept of integration, therefore, encourages the cultivation of difference. However, the report focuses almost exclusively on what happens **after** immigration to Canada; it is as though this difference should be constructed in a Canadian setting without drawing extensively upon past experience. The terms "heritage language" and "heritage culture" indicate that something is to be retained from the past, but since heritage culture is defined as "the development of an ethnic group **inside** Canada," (ibid., emphasis added) it would appear that immigration is an event that rather clearly demarcates the past from the present.

Certain unexamined assumptions may be at work when the act of immigration is visualized as a kind of rebirth process, in which an old life is discarded and replaced by a fresh start full of hope and expanding horizons. Whereas early immigration to Canada was dominated by peoples of Northern European origin, followed later by Eastern and Southern Europeans, at present the majority of immigrants come from the so-called Third World countries. In the global village of today, the "sophisticated" metropolitan centres of Northern Europe and North America which receive immigrants are thought of as the nerve centres of "advanced" nations. This First World is contrasted with the birthplaces of the majority of immigrants, the "underdeveloped" nations and regions (including the Canadian North), that are associated implicitly with poverty, dirt and ignorance. There is sometimes an unspoken understanding that immigrants should be grateful; that their movement across the boundary away from dirt and disorder into civilization should be almost all gain and little loss. It is this tacit assumption that leads to an acceptance of the idea that although "difference" can be encouraged through an active promotion of multiculturalism, it should be something that is created inside Canada, and largely disassociated from the hardships and assumed ignorance of life before migration. In teaching about multiculturalism, therefore, students and clinicians need to be made aware of many factors: the history of migration patterns to Canada; the current political, economic and demographic reasons for the official encouragement of immigration to Canada; the numerous conditions that lead to emigration from one's birthplace; and the factors, most particularly lack of employment or discrimination in the host society, that are contributory to ill health. The Task Force Report on Mental Health covers each of these points in some detail.

THE CULTURED BODY

Over the past twenty years, and lately with increasing frequency, some researchers have questioned the validity of a health care model in which the body is visualized as a stable unit, firmly encased by the skin, independent of society and culture, and even of the workings of the mind. Although an analytic approach to the body has been and continues to be very powerful, an approach in which cultural beliefs and practices are visualized in a dynamic interrelationship with biology has also been found to be necessary. When this dynamic approach is used, the emphasis is less upon final common pathways at the cellular level, and more upon the way in which the physical environment, the societies in which we live and cultural ideas about health and illness, influence the incidence and management of illness, its subjective experience and therapeutic outcomes.

Although culture is a concept which is notoriously difficult to define, it is nevertheless very useful when trying to describe and account for some of the characteristic features of different groups of people. The definition suggested by the anthropologist Geertz is a useful starting point. According to him, culture is "an historically transmitted pattern of meanings embodied in symbols, a system of inherited conceptions expressed in symbolic form by means of which [people] communicate, perpetuate and develop their knowledge about and attitudes towards life" (Geertz, 1973). The symbolic forms which Geertz refers to include language, ideas, behaviour and material artifacts.

These beliefs are not merely layered over a **biological reality like** icing on a cake, nor can they be stripped away to reveal the "real" physical problems underneath. Cultural beliefs and practices function in a dynamic and interdependent relationship with biology, which in turn produces an effect on the epidemiology of disease, and also on the subjective understanding of illness, including the meanings which are attributed to illness episodes.

Socialization into a culture involves the learning of an appropriate language. However, being, for example, Chinese, Nicaraguan or Inuit is not limited to language use. We are all **embodied** in a culture: our sense of being in the world is such that subjective sensations, unconscious and partially conscious behaviour, ideas about individuality, mind, emotions, morality, values and behaviour are all largely culturally produced. Central to becoming a cultured human being is the development of an awareness of a sense of self which is initially accomplished in primary social groups, and later in school, work, and community settings.

Early socialization has a profound impact on the subjective experience of one's body. For example, an infant who spends most of its time during the first few months in close proximity to another human being will learn to interpret ideas about body boundaries, autonomy and independence in a different way from an infant which sleeps and naps in its own room away from other people (Caudill, 1976). Later on, with language acquisition, a child learns how to give culturally appropriate labels to subjective physical sensations, how to interpret and vocalize discomfort, distress, pain, and happiness, which is then in turn reinforced through participation in primary and secondary social groups.

Research in psychology has demonstrated that losses, such as those which occur with immigration, including loss of loved ones, material goods, or a linguistic community have a negative effect on health, as does a lack of social support, or repeatedly being subjected to racist or sexist prejudices which then lead to chronic unresolved feelings of anger or fear (Krieger, 1990). These and other negative emotional states influence the basic biochemistry of the body: the immune system, the autonomic nervous system, and so on (Bolles & Fanselow, 1982). At the level of the immune system, we are talking about physical changes which are probably universal, but the moment there is an effort to contextualize and understand feelings such as anger or fear in the daily lives of individuals, then we are in the domain of culture. Grief, pain, lack of self-esteem, anger, sadness or happiness are embued with various meanings and understood and dealt in various ways depending upon cultural context.

All cultures have developed explanatory systems which account for the occurrence of distress and illness, and these explanatory systems provide the framework on which individual illness behaviour and medical knowledge and practices are built (Lock & Scheper-Hughes, 1990). They also provide a necessary attempt to bring a sense of order and control to the experience of the illness. Distress is experienced everywhere as both an emotional and a physical event, but culture has a profound influence on how it is recognized, labelled and managed (Beiser, 1985; Kleinman, 1982; Lock, 1980). When we think about the body scientifically, we tend to think of it as like a machine, or as an aggregate of cells and molecules. But it also is a medium for communication. In fact, the body is most frequently used symbolic medium with which belonging to social groups is expressed. Because most cultural explanatory systems encourage an understanding of illness as having its origins in cosmological, social, moral or familial disruptions, it follows that, in general, people understand their own aching and painful bodies, not simply as representing biological breakdown, but also metaphorically, as an expression of the end result of ongoing psychological or social problems (Helman, 1988; Lock, 1990). In biomedical settings, it has been shown many times that although the encounter between health care practitioner and patient may be limited to the relief of physical symptoms, the patient nevertheless remains very concerned about possible social origins and implications of illness episodes (Harris, 1989; Williams & Wood, 1986).

In North American culture, the dominant idiom for the expression of distress is by means of "psychologization." Suffering is thought to produce unwanted effects on the moods, thoughts and feelings of individuals. Severity of distress is measured by its impact on mental functioning and its disruption of an internalized coherent sense of self (Kirmayer, 1989). Largely as a result of the influence of psychiatry and psychology, it has become usual for us to think of distress in a rather individualized idiom, as something which happens mostly in our heads. Even when using the concept of "stress" or psychosomatic explanatory models, it is still common in both clinical settings and daily life to focus on either the mental functioning of patients, or on physical symptomatology. Very often, however, these two sides of the problem are not pieced together (Kirmayer, 1988; Young, 1980). Because distress is individualized, major contributory factors, social and political, may well be ignored.

In contrast to the "psychologized" explanations commonly used in clinical settings in North America, in the majority of cultures, emphasis is given to somatic changes, and the impact of distress on individual emotional states is played down, or may go virtually unrecognized. This means that physical sensations of all kinds are directly associated with perceived problems in the social order, without mediation through the Western cultural construct of the "psyche." Culture functions to pattern these associations so that some specific sensations and body organs take on metaphorical significance, while others are not invested with much emotional content (Littlewood & Lipsedge, 1985; Lock, 1980; Lock & Dunk, 1990; Tousignant, 1984; Obeyesekere, 1985). The body is readily recognized as a medium for the expression of political and social injustices. In pluralistic health care settings, patients and health care providers are at considerable risk, not merely of misunderstanding each other because of language barriers, but of completely talking past each other, of being frustrated and perplexed as to why great importance is attributed certain symptoms and feelings, while others go unrecognized or ignored.

Culturally sensitive health care can only be undertaken by asking patients to talk about their illness, to create a narrative, most particularly about what they think caused the problem, and what meaning it has for them (Kleinman, 1988). This exercise has been termed a "narrative reconstruction" (Williams & Wood, 1986). Certain key terms which link states of mind and body and indicate feelings of distress, such as "stress," or the state of one's nerves (*nevra* or *nervios* in Greek or Spanish), or chronic fatigue are often useful starting points for an exercise in social "free association" to be undertaken by the patient. This obviously takes time and patience, and is not easy to accomplish given the present structure of the health care system.

Because of the complexity of the concept of culture, the number of ethnic groups involved and time constraints, health care professionals cannot possibly hope to have the relevant information, language ability or the necessary experiential base to enter into the life-worlds of patients who come from the many different cultural backgrounds present in Canada today. It follows, therefore, that in clinical practice one must think **first of all** of the patient as an individual, and as part of a primary social group, rather than as a member of a particular ethnic group or culture (even though these concepts may well turn out to be important once the details of the case have been narrated by the patient). When a meaning-centred approach is used, in which the patient narrative is given due attention, the human **experience** of sickness takes center stage, rather than a rapid search for the correct diagnostic category. Reconstructed illness narratives, replete with beliefs about responsibility and morality, open the door directly into the culture of the patient. Listening with an open mind and without putting a hasty label on the problem is essential. However, this is only half the exercise, because if the patient narrative is simply used in order to obtain better compliance, then very little has been achieved. It is necessary to enter into a dialogue where unexamined values, assumptions and gaps in knowledge on **both** sides are scrutinized. In particular, assumptions need to be explored in connection with family structure and dynamics, independence and autonomy, allocation of responsibility and the relationship of mental with physical states. This is the starting point for culturally sensitive health care, and it should be incorporated into all health care education beyond that of the basic sciences.

TEACHING ABOUT CULTURE AND HEALTH

On the basis of fourteen years of experience of teaching about the relationship of culture to health and illness, it is apparent to me that students who have taken courses in anthropology, particularly medical anthropology, before starting their training in medicine or nursing, are much more able to grasp the importance of paying attention to cultural difference in health care settings. Prerequisites in anthropology or certain courses in sociology, geography or history should be encouraged much more strongly than is presently the case. These are the disciplines that promote understanding of cultural relativism and difference.

During all stages of basic medical and nursing education, courses which incorporate materials relating to culture and health, comparative ethics, the history of medicine, nursing and social work, and the comparative study of medical knowledge should be required. By the end of their basic training, students should have learnt in some detail how patients bring to health care settings culturally informed perspectives which influence their behaviour and expectations in these settings. Students should have read several relevant ethnographics, in order to better understand the way in which ideas about health and illness are intricately related to wider cultural contexts. They should also have learnt about cultural variation in connection with the concepts of the family, the individual, and the meanings associated with birth, death and the various stages of the life cycle.

In addition, students need to be made aware that they will not be able to "cure" many of the problems brought to them in primary care settings because many of these are multifactorial, non-specific illnesses, for which there is no simple diagnosis and cure. It is important to acknowledge that a large number of problems brought to medical professionals have major political and economic components often relating to poverty and discrimination, which health care professionals can do little to alleviate directly. Inappropriate medication of distress when no disease can be diagnosed should be discouraged, and team work and an ongoing engagement with community organizations of all kinds is necessary in a culturally sensitive approach to health care.

It is equally important that students learn that contemporary medical knowledge is a product of the Western philosophical heritage, and that there are often other ways of thinking about the body which, while they do not always involve technical mastery over biological breakdown, have other kinds of therapeutic advantages. Students should have explicitly examined the way in which value judgments are necessarily incorporated into a large number of medical decisions, and should be aware that there are gaps in scientific knowledge about the body which need to be openly acknowledged. This kind of training should be team-taught so that basic scientists, clinicians, anthropologists, medical ethicists present their different points of view. It is obviously necessary to teach an approach such as this in a sensitive way, so that the student is not left feeling frustrated and helpless by uncertainty. On the other hand, medical education to date has tended to gloss over inevitable deficiencies in biomedical knowledge, and has at times asserted authority in the name of science where it was inappropriate. The ultimate objective is to combine the practice of good technological medicine with a culturally sensitive approach to health care. Such an approach means that where cultural beliefs can be clearly established as creating genuine health hazards, then patients should be informed that such is the opinion of the health practitioner and why.

Beyond this, practitioners should remain open to negotiation and compromise.

Testing student knowledge on information of this kind should rely as little as possible on the use of multiple choice questions. The very process of selecting information to place into appropriate boxes, or the equivalent, works in opposition to the kind of flexible open-minded and contextualized approach which is at the heart of a multicultural approach to health care. Essay questions or short-answer questions which require students to demonstrate that they are aware of the complexity of the issues involved are much more appropriate.

Research projects, rotations and internships in which students work abroad, in rural areas, or in immigrant communities should be encouraged. If graduate students in the social sciences can be paired with students in the health sciences, so much the better. One of the most important parts of training as an anthropologist is the process of immersion in another culture in order to carry out what is known as "field work." Field work forces students to examine their own assumptions and unquestioned values, and if made integral to health care training, could provide invaluable experience.

At the postgraduate level, there should be regular workshops and seminars for students in which speakers representing various ethnic groups and Aboriginal peoples are called upon, and in which special topics relating to immigration, medical interpreters, or the anthropology of the body are considered. Above all, there should be a close link between theory and clinical practice, and between social scientists, health care professionals and community organizations of all kinds.

Finally, a great deal more careful research into the relationship of culture and health needs to be done which should be coordinated to some extent throughout Canada to facilitate exchange and cooperation so that feedback can be systematically integrated into the training of students and clinicians.

REFERENCES

Beiser, M. (1985). A Study of Depression among Traditional Africans, Urban North Americans, and Southeast Asian Refugees. In A. Kleinman & B. Good (Eds.), *Culture and Depression* (272-98). Berkeley: University of California Press.

Bolles, R.C. & Fanselow, M.S. (1982). Endorphins and Behaviour. *Annual Review of Psychology, 33,* 87-101.

Canadian Task Force on Mental Health Issues Affecting Immigrants and Refugees. (1988). *After the Door Has Been Opened: Mental Health Issues Affecting Immigrants.* Ottawa: Multiculturalism and Citizenship Canada.

Caudill, W. (1976). Everyday Health and Illness in Japan and America. In C. Leslie (Eds.), *Asian Medical Systems* (159-77). Berkeley: University of California Press.

Cooper, R., & David, R. (1986). The Biological Concept of Race and Its Application to Public Health and Epidemiology. *Journal of Health Politics, Policy and Law, 11,* 97-116.

Corin. E.E. (1990). Facts and Meanings in Psychiatry: An Anthropological Approach to the Lifeworld of Schizophrenics. *Culture, Medicine and Psychiatry, 14,* 153-88.

Duster, T. (1990). *Backdoor to Eugenics.* New York: Routledge.

Geertz, C. (1973). *Interpretation of Cultures.* New York: Basic Books.

Good, B. & Delvechhio Good, M.-J. (1981). The Meaning of Symptoms: A Cultural Hermeneutic Model for Clinical Practice. In L. Eisenberg & A. Kleinman, (Eds.), *The Relevance of Social Science for Medicine* (165-97). Dordrecht: D. Reidel.

Good, B., & Kleinman, A. (1985). Culture and Anxiety: Cross Cultural Evidence for the Patterning of Anxiety Disorders. In H. Tuma & J. Mazur (Eds.), *Anxiety and the Anxiety Disorders* (297-324). New York: L. Earlbaum.

Gould, S.J. (1979). *Ever Since Darwin: Reflections in Natural History.* New York: W.W. Norton.

Harris, G. (1989). Mechanism and Morality in Patients' View of Illness and Injury. *Medical Anthropology Quarterly, 3,* 3-21.

Helman, C. (1988). Psyche, Soma, and Society: The Social Construction of Psychosomatic Disorders. In M. Lock & D. Gordon, (Eds.), *Biomedicine Examined* (95-122). Dordrecht: Kluwer Academic Publishers.

Kaufert, P. (1990). The Boxification of Culture: The Role of the Social Scientist. *Culture, Santé, Health. 7*,139-48.

Kirmayer, L. (1988). Mind and Body as Metaphors: Hidden Values in Biomedicine. In M. Lock & D. Gordon (Eds.), *Biomedicine Examined* (57-93). Dordrecht: Kluwer Academic Publishers.

Kleinman, A. (1982). (1982). Neurasthenia and Depression: A Study of Somatization and Culture in China. *Culture, Medicine and Psychiatry, 6,* 117-89.

— —. (1986). *Social Origins of Distress and Disease: Depression, Neurasthenia in Modern China.* New Haven: Yale University Press.

— —. (1988). *The Illness Narratives.* New York: Basic Books.

Krieger, N. (1990). Racial and Gender Discrimination: Risk Factors for High Blood Pressure? *Social Science and Medicine, 30,* 1273-81.

Littlewood, R. & Lipsedge, M. (1985). Culture-bound Syndromes. In G. Granville-Grossman (Ed.), *Recent Advances in Clinical Psychiatry, No. 5* (105-42). Edinburgh: Churchill Livingstone.

Lock, M. (1980). *East Asian Medicine in Urban Japan: Varieties of Medical Experience.* Berkeley: University of California Press.

— —. (1986). Ambiguities of aging. *Culture, Medicine and Psychiatry, 10*(1), 23-46.

— —. (1990). On Being Ethnic: The Politics of Identity Breaking and Making in Canada, or *Nevra* on Sunday. *Culture, Medicine and Psychiatry, 14,* 237-54.

Lock, M., & Gordon, D.R. (Eds.) (1988). *Biomedicine Examined,* Dordrecht: Kluwer Academic Publishers.

Lock, M., & Scheper-Hughes, N. (1990). A Critical-Interpretive Approach in Medical Anthropology: Rituals and Routines of Discipline and Dissent. In T.M. Johnson & C.E. Sargent, (Eds.). *Medical Anthropology: Contemporary Theory and Method* (47-72). New York: Praeger Publishers.

Lock, M., & Wakewich-Dunk, P. (1990). Nerves and Nostalgia: Expression of Loss Among Greek Immigrants in Montreal. *Canadian Family Physician, 36,* 253-58.

Obeyesekere, G. (1985). Depression, Buddhism, and the Work of Culture. In A. Kleinman & B. Good (Eds.). *Culture and Depression* (134-52). Berkeley: University of California Press.

Tousignant, M. (1984). *Pena* in the Ecuadorian Sierra: A Psycho/
    Anthropological Analysis of Sadness. *Culture, Medicine
    and Psychiatry, 8,* 381-398.
Weissman, A. (1990). Race-Ethnicity. A Dubious Scientific Con-
    cept. *Public Health Reports, 105,* 102-103.
Weisz, G. (1990). *The Social Science Perspective on Medical Ethics.*
    Philadelphia: University of Pennsylvania Press.
Williams, G., and Wood, P. (1986). Common-sense Beliefs about
    Illness: A Mediating Role for the Doctor. *The Lancet, 20,*
    1435-37.
Williams, R. (1973). *The Country and the City.* New York: Oxford
    University Press.
Williams, R. (1976). *Keywords: A Vocabulary of Culture and Society.*
    London: Fontana.
Wright, P.W.G., & Treacher, A. (1982). *The Problem of Medical
    Knowledge: Examining the Social Construction of Medicine.*
    Edinburgh: University of Edinburgh Press.
Young, A. (1980). The Discourse on Stress and the Reproduction
    of Conventional Knowledge. *Social Science and Medicine,
    14B,* 133-46.
Zoborowski, M. (1969). *People in Pain.* San Francisco: Jossey-
    Bass.

- 10 -

What is Experiential Learning?

Basanti Majumdar

In today's increasingly complex and multicultural society, health care workers must develop cultural sensitivity in order to provide holistic care to patients as well as to prepare themselves for participation in health care teams at community, national and international levels. The transfer of technical skills without a conceptual framework that recognizes cultural differences is inadequate. Currently, there is both an increasing number of international students in North American programs and increasing opportunities for international work experience for graduates (Filerman, 1986). Such increases, coupled with growing societal diversity, make cultural sensitivity in health care a priority.

In the context of health care education, learners must be given an opportunity to identify and clarify their own values in order to prepare them for making moral and ethical decisions. Health education curricula, however, have tended to "emphasize the development of cognitive abilities, such as analytical thinking and ability to conceptualize, rather than the affective domain that includes the examination of values and their influence on decisions and behaviours" (Arosker, 1977). Consequently, health professionals may "base complex value decisions on intuition, emotions, or policies or precedents, with very little awareness of the consequences or impact of these decisions" (ibid.). Educators have an obligation to provide "learning opportunities specifically designed to help individuals systematically identify, explore and develop their personal values" (Uutal, 1984) as the first step in developing cultural sensitivity.

Experiential learning workshops are useful in evaluating and understanding existing levels of personal cultural awareness (Majumdar & Hezekiah, 1990). Experiential Learning (EL) is learning through experience. It is an active approach to education in which knowledge is linked to the unique experiences of each learner. The process entails an integration of knowledge and doing in which both are repeatedly transformed. EL should have been part of every educational curriculum long ago. The purpose of EL is to assist a person to reflect on old and new ideas, beliefs and values. These activities help the participants to shift from their "old me" to "new me" by stating "where they are" at the point of entry and through the activities introduce themselves to new and more appropriate approaches in the old or a new solution (Kohls, 1984).

A successful integration of knowing and doing in EL incorporates the following general principles and strategies: 1) concreteness (the learning strategies must be based on the student's own concrete experience); 2) involvement (learning that involves the "whole" person through a range of modalities (cognitive, affective, kinaesthetic, attitudinal and behavioural) is more effective); 3) dissonance (when learners temporarily face dissonance, they rethink their knowing, reshape their doing, and move towards a deeper level of understanding. Points of dissonance may be between theory and practice, cognition and emotion, expectation and reality, and "should" and "must"); 4) reflection (when the learners have the ability and opportunity to step aside and think about their experience, they will be able to abstract new meaning and knowledge relevant to other experiences).

EL strategies utilize the underlying principles of Gestalt-insight. Here, the learner faces confusion provided by a problem. Through restructuring his/her perceptions, the student attains new insight and learning (Boydell, 1976).

Various techniques may be employed for this type of learning: 1) lectures; 2) discussions/workshops; 3) case studies/role play; 4) games/drama/song; 5) experiential exercises/structured experiences; and 6) field experience.

Group 5, experiential exercises and structured experiences, covers a variety of activities; these exercises have in common the participants' engagement in an activity. These may be simulated exercises based on subject matter or on human relations. Or they may be real issue exercises, based on "this group" issues or exercises giving the individual self-insight. Various integrations of the above formats will be considered in the section below on "Design for Cross-Cultural Learning."

The objectives of each activity must be clearly identified. It should be clear to the participants that the focus of the session is gaining knowledge, developing skills or attitudes relevant to reflect on the values of self, group, a society or a specific community or a problem. Activities should have a clear outline, including stated objectives, equipment, playing rules or process and evaluation. The number of participants, time, type of place and assistance for the activity should be considered.

The activity leader and the assistant leader must keep an eye on the following areas as the activity continues and at the end of the game:

- how the activity influences the participants;
- what happens to the individual participants and the group (expression of their verbal and non-verbal clues);
- what different communication patterns evolve between participant groups; and
- how the groups (individuals) reflects on their old and new values.

It is essential to debrief the activity sessions with the participants and to discuss with them identified issues so that they can relate the learning with the predetermined objectives and new ideas or learning beyond the identified objectives. Specific feelings of individuals, such as frustration, confusion, anger, etc. should be dealt with within the group before terminating the session. It should be emphasized that such emotions are necessary for self-education and group process.

A possible shortcoming of participatory learning could be that participants feel dissatisfaction because they perceive such sessions as "fun" and lacking any objective. Therefore, these activities should be carefully administered so that they reflect on learning as a social act. The process should provide the student with an opportunity for reflection of self, self within a group and group behaviour.

Finally, the principles of EL should be explored. They are as follows:

1. **Empowerment:** The learning process should be an empowering action process.
2. **Learning and Reflection:** Learning is a continuous and life-long activity. It causes us to reflect on what we have done in order to improve on what we are going to do.

3. **History and Analysis:** Each learner has a life history that is rich in experience, knowledge and skills.
4. **Change:** Learning means changes in understanding, knowledge, attitude, feelings or skills.
5. **Collective Learning:** Everyone is learning together; new knowledge is created and old knowledge is re-created into new understanding; the knowledge and learning is a collective effort.
6. **Strategy and Action:** Paternalistic teaching methodologies create dependency and apathy. Activity-oriented learning provides concrete learning experiences with the opportunity for reflection, analysis and action (Cuso, 1988).

These principles are essential in developing positive attitudes towards multicultural concepts and in creating attitudinal changes for the understanding of a multicultural outlook.

Rogers (1969) pointed out that the total learning includes both intellectual and emotional level of the learner which seems particularly relevant to learning multicultural concepts. This theory is based on the pedagogic method, which can be described as follows: an exercise, selected and presented by a facilitator, permits the participants to experience a certain situation (Phase I); to detect a series of problems (using a theoretical framework, if necessary), and analyse their causes and consequences (Phase II); to search for possible solutions (Phase III); and to test these solutions (Phase IV), either in an intermediate way that returns the participants to a deeper investigation of the problems or in a definite way that brings the participants to the selection of a new theme of research (Figure 1).

Kolb (1984) describes how individuals construct abstract presentations from concrete experiences, which direct subsequent actions from concrete experiences, which direct subsequent actions in similar situations. He states that learning is the process whereby knowledge is constructed through the transformation of experience. Learning is a life-long process resulting from continual person-environment interaction and involves feelings, perceiving, thinking and behaving. These are the essential components of cultural awareness.

Kolb's model of experiential learning is based on the problem-solving process. The model includes both active and passive, abstract and concrete learning. This EL cycle has four stages: (1) Concrete experience followed by (2) reflective observation, which leads to (3) the formation of abstract concepts and generalizations which progress to (4) active experimentation in which

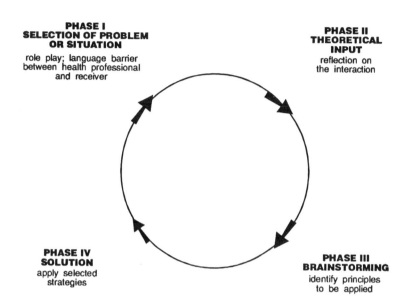

PHASE I
SELECTION OF PROBLEM
OR SITUATION
role play; language barrier
between health professional
and receiver

PHASE II
THEORETICAL
INPUT
reflection on
the interaction

PHASE IV
SOLUTION
apply selected
strategies

PHASE III
BRAINSTORMING
identify principles
to be applied

Figure 1: Pedagogic Method of Experiential Learning,
(Adapted from Rogers' (1969) description of four phases.)

generalizations are tested and new hypotheses are developed to be tested in future concrete experiences. An excellent example of the concrete experience proposed in Kolb's theory is the game "Bafa Bafa" (Shirts, 1977). In this game, participants are divided into two groups, each with their own distinctive culture. During the exchange of group members, attempts are made at interpreting and understanding each other. After the game, participants can reflect on how they played and share their perception of the experience highlighting their feelings (stage 2) and examine the reasons behind their behaviour (stage 3). Finally, it is explained to the participants that such interactions are successful when they occur on neutral ground and are free of past experiences (stage 4).

Cultural sensitivity is essential in understanding multicultural concepts. The underlying principles of EL make it particularly suitable for teaching cultural sensitivity. Just as each individual possesses a unique personality, the sum of these individuals (a group) has its own distinct culture. Chen (1990, 257 as cited in Nwanko, 1991) states that "to be competent in intercultural interaction, individuals must communicate effectively and appropriately." Understanding and accepting that various cultures communicate with one another and their environment in different yet valid ways is essential in the teaching-learning process. On the one hand, sensitivity to variations in cultural style enriches this interaction. On the other hand misunderstanding of behavioural style results in:

- erroneous estimations of a student's or a cultural group's intellectual capabilities;
- misjudging students' language abilities (teachers often use their own language or dialect as the norm);
- misreading of students' achievement in academic subjects such as creative expression, and
- difficulty in communicating and establishing rapport.

Teachers' expectations and the accompanying teaching behaviours influence and are influenced by students' performance. In the teaching-learning interaction, this has led to a lower performance of racially, ethnically and economically different students. A multicultural education system should be influenced by cultural sensitivity in the development of both its curriculum content and the delivery of its instructional services. The following is one example of how cross-cultural learning may be accomplished through EL methodology.

DESIGN FOR CROSS-CULTURAL/ MULTICULTURAL LEARNING MODEL

This learning model proposed by Sikkema & Niyekawa (1987) has two overall objectives: (1) cross cultural: to cause students to become multiculturally oriented by developing the capability to adapt and function competently in cross-cultural circumstances and (2) personal: to cause them to become more tolerant, flexible and creative through a different understanding of themselves in relation to others and the world. The proposed cross-cultural learning design accomplishes these objectives through the following processes: by recognizing and amending personal and cultural biases in perception and interpretation of values and behaviour; by cultivating sensitivity to cultural differences and ability to appreciate the validity of various values and means of meeting life's situations; and by cultivating creativity through recognition of other ways to solve problems. There are three components of this learning model.

I. Pre-field Seminar

The purpose of the pre-field seminar is to help learners acquire an intellectual understanding of cultural and personal awareness. Pertinent theoretical information on cross-cultural learning is provided. Such an emphasis on cognitive learning allows for the analysis and understanding of the actual field experience through a framework. During the pre-field seminar, a mental attitude in which learners assume an active role in the next phase is encouraged.

II. Field Experience

This component provides the experiential complement to the cognitive learning acquired in the previous phase. The purpose is to experience culture shock: "The students go to an essentially unknown culture with, desirably, the fewest possible preconceptions about how people there behave and what their values and customs are. As the students attempt to find their way in that culture and encounter the problems and ambiguities involved, they experience culture shock" (Sikkema & Niyekawa, 1987). Instead of real field experience, learners may play "Bafa Bafa". (Shirts, 1977)

A crucial element of the model is the process of resolving this culture shock. The learners are assisted to face the psycho-social and philosophical differences between their own culture and that of the new one. The author would like to re-emphasize here that, it is essential to debrief the learners before they leave the session. The learners must not leave with unresolved strong feelings.

III. Post-field Program

This component of the model provides the time necessary for reflection and internalizing the new learning once the learners are back within their usual environment. It is composed of a seminar and two learning summaries.

The seminar allows for retrospective analysis of the field experience and a consolidation of affective and cognitive learning. The first summary is a recording of basic learning and is written one month after phase II. The second summary, within which the learning experience is evaluated, is written six months after the field experience. The learners identify changes in their attitudes and the new insights they have acquired. They examine how the learning experience has influenced their encountering cross-cultural and other circumstances at present.

A number of factors have led to a resistance to EL, such as budgetary restraints and lack of administrative and/or faculty support. Secondly, EL has been derogated as being non-scholarly and "merely vocational." Society continues to be influenced by epistemology. Cognitive education is seen as scholarly. However, to understand one's total environment, experience must be brought to awareness and comprehended in its affective complexity. Besides reasoning and logic, intuition is necessary for full knowing. Finally, EL requires the teachers to use non-traditional and possibly unfamiliar teaching methods. Often these imply a shift in power from that of control (traditional teaching strategies) to one of mutual openness and respect. This may lead to feelings of being threatened and to resistance. To overcome such resistance, teachers need to be trained and willing to deal with affect as well as cognition in the teaching-learning process.

CONCLUSION

Everybody is assumed to be capable of all kinds of behaviour (i.e., everybody is capable of learning). But, as stated by John Dewey (1987), this process can be painful. No one can enter a new world without forsaking an old one. New ideas and feelings may be exciting, but the newly acquired knowledge and experience may "rub up" against long-held beliefs and principles (Majumdar, 1990). Kolb and Fry (1977) suggest that everybody, if they are to acquire learning (by changing their behaviour or beliefs in some way) will need four different kinds of ability. They must be able to involve themselves in new experience, observe and reflect on that new experience from different perspectives, create concepts that integrate observations into logically sound theories and use them to make decisions and solve problems (Christopher, 1987).

To increase knowledge and understanding of ethnic groups and cross-cultural interactions, the technique of direct experience is more effective than presenting factual information (Mio, 1989). Depth of experience is a key factor in cross-cultural sensitivity. This does not imply that breadth of experience with minority groups is useless. Cross-cultural contact should accompany academics through innovative teaching strategies. Experiential learning methods provide various techniques to increase cultural sensitivity experientially.

Cultural awareness includes insight into our own cultural beliefs and biases. Because it is our culture, it is our own beliefs and values that filter what we see and hear. Therefore, we restrict our thoughts to when and what we teach and how communicate with others (Majumdar & Hezekiah, 1990). Cultural awareness is acquired by developing a special sensitivity to ourselves and to each other, through constant reflection on our own behaviour, on what we believe and why, and on what we are teaching and how we communicate.

REFERENCES

Arosker, M. (1977). Ethics in the nursing curriculum. *Nursing Outlook*, 25(4), 260-64.

Boydell, T. (1976). *Experiential Learning* (Manchester Monographs: 5, 23-25). Dorset, England: Direct Design Ltd.

Christopher, E. (1987). Academia: A Cross-Cultural Problem. *International Journal of Intercultural Relations*, 11(2), 191-206.

CUSO Education Department. (1988). *Basics & Tools: A collection of popular education resource and activities.* (113, 116-117, & 142).Ottawa.

Dewey, J. (1975). *Experience and Education.* New York: Collier Books.

Filerman, G.L. (1986). Canadian universities and international health. *Health Management Forum.* Spring, Vol. 7, 4-16.

Kohls, L.R. (1984). A Traditional Approach to Developing cross-cultural preparedness in adult education training orientation and briefing. *International Journal of Intercultural Awareness*, 11(1), 89-106.

Kolb, D.A. (1984). *Experiential Learning.* Englewood Cliffs, New Jersey: Prentice-Hall, Inc.

Kolb, K. and Fry, R. (1977). Towards an Applied Theory of Experiential Learning. In Cooper, C.L., *Theories of Group Process*, 33-57. London: John Wiley.

Majumdar, B. (1990). *Learning Can Be a Social Act & It Can Be Fun.* Unpublished. School of Nursing, McMaster University.

Majumdar, B., & Hezekiah, J.A. (1990). Professional Ideals Versus Personal Values: Some Observations on Transcultural Health Issues. *Sante, Culture, Health, 12*(1), 33-40.

Mio, J.S. (1989). Experiential involvement as an Adjunct to Teaching Cultural Sensitivity. *Journal of Multicultural Counselling and Development, 17*(1), 38-46.

Nwanko, R.N. (1991). Communication and social values in cross-cultural adjustment. *The Howard Journal of Communication, 3*(1 & 2), 99-111.

Rogers, C.R. (1969). *Freedom to learn.* Columbus, Ohio: Charles E. Merrill Publishers.

Shirts, R.G. (1977). *BaFa BaFa: A Cross-Cultural Simulation.* Del Mar: Simile II.

Sikkema, M., & Niyekawa, A. (1987). *Design for Cross-Cultural Learning.* Maine: Intercultural Press, Inc.

Uutal, D. (1984). Values education: Opportunities and imperatives. *Nurse Educator,* Jan.-Feb., 9-13.

- 11 -

Cultural Perspectives in Chronic Illness

Enid Collins

Chronic illness has a significant impact on the lives of individuals and families. Coping with chronicity involves lifelong alterations in lifestyle. Whether chronicity occurs during childhood as a result of birth defects, or during adulthood with the onset of diseases such as diabetes and hypertension, individuals and families have to cope with many crises that begin with diagnosis of the disease and continue with periods of stabilization that are interspersed with periods of exacerbation of disease symptoms. This chapter will examine the impact of chronic illness within the sociocultural context, with particular emphasis on the coping strategies of individuals and families at different stages of illness. Case studies of actual chronic illness situations will be used to demonstrate application of the concepts.

Health care providers are faced with an enormous challenge to respond to the needs of culturally diverse clients. If they are to achieve the ultimate goal of preventing or delaying disease in high risk populations and decreasing the rates of morbidity and mortality associated with chronic diseases, health care providers must ensure that their care is based on a consideration of cultural factors.

Coping strategies that are developed are determined within the cultural context of individuals and families. Beliefs about health and illness, such as what caused the disease, treatment, modalities that constitute cure, and spiritual beliefs will inherently determine how clients respond to, and follow through with, therapeutic regimes. Interacting within family support systems are cultural determinants that influence the outcomes of chronic illness. These factors must be considered by health care practitioners in order to assist individuals and families to develop effective coping strategies through the various phases of chronic illness.

DEMOGRAPHIC FACTORS

Changing societal trends have led to new disease patterns. Advances in health care and developing technologies have contributed to increased longevity. As the population ages, the incidence of chronic illness increases. Hanson (1987) identifies that the elderly population is more prone to chronic conditions than the population in general. An increased incidence of arthritis and hypertension are among the leading conditions affecting those over 65 years old. Among the chronically ill elderly, the ethnic mix is changing to reflect the multicultural mix in society. Hanson (1987) identifies the growing numbers of elderly non-white people in the population.

Genetic and other childhood diseases that are major killers of children are now responding to more effective treatment modalities. Those with chronic diseases such as cystic fibrosis, juvenile onset diabetes and sickle cell disease are now living into adulthood and are themselves becoming parents. Bio-sociocultural variations are a significant factor in the determination of chronicity among ethnic groups. Conditions such as Tay-Sach's disease, thalassaemia and sickle cell disease are common among some ethnic groups (Masi, 1988c), as are other chronic illnesses infrequently found in found in the general population. Other factors may complicate the health status of some ethnic groups and render them vulnerable to the effects of chronic illness. Morse et al. noted that Southeast Asian refugees may have "poor nutritional status as a result of lack of food in the refugees' homeland and in the refugee camps and the problem may be further compounded after arrival in Canada by difficulty in adjusting to Canadian food" (1988, 2047). Some chronic diseases that are found across various cultural groups carry varying risk factors in specific ethnic groups.

Among Blacks, the incidence of hypertension is twice that of whites. The disease develops earlier in life in Blacks and more often results in malignant hypertension. In general, hypertension among blacks carries a higher risk of mortality and morbidity (Boyle & Andrews, 1989). According to Masi (1989a), there is a need for physicians to develop a greater awareness of inherited disorders that are ethnic related. This is true especially for those physicians who work in communities where there is a high percentage of ethnic people. It is also true for all health care professionals who provide care for individuals of different ethnic groups who may be prone to chronic diseases that are unfamiliar to them. The author recounts a situation where a nurse's lack of knowledge of cultural characteristics made a difference in a complex situation. The client, a 13-year-old girl, was admitted to a paediatric acute care ward. Her diagnosis was sickle cell thalassaemia disease. Her features were oriental; her nationality was Jamaican. The admitting nurse was not only unaware that people of Chinese origin lived in Jamaica, but was also unaware of the biocultural transmission of the disease.

FRAMEWORKS TO ADDRESS CHRONIC ILLNESS

Because of the complex, multifaceted ongoing nature of chronic illness, health practitioners need a framework within which to address problems from a holistic perspective.

In identifying a working definition of chronic illness, many writers have drawn on the 1956 definition that was "proposed by the Commission on Chronic illness 1956" (Diamond & Jones, 1983, 33). This definition focuses on "impairments or deviations from normal" characterized by permanent residual disability, non-reversible pathological alteration, requiring training or rehabilitation and long term supervision and or care (Glaser & Strauss, 1975). This definition remains workable and still appears in the literature through the 1980's, however, it is problematic since it emphasizes only physiological abnormalities (Diamond & Jones, 1983).

More holistic definitions have evolved to address the multifaceted nature of issues related to chronic illness. This author subscribes to a more holistic definition such as the one proposed by Diamond and Jones. This model states that "interactions of clinical, personal and social definitional systems can be conceptualized as major determining patterns of behaviour (disability) of individuals with chronic illness" (1983, 37). The clinical dimension focuses on anatomical or physiological manifestations. Personal definitions focus on the meaning of the illness to the individual and the way the person defines himself or herself. The person's age, sex, cultural and social expectations, perceived loss of functional capacity and changes in lifestyle, activity, and roles have an impact on the meaning attached to illness. Social definitions are " based on the expectations of behaviour ingrained in others through socialization process that occur in all culture and societies". This dimension includes the implicit and explicit definitions made by others in the family and social network, as well as other systems such as employers, health care workers, and workers in social and welfare benefits offices.

This definition presents a more holistic perspective, which allows health care practitioners to consider the totality of the experience of chronic illness within the sociocultural context of the individual and family. Many health care practitioners view the responses to chronic illness from their own cultural position, which is often dominant Anglo Saxon, as well as the subcultural context of the healing professions, which is often the Western scientific model. The tendency is to stereotype the presenting or expected behaviour of chronically ill persons according to the expectations of such behaviours as it is anticipated within the dominant culture, or at the other extreme, to attribute all behaviours to a person's cultural context without consideration of all the interrelated dimensions of chronic illness. It is a reality that the manifestations of chronic illness are expressed within the cultural context, however, the severity of pathophysiology must be considered in dealing with clients' responses. Interpretation of client verbal and non-verbal behaviour, may stem from health care workers lack of understanding of cultural differences. They may attribute meanings to client's behaviour other than those intended by clients. In studying disability behaviour among more than 2000 clients applying for social benefits, Brodsky concluded that "no deviant disability behaviour was observed that was typical for the members of any cultural group" (1983, 92). It was noted that cultural stereotypes of disability behaviour were not supported by data, and that, "examples of unique and extreme disability behaviour were seen as frequently among many ethnic groups including persons of Northern European ancestry as among those of Oriental Mediterranean or other racial and ethnic backgrounds" (1983, 92). These findings are of importance in chronic illness situations, since health care providers should be aware of interpreting clients' behaviours solely on the basis of cultural perceptions, but should consider the interrelationships of pathological manifestations. According to

Brodsky's finding a substantial part of peoples behaviour can be determined by chronic illness, but if there is no disease present, the assumption can be made that behaviour is a result of personality or sociocultural factors.

Chronic illness may be gradual or sudden in onset, and requires the person to make major adjustments in lifestyle, roles and relationships. Furthermore, these adjustments continue over the lifespan. Hanson (1987 cites Strauss and Glaser (1975) in identifying tasks that families with chronic illness must accomplish. These include: 1) preventing and managing crises; 2) managing treatment regimens; 3) controlling symptoms; 4) adapting to temporal and role disruption; 5) learning to handle the disease course and trajectory; 6) overcoming social isolation; and 7) managing financial needs. These tasks provide a framework for understanding how families react to and deal with chronic illness within the sociocultural context.

Families faced with chronic illness deal with crisis continually. The diagnosis of a chronic illness may be made after the gradual onset of symptoms, or suddenly, with little warning. After the initial diagnosis, periods of intermittent crises occur either as a result of the progression of existing symptoms, or the appearance of new ones. The responses of individuals and families to crises are closely related to their beliefs about illness and its causation and cures. An individual or family may believe that the symptoms of disease are caused by supernatural powers or as punishment for previous wrongdoing. For example, Morse et al. (1988) notes that among some Southeast Asian groups, persons afflicted with a chronic illness may associate its causation with supernatural forces which include punishment for previous violation of a taboo. Alternative healers may be sought who are thought to understand the forces involved and can intercede on behalf of the ill individual (Masi, 1988b). Health care workers may see clients at the onset of the crisis before they have sought help from alternative healers, or the clients may see the healers on an ongoing basis. It is important that health care practitioners become aware of the client's system of beliefs in assisting them to cope with crisis situations.

The following clinical situation encountered by the author is an example of a crisis that created a conflict between the caregivers and the family. An only child of a South Asian Family had become unconscious after aspiration of some swallowed pea seeds. The family, reassured by their religious leader that the child would regain consciousness, kept a daily vigil by her bed.

The child's birthday was the appointed day that she would regain consciousness. When this did not happen, the family reacted with an extreme emotional outburst. Throughout the time that the child was hospitalized many staff members voiced their feelings that the religious leaders were not being honest with the family; as well, they felt that all the family members present were a hinderance to care. The child remained unconscious for several months, the parents continued to hope for a change in her condition and the staff continued to express anger at what they perceived to be irrational behaviour on the part of the family.

The initial crisis that arises from a diagnosis of a chronic illness signals the onset of major ongoing adaptations. The intensity and frequency of subsequent crises depend on a number of factors, such as the course of the disease, response to treatment, and the willingness of individuals and families to follow the prescribed regimens. Treatment regimens require families to engage in managing complex protocols such as administration of medication, modification of diet, management of surgical incisions. They also have to plan for repeated assessment procedures such as venipuncture to obtain blood samples. The management of complex treatments goes hand in hand with symptom management and control. Maintaining these treatment protocols can be challenging as well as frustrating for clients and their families. Health care professionals feel challenged when behaviours of clients are perceived as non compliant. Clients who act in accordance with their beliefs about health and illness may modify treatments to fit their perception of effective management strategies. Conflicts that arise as a result of such beliefs or from misunderstanding arising from ignorance or language barriers are major sources of non-compliance among chronically ill clients and their families.

When protocol requires treatment through taking medications, these may be taken with or substituted by, various home remedies or over-the-counter drugs. In their study of "Curanderismo," the folk medical system of traditional Mexican and Spanish American communities, Scheper-Hughes et al. (1983) found that among these groups a number of folk remedies and over-the-counter drugs were taken to treat illness and symptoms such as bronchitis, colds, fevers, to act as diuretics, to settle the stomach, purify the blood, or ameliorate heart conditions. Home remedies were only part of their way of managing symptoms. They also relied on regular medical systems and received most of their primary care from physicians, clinics and hospitals. When alternative approaches to treatment of chronic illness are taken, these may lead to illness, addiction or neutralise the effects of prescribed treatment. For example, diuretic teas taken with antihypertensive medications may lead to hypotensive episodes. Another problem with the management of medication regimes arises when over-the-counter drugs are taken for other than their intended effects. Mitchell notes that among Jamaicans, over-the-counter drugs are widely used and that problems arise because they are used in "congruence with popular medical concepts" (1983, 40). For example, antacids may be taken for arthritic pains because they cut gas, bitter tonics for diabetes because they clean the blood, or inhalants for hypertension because they cool the head. Exacerbation of symptoms would obviously arise if these remedies were substituted for prescribed medical treatment. The manifestation of overt symptoms are of significance in the way that they are interpreted and managed by some cultural groups. For example, among Jamaicans the absence of symptoms means the absence of disease, so, for those chronic diseases such as hypertension that tend to be intermittently asymptomatic, the tendency is to discontinue medications when no symptoms are present. A common approach in management of antihypertensive medications is to take them when severe headaches are present (Mitchell, 1983).

In a situation that the author encountered clinically, a child was receiving chemotherapy treatments and as a result had mouth ulcers. When the mother was asked by the nurse what she did for the ulcers, she volunteered that, on the advice of a neighbour, she had substituted potassium chloride mouth washes for prescribed sodium bicarbonate treatment. The mother thought that she was doing her best to increase the child's comfort but had no idea of the possible consequences of potassium imbalances. Ongoing assessments that involve blood taking for laboratory tests is part of the process of management of chronic disease symptoms. Some groups such as Southeast Asians miss appointments because of they resist venipuncture which is associated with fear of upsetting the hot cold balance of the body. They may also display resistance because of their experience with the military's need for blood (Morse, et al., 1988).

Pain is a symptom of chronic illness that is commonly manifested in a number of diseases such as arthritis, chronic back problems and cancers to name just a few. When chronic illness is present, pain persists for prolonged periods, increase in severity often is minimally relieved by therapeutic regimes and may be aggravated by some treatment modalities. Manifestations of pain vary widely, with different cultural groups: for example, people of Greek and Italian origin are often vocal in expression of pain, while Chinese people are known to be less expressive of such feelings.

Manifestations of symptoms of chronic illness, when considered in the cross-cultural context, can lead to problems for the client and family, the health care providers and larger systems. Even within a single culture, wide variations of belief systems and practices may occur. Within some groups, chronic illness resulting from genetic or birth-related defects may be considered a curse that has been supernaturally inflicted as punishment for previous wrongdoing.

Having such a child may cause shame to the family so they may choose to keep the child within the confines of the family. An example of this was recently publicized in Miami where a woman kept her retarded child locked in a room and fed the young woman through slots in the wall. When the case came to light as a result of neighbours hearing peculiar noises, the retarded woman was 23 years old. When the mother was arrested, she claimed that she had done the best for her child and had no help from the system. Although the cultural component was not emphasized in the media, it is likely that socioeconomic or subcultural factors played a part. The mother was portrayed by the media as an elderly black woman living in depressed inner city housing in Miami.

It is well known that symptoms of some diseases are stigmatized among some cultural groups. Consequently members suffering from these diseases may be kept within the family, with the result that treatment is denied to the ill individual. According to Lin (1983), among Chinese communities all over the world, mental illness and related strategies for coping are managed within the family. Reporting findings of research carried out in Vancouver, it was observed that Chinese families have distinctive patterns of dealing with serious psychiatric illness that follow five distinctive phases. During the first phase, which may last as long as 10 to 20 years, attempts are made by the family to influence abnormal behaviours of sick family members by using various remedies. These practices stretch the means and resources of the family to the limits. In the second phase, the help of trusted friends and elders is enlisted. In the third phase, outside helpers such as herbalists, physicians or religious leaders treat the person's psychotic symptoms but they are still kept within the family. During the fourth phase, the person is labelled mentally ill and is treated by trusted outside agencies or physicians Labelling means that the family is stretched to its limits. During the final stage, "the hope of recovery of the sick person fades and the psychological and financial burden of caring for a mentally-ill family member becomes unbearable, it is then that phase five, the final phase of rejection and scape-goating sets in. The family gives up hope and is reconciled with its fate of having a mentally-ill patient in its care for the rest of the patient's life, or the patient is kept far away in a mental hospital so that the family no longer has to think about him or her" (ibid., 60-61).

The findings of Dr. Lin's research provide a poignant example of a cultural system of beliefs that has implications for the ill individual, the family, the health care system and the community as a whole. Decisions about the management of symptoms are not an individual but a family responsibility. The course of action pursued places major strains on the family. When the sick person's condition does not improve that person is scapegoated and ostracized. One cannot help but wonder about whether guilt is raised in those family members, whose efforts are not rewarded by the improvement of the condition of the family member. This begs the question of whether some cultural models of caring contribute to undue stress within families. members. Health care practitioners need to be alert for indicators of stress and to assist families in a realistic way without negating their commitment to cultural beliefs.

When an individual family member develops a chronic illness, established role relationships within the system are greatly affected. The sick role assumed by the ill person is derived from the cultural context of the family and sociocultural community. Within some cultural communities the family is a major social network. When a person is ill , he or she may seek advice or use advice given by family members as an adjunct to the advice provided by health care practitioners. Some approaches used by Vietnamese families cited in Orque et al., (1983) suggest the extensive influence of the family. Health is viewed as a family responsibility. The family, will go to great lengths to cure the relative before seeking outside help. A mentally ill Vietnamese patient may postpone seeking professional help because his illness may be interpreted as the family's failure to fulfil it's obligation towards him.

While mutual support within the family is desirable, a decision to delay seeking outside help for the sick individual may result in exacerbation of symptoms, as well as considerable strain on the family's resources. In some cultural groups the question of who makes decisions on behalf of the ill person is complex. In North American health care systems, the rights of the individual to be informed and to make decisions about care is the norm. In some cultures, however, the decision about seeking help may be made by the individual's family, perhaps because of his or her status or the belief system within the family. The chronically ill person may be excluded from the decision making, with or against his or her wishes. The effect of exclusion of the ill person can be devastating as will be demonstrated in a case study that be discussed later in this chapter.

Health care practitioners need to be aware of the behaviour norms with respect to the elders in some families, such as Chinese, Vietnamese and West Indian families. Older people from these cultures may not divulge information to persons who are young. For example, an elderly black woman from Barbados refused to give information when questioned by a young intern who addressed her by her first name. She later confided to a black nurse who was closer to her own age that the intern was younger than her son and that he had no respect.

Extended family and kinship networks among some ethnic groups unquestionably provide support for chronically ill family members, however, when families isolate themselves from community supports, the emotional and physical toll on family members can lead to increased stress. Bonar (1985) cites a study by Fandetti and Gelfand done in 1976 in which researchers examined the attitudes of Polish and Italian respondents toward services and caring for elderly relatives. The majority of respondents agreed that elderly relatives should live with families rather than on their own or in institutions. Bonar notes that when individuals are chronically ill or bedridden, families are faced with difficult problems that can affect their whole life when they try to provide continuous care 24 hours a day. They often face major conflicts that may arise from their own value orientation of loyalty to older family members and the necessity to meet their own needs.

The course of chronic illness varies considerably with different diseases. Whether the onset is acute with a rapid downward course, or whether it is ongoing with asymptomatic periods interspersed with periods of symptom exacerbation, individuals and families require major adaptation in lifestyle. The coping strategies developed are determined within the cultural context. People may perceive the meaning of illness to be from supernatural causes, or may turn to religious practices. The family's religious leader, minister, priest, rabbi or shaman may be a constant source of support for the sick person, and should included in the caring team. Religious rituals may be part of the coping strategies and should not be discouraged. The following anecdote exemplifies a situation where the nurse, unaware of the cultural significance of a terminally ill client's behaviour, made a decision that was not in the client's best interest. Fortunately, with the intervention of a culturally aware colleague, the decision was reversed. Mrs B., an elderly West Indian woman had terminal cancer. Each night she engaged in lengthy monologues reciting several names. The woman's monologue disturbed the other client who was in the room. The nurse interpreted her behaviour as confused hallucinations and it was decided that the woman's bed should be placed in the hall where she would not disturb the other person. Upon investigation by a nurse from the woman's culture, it was discovered that the client had eleven children and several grand children who she named in her nightly prayers.

Another commonly acknowledged coping strategy in dealing with chronic illness is that of seeking normalization of individual and family life. In the normalization process, people attempt to cope and lead as normal a life as possible, while maximizing their potential within the limitations of their illness. A case study illustrating the normalization process within the cultural context will be discussed later in the chapter.

An inevitable part of the chronic illness trajectory, is that of recognizing the inevitability of death. The booklet *Caring Across Cultures - Multicultural Considerations in Palliative Care* (1988) grew out of the recognition that nurses in the Saint Elizabeth Visiting Nurses Association, Metropolitan Toronto area, are increasingly faced with the need to care for clients from a number of ethnic groups in palliative care situations. This work cites a list of religious beliefs and practices which are essential knowledge for nurses in order for them to provide culturally sensitive care. For example, in the Hindu religion "women wear a nuptial thread on the neck and sometimes a red mark on the forehead....a male may wear a sacred thread around the arm indicating attainment of adult religious status" (25). When car-

ing for the dying patient the nurse should be aware that these
should not be removed from the body. A number of traditional
symbols worn by persons of the Sikh religion are also identified.
These should be left on the bodies of dying persons.

The last two tasks identified by Diamond and Jones's model
of family adaptation to chronic illness are overcoming social
isolation and managing financial needs. Regardless of the socio-
economic class or cultural group, stresses arising from long-
term care of a chronically ill family member are very real. Within
the dominant Anglo-Saxon culture, care-givers and clients alike
suffer much hardship and social isolation. Care-giver stress is
becoming a major issue to be addressed by health care workers.
It is beyond the scope of this paper to address this problem.
Within ethnic communities strong kinship, family ties and mutual helping and sharing is often the norm.

Taken to the extreme, however, families can assume an increasing burden for the care of chronically ill family members
while refusing to accept help from outside resources. For the
family, the financial and emotional burdens can be severe in
some cases, as for example, the findings of Dr Lin's research
reveal with Chinese families.

IMPLICATIONS FOR HEALTH CARE PRACTITIONERS

The long term and multidimensional nature of chronic illness
bring clients, their families and health providers together in
complex relationships over extended periods of time. During
periods of crisis, the chronically ill individuals and their families may be in acute care settings where they are subjected to the
many institutional rules and regulations that may present conflicts to their cultural beliefs and values. During non-crisis
periods, individuals and families are expected to manage the
impact of illness on all aspects of their lives, which include
managing complex treatment protocols, dealing with disease
symptoms, managing demands of living and meeting role expectations. The family and community becomes the central locus of
care. It is critical that the interrelatedness of the many dimensions of life be considered. In suggesting effective strategies for
cross-cultural care Anderson advocates a "mutual participation
model ....in which the patient's and families beliefs are seen as
legitimate" (1987, 9). Health care practitioners who accept the
centrality of the client and family as the major part of the team

must be cognizant of the clients and families cultural beliefs and values, but must also be aware of their own cultural and subcultural orientation. Health care practitioners are influenced by the values derived from their own cultural and ethnic background as well as those of the professional and health care system subcultures. Recognizing how these value orientations are similar, or different from their clients' values, and responding to clients' cultural orientation is a basic principle underlying mutual participation with clients.

Another important principle is the need to develop awareness of differences within and across cultures, which might be related to variables such as socio-economic class, level of education and the numbers of years since migration. By developing awareness of such differences, health care practitioners are able to focus on individuality and to avoid stereotypes. Important areas that should be explored from the point of view of recipients of care within a cross-cultural context include beliefs about health and illness, the influences of family orientation on decision making patterns, strategies in coping with chronic illness and support systems within the ethnocultural community and the larger community. In situations of chronic illness, continuity of care between different levels within the health care systems is vital to maintaining multiple relationships between health care practitioners, clients and families.

Communication can be fraught with difficulties, often due to language barriers and construction of meaning when interpreted in the cross-cultural context. The use of interpreters is often essential in such circumstances. Their role takes on particular significance in chronic illness situations where the interpreter and clients are from the same cultural group, and the health care practitioner is not. The interpreter may convey meanings within the cultural context, for example, giving information to make the clients "look good," or not revealing to the health care provider information that may be embarrassing to the client and family.

THE MUTUAL PARTICIPATION MODEL: A CASE STUDY

Another important dimension of developing the mutual participation model in dealing with chronic illness is the need for health care practitioners to recognize the expertise of clients and their families from a cultural perspective, as well as their need to become the experts in management of their own situation and to be a part of the ongoing education process. The following case study exemplifies the mutual participation model.

Tom (not his real name), aged 42 years, was diagnosed with sickle cell disease at the age of 12 years, and came to Canada from Jamaica in 1971. He has four sisters, two of whom have sickle cell trait and three brothers, of whom all have sickle cell disease. One brother died of sickle cell related complications one winter after prolonged exposure from walking a long distance in the cold. Tom's father died of hypertension and his mother, currently living with him, has diabetes and sickle cell disease.

Tom is very knowledgeable about his disease and its management. Over the years he has managed his disease and has been gainfully employed. He has had many episodes of illness related to sickle cell crises and other complications. He talks about his early days in Canada when he went to hospitals and the doctors and nurses knew little about his disease. He now receives supervision in a major medical centre and is happy with the treatment received from doctors and nurses. They respect his opinions and give him the freedom to make decisions about his care. Tom has a crisis prevention protocol that consists of hydration, oxygen therapy and analgesics. Tom expressed that his greatest fear is of pain during crisis episodes. He states that he is glad that his doctors allow him to take medications at home without worrying about him becoming addicted. Within the last few years he has had decreased vision in both eyes as a result of retinal detachment following vaso-occlusive crises.

Tom is actively involved with the Sickle Cell Association. He participates in education sessions with various groups including health care providers, teachers and students in schools with large numbers of black students. He finds that he can relate and respond to many concerns of students about sickle cell disease such as causation of disease, concerns about marriage and childbearing, and for some students, management of symptoms and concerns about addiction arising from the use of analgesics.

Respecting the cultural background of the client and the knowledge gained from years of adaptation is a dimension that can be satisfying for the client, but can provide valuable education opportunities that can ultimately enhance outcomes in chronic illness situations.

ETHICAL DILEMMAS: A CASE STUDY

Clinical practice situations involving chronic illness present multiple challenges, some of which may arise from the cultural context. These challenges may result in ethical dilemmas involving families and health care practitioners. This case study raises many ethical issues. The family was encountered recently by colleagues in an acute care setting.

The G. Family

The family came to the attention of the health care team when Connie, the oldest girl at 8 years, was diagnosed with chronic myelogenous leukaemia. Sally, who was 6 years old, and the second girl, was later to become a bone marrow donor for Connie; Jamie, a boy of 5 years, was well. The G. family was of East Indian background. The parents' exact ages were not known, but they were apparently in their mid-40s, with the mother appearing slightly older. The father appeared culturally more Westernized and fairly well educated. He assumed child caring roles on and off while his wife worked. At the time of the encounter, both parents were working outside the home, he in a skilled job, and she in an unskilled job.

The family's exact religion was not known but they were often accompanied by a spiritual leader who was dressed in white with flowing white hair and beard.

At the time of Connie's diagnosis, the physicians decided on a treatment protocol that involved a bone marrow transplant. It was decided that the treatment should be done immediately in order to minimize the risk of the disease converting to an acute, more aggressive type of leukaemia. In discussing the diagnosis and treatment plan with the family, the father was ready and willing to work with the health care team in gaining information and in involving Connie and the other children. The mother, on the other hand, refused to cooperate with the health team. She refused to discuss Connie's diagnosis and treatment. She often repeated the response that it was in God's hands. She insisted that Connie, and the other siblings, not be given any information. The father, although willing to work with the health team and to involve the children in preparation for hospitalization and treatment, was ineffective in having the wife change her position. She was over protective of Connie. Each time nurses attempted to communicate with the child, she intervened insisting that she should not be given information, and that God would take care. She spoke to the child in hushed whispers and insisted that she not be told her diagnosis. She eventually told her that she had leukaemia, but refused to say the word cancer.

The parents did give consent for Connie to have a bone marrow transplant, and the 6-year-old sister was determined to be a suitable donor. The health care team went ahead with the procedure even though the child had little preparation and was given no information. The transplant was successful in the physiological sense, however, Connie who prior to her illness was a healthy outgoing child, manifested dramatic behavioural changes. She displayed hysterical behaviour, and had many psychosomatic symptoms which were often supported by the mother who talked about her own illness. Connie talked of committing suicide. Nurses who cared for the child during hospitalization expressed anger and frustration in not having any input in decisions about the child's preparation prior to surgery, and having to deal with the aftereffects of the child's behaviour.

Analysis of this case raises many issues involving the cultural dynamics of this family's situation. It is obvious that the cultural and belief system very strongly influenced the decisions that were made in dealing with the child's illness. The mother, with a strong belief in the supernatural, was the primary decision maker. Even though the father was at another level of acceptance of Western medicine, he was not a major influence in the decisions about his daughter's care.

The ethical principles of autonomy and justice had an impact on making decisions about the rights of the 8-year-old child, as well as the rights of the father to have input in the decision making about the treatment of his child. The mother's belief system was a major consideration by members of the health care team not to provide adequate preparation for the child, who suddenly went from being well to experiencing major treatment procedures involving prolonged hospitalization with stringent isolation procedures.

In North American health care system, the right of individuals to have information underlies the major health care practice decisions. In this situation, the cultural belief of one member of the family determined the decision making. Dilemmas arising from the cultural context often confront health care practitioners when dealing with chronic illness situations. The influence of culture is a major determinant of outcomes, but they cannot be considered in isolation from other factors. In this situation, decision making based on the principle of beneficence, where the greatest good for the greatest number is considered, may have resulted in a more positive outcome. To return to the model of Diamond and Jones (1983), which advocates an integrated approach involving the interaction of clinical, personal and social definitions of chronic illness, it is obvious that in the case of the G family the clinical dimension was given precedence over other dimensions with a consequently disastrous outcome. Health care professionals should consider the need for consultation and collaboration with professional colleagues when making decisions in situations involving complex cultural systems.

SUMMARY

This chapter espouses the belief that chronic illness influences all dimensions of the lives of both the ill individual and their families. The interrelationships of clinical physiological and sociocultural factors must be considered. In responding to the needs of individuals and families affected by chronic illness, health care practitioners must consider the interrelatedness of cultural influences that arise from the cultural beliefs of clients and their families as well as of their own cultural beliefs and those beliefs and values that arise from the professional and health care systems of the dominant cultural group.

REFERENCES

Anderson, J. (1987). The cultural context of caring. Canadian *Critical Care Nursing Journal, 8* (6), 7-15.

Bonar, R. (1985). Multicultural issues in old age. *Multiculturalism, 8* (2), 113- 15.

Brodsky, C. (1983). Culture and disability behaviour. *The Journal of Western Medicine, 139* (6), 88-95.

Boyle, J., & Andrews, M. (1989). *Transcultural concepts in nursing.* Glenview, Ill: Scott Foresman.

Curtis, J., & Benjamin, M. (1986). *Ethics in Nursing.* New York: Oxford University Press.

Diamond, M. & Jones, S. (1983). *Chronic illness across the life span.* Norwalk, Ct: Appleton-Century-Crofts.

Hanson S. M. (1987). Family nursing and chronic illness. In L.M. Wright & M.Leahey (Eds.), *Families & Chronic Illness,* (2-32). Springhouse: Springhouse.

Health Consultation. South East Asian Community. Toronto: City of Toronto Department of Public Health.

Lin, T. (1983). Psychiatry in Chinese culture. *The Journal of Western Medicine, 139*(6), 58-63, 199.

Bradley, H. A., Leishman, M., Lemmon, B. E., Lundy, M. J., Mildon, E. L., Snape, H. A. & Wiggan, C. G. (1988). *Caring across cultures: Multicultural considerations in palliative care.* (1988). Toronto: Saint Elizabeth Visiting Nurses Association.

Maduro, R. (1983). Curandersimo and Latino views of disease and curing. *The Journal of Western Medicine, 139* (6), 64-70.

Masi, R. (1988a). Multiculturalism, medicine, and health: Part III: Health beliefs. *Canadian Family Physician, 34,* 2649-53.

— —. (1989b). Multiculturalism, medicine and health: Part IV: Individual considerations. *Canadian Family Physician, 34,* 69-72 .

— —. (1989c). Multiculturalism, medicine and health: Part V: Community considerations. *Canadian Family Physician, 34,* 251-54.

Mirdal, G. (1988). The interpreter in cross-cultural therapy. *Institute of Clinical Psychology, 26,* 328-33.

Mitchell, M. (1983). Popular medicine concepts in Jamaica and their impact on drug use. *The Journal of Western Medicine, 139* (6), 37-43.

Morse, J., Edwards, A., & Kappagoda J. (1988). The health care needs of South East Asian refugees. *Canadian Family Physician, 34,* 2405-9.

Orque, M., Bloch, B., & Monrroy, L. (1983). *Ethnic nursing care: A multicultural approach.* St Louis: Mosby.

Scheper-Hughes, N. & Stewart, D. (1983). Curenderismo in Taos County New Mexico - A possible case of anthropological romanticism? *The Journal of Western Medicine, 139* (6), 64-70.

Spector, R. (1985). *Cultural diversity in health and illness.* Norwalk, Ct: Appleton-Century-Crofts.

Strauss, A., & Glaser, B. J. (1975). *Chronic illness and the quality of life.* St. Louis: Mosby.

Acculturation of Food Habits

M.M. Krondl
D. Lau

The process of food selection by human beings is part of a complex behavioural phenomenon shaped by many factors (Lau et al., 1984). The association between food and health is often intertwined with social, cultural and historical influences. Foods have in common that they provide energy and nutrients that are essential for life. One may assume that optimal nutritional health can be achieved when there is abundant food. However, this is not necessarily the case. In the modern world, even those who have access to a plentiful food supply, may experience social forces and technological factors that affect food patterns and that result in unbalanced diets associated with chronic diseases. This chapter will discuss how food habits develop, how their change is influenced by acculturation and what the potential impact of dietary acculturation is on health.

FORMATION OF FOOD HABITS

Food practices usually form a specific pattern; they are repetitious and thus are called food habits or foodways. They develop as a result of food availability, cultural traditions and individual decisions.

ENVIRONMENTAL INFLUENCES

The environment allows access to food, which in turn establishes the type of diet of the indigenous population. Archaeological evidence has provided us with information on the dietary habits of prehistoric man. All humans were hunters and gatherers until about 10,000 years Before Present (B.P.). In time, as vegetation was depleted and animal population dwindled, search for food led to the development of the migratory lifestyles. Eventually, as people learned to domesticate plants and animals, the food supply became more stable and abundant. Further improvement in agricultural practices allowed increased control over plant and animal production. Although this process made available a large quantity of food, it decreased food product diversity (Bryant, Courtney, Markesberg, Dewalt, 1985). Different regions adapted production of dominant food types which became characteristic for the food patterns of the inhabitants. Thus some populations of the Orient are referred to as rice eaters. Many of those inhabiting some European countries are described as wheat eaters, and those in some parts of South America and Africa as corn eaters. Cereals represent the basic component of the food patterns of most of the world; they are the sources of complex carbohydrates that provide most of the food energy intake. Industrialized countries such as Canada do not depend on cereals alone, but often also on foods of animal origin (Krondl & Coleman, 1986).

Yoshida (1981) analysed food consumption data of 27 countries using 11 food categories, and was able to identify several clear-cut trends in global food consumption. The European-American pattern is characterized by foods such as meat, milk, milk products and fruits while the Asian-African pattern is represented by the predominance of cereals and generally by lower energy consumption. Regional food consumption patterns are determined by what food items are available. For instance, in the Ivory Coast and Brazil taro, a source of non-cereal carbohydrates is typical, while in postwar Germany, potatoes were a staple. In Japan, Greece, Italy, Spain and Israel, fish and vegetables dominate the diet. People who live along coastal areas usually supplement their diet with fish, shellfish and other marine products.

FOOD COMBINATIONS IN A MEAL

Most foods are not eaten singly but are combined into a composite dish and/or used together as part of a meal. The significance of food combinations in the food-selection process was established by Lau (1985) by using the method of personal constructs (Kelly, 1975). Niewind, Krondl and Van't Foort (1986) illustrated the important role of culture in the development of different concepts of food compatibility by comparing the food combination patterns of Chinese, European and West Indian women. This study indicated the West Indian women tended to be the least restricted in their options for food combinations.

Chinese and European women seemed to have more specific rules for what were considered appropriate food combinations in a meal. In this study, vegetables contributed most to the cultural variance in food compatibility, as compared to starches and beverages. Differences in food combination patterns between the three groups of women were more pronounced than were similarities, indicating that each culture has its own way of combining foods leading to different dietary patterns.

FOOD PERCEPTIONS

Undoubtedly collective food memory and, thus, ethnicity is important in determining what people eat. However, food habits of ethnic groups are individualized (Hrboticky & Krondl, 1985). The frequency with which a particular food is selected for consumption is to a large extent determined by a set of food-related internalized stimuli. These have been categorized as cultural, social and personal food choice determinants or food perceptions (Krondl & Lau, 1978; Lau, Krondl & Coleman, 1984). A person can rate a particular food according to its specific satiety value (Chong, Holowaty, Krondl & Lau, 1976), or label it as to its association with illness, discomfort or intolerance (Zimmerman & Krondl, 1986). The memory of flavour and other sensory factors (Olson, 1981) as well as the degree of experience or acquaintance with the food or mental barriers that the food must pass before it is accepted for consumption. Beliefs about healthfulness (Ludman & Newman, 1984; Sheppard, 1988; Chau, Lee, Tseng and Downes, 1990) and knowledge of the social factors—price, prestige and convenience—will also be considered in the food acceptance process (Raeburn, Krondl & Lau, 1979). Preferences for specific foods are passed on from generation to generation, forming traditions within families and communities. For example, the preference for chili peppers by some humans was well documented by Rozin and Schiller (1980).

DIETARY ACCULTURATION

The term "acculturation" means the process by which a person gradually accepts and takes on some habits and traits from another, often dominant, culture. Dietary acculturation is one of the many behavioural consequences of immigration. New food-use patterns develop through the rejection of traditional items and the acceptance of culturally new foods. The impact of this process of dietary acculturation on health is related to the balance achieved between nutritionally sound and nutritionally questionable food-use changes. The rate and degree of adaptation by immigrants to the diet of the dominant cultural group will differ according to their ethnic origin and personal background. It depends upon their desire and opportunity to assimilate and upon the degree that they are influenced by tradition and by family values. Immigrants who have personal values that are very different from their host country will change their lifestyle and dietary patterns more slowly than those who have more similar values. Inevitably, however, changes in dietary patterns will occur in any ethnic group or among any individuals arriving to a new country. Even though certain traditional practices are retained intact, some new foods and food-related manners will be adopted (Grivetti and Paquette, 1978). In a study of Southeast Asian (Cambodian and Laotian) refugee families living in the United States, Story and Harris (1989) reported that high-status foods in the country of origin remain highly preferred and are frequently consumed. Fresh fruits, meats and soft drinks are high-status foods in Southeast Asia. Steak, infrequently eaten in the homeland, was reported to be the food most preferred among Vietnamese refugees living in the United States (Crane & Green, 1980). The price of food may also affect the pattern of food changes in the new country. Foods such as fish, shellfish and duck are more expensive in the United States than in Vietnam and are eaten less often by the Vietnamese living there, while cheaper foods such as eggs, sweet snack foods, sodas, butter and margarine, are consumed more frequently (Tong, 1986). The extent of dietary change is largely related to the length of exposure to the new cultural environment (Bavly, 1966; Ho, Nolan and Dodds, 1966; Duyff, Sanjur and Nelson, 1975; Yang & Fox, 1979; Freedman & Grivetti, 1984). However, other factors of acculturation, such as ability to speak the new language (Hrboticky & Krondl, 1985; Chau et al., 1990) and social contact with members of the new culture (Gupta, 1975) may be important.

Generally, young immigrants are more likely than older ones to change their food habits (Wenkam & Wolff, 1970; Cominsky, 1977; Story & Harris, 1989). Furthermore, this process may be easier for males than for females who have more knowledge and experience with traditional cuisines (Katona-Apte & Apte, 1980).

Changes in food habits also proceed more rapidly in families with children, especially with those between the ages of 10 to 16, who interact extensively with non-ethnic peers and introduce new foods to the family (ibid.; Story & Harris, 1989).

HEALTH RISKS OF DIETARY ACCULTURATION

Dietary factors that have been epidemiologically linked to chronic diseases in affluent societies include the overconsumption of food energy, fat and simple sugars that can lead to obesity, diabetes mellitus, cardiovascular diseases and certain cancers; excessive intake of sodium or salt-cured or pickled foods leading to hypertension or stomach cancer; and the inadequate consumption of some foods or nutrients that may protect against cardiovascular diseases, cancer or osteoporosis, such as vitamin A or carotenoids, vitamin C, potassium, calcium, fibre and complex carbohydrates, fruits and vegetables (US Department of Health and Human Services, 1988; Committee on Diet and Health, 1989).

Kumanyika (1990) in a review of issues related to diet and chronic disease for minority populations in the United States suggested that nutrition interventions based on increased consumption of fruits, vegetables and dietary fibre and decreased consumption of saturated fat can result in reduced chronic disease risk in these minority communities, which include immigrants.

In a well-cited study, Tillotson et al. (1973) document the negative impact on the epidemiology of coronary heart diseases and stroke of immigrant Japanese men living in Japan, Hawaii and California when they adopted a Western diet.

Hrboticky and Krondl (1984) studied Chinese adolescent boys and indicated that immigration to a Western country such as Canada may have nutritionally undesirable effects. Flavour ratings of the Chinese immigrant boys reflected a stronger liking of desserts, snacks, fast foods and soft drinks on acculturation. This change in the perception of flavour and the prestige of sweet and salty foods, eaten mainly for pleasure, may enhance nutritionally undesirable changes in the immigrants' food habits. Food-use frequency data from the same study (ibid., 1985) indicated a general trend towards the higher use of highly processed foods and lower food variety within the vegetable food group. Dietary acculturation changes at adolescence, especially those involving an increased use of processed foods high in refined sugars and fat, should be of concern if found to persist into adulthood.

New immigrants should be encouraged to maintain their traditional dietary patterns if they include foods that are in accordance with the host country's nutrition recommendations. The 1990 Canadian Nutrition Recommendations (Health and Welfare Canada, 1990) aim at the reduction of some energy sources, particularly fats high in saturated fatty acids, to decrease the risk of chronic diseases for all Canadians (Murray & Beare-Rogers, 1990).

Nutrition misinformation can lead new Canadians into making food and health choices that may have serious consequences. The diets of most Southeast Asians are high in sodium and potassium (Ziegler, Sucher and Downes, 1989), which may place them at a higher risk for kidney diseases. Nutrition education regarding general nutrition issues, preparing North American foods and the nutritional quality of specific foods should be addressed to new immigrants so that they can make informed decisions about adopting new foodways and making healthy food choices in a new environment (Story & Harris, 1989).

CONCLUSION

In general, food habits are shaped by available foods. Changes in food patterns reflect improved access to foods due to advanced methods of food production, processing and marketing. The shrinking globe and increased local food variety has helped to reduce intercultural differences in food patterns. Nevertheless, foods have their specific meanings by way of family traditions, social norms and cultural beliefs and these food perceptions contribute to the maintenance of established foodways. Immigration represents a case of accelerated induction of food habit changes.

Newcomers to a host country may gradually adopt new life values and adapt to the food patterns of the dominant culture. The North American (Western) dietary pattern may pose potential health risks to immigrants, especially those from the eastern cultures, who are unaware of the possible nutritional and health threats within their new environment.

Although many studies have described food habits and their characteristics, they have not succeeded in explaining how food habits change (Parraga, 1990). Little research has been conducted to determine the extent of change in the diets of immigrants after they arrive in Canada. A challenge to health professionals is to establish a monitoring system that will ensure the optimal nutrition and health status of the ever-increasing multicultural population in Canada.

REFERENCES

Bavly, S. (1966). Changes in food habits in Israel. *Journal of American Dietetics Association, 48,* 488-95.

Bryant, C.A., Courtney, A., Markesberg, B.A., & Dewalt, K.M. (1985). Diet and human evolution: Are we what they ate? *In The Cultural Feast: An Introduction to Food and Society* (5-32). St. Paul, MN: West Publishing Co.

Chau, P., Lee, H.S., Tseng, R., & Downes, N.J. (1990). Dietary habits, health belief and food practices of elderly Chinese women. *Journal of American Diet Association, 90* (4), 379-80.

Chong, R., Holowaty, M., Krondl, M., & Lau, D. (1976). The effect of culturally determined satiety meaning on food practices. *Journal of Canadian Dietetic Association, 37* (4), 245-49.

Committee on Diet and Health, Food and Nutrition Board, Commission on Life Sciences National Research Council. (1989). *Diet and Health. Implications for reducing chronic disease risk.* Washington DC; National Academy Press.

Cosminsky, S. (1977). Alimento and fresco: Nutritional concepts and their implications for health care. *Human Organization, 36,* 203-207.

Crane, N.T., & Green, N.R. (1980). Food habits and food preferences of Vietnamese refugees living in Northern Florida. *Journal of American Dietetic Association, 76,* 591-95.

Duyff, R.L., Sanjur, D., & Nelson, H.P. (1975). Food behaviours and related factors of Puerto Rican American Teenagers. *Journal of Nutrition Education, 7,* 99-107.

Freedman, M.R., & Grivetti, L.E. (1984). Diet patterns of first, second and third generation Greek American women. *Ecology of Food and Nutrition, 14,* 185-204.

Grivetti, L.E., & Paquette, M.B. (1978). Non-traditional ethnic food choices among first generation Chinese in California. *Journal of Nutrition Education, 10,* 109-12.

Gupta, S.P. (1975). Changes in the food habits of Asian Indians in the United States: A case study. *Sociology and Social Research, 60*, 87-99.

Health and Welfare Canada. (1990). *Nutrition Recommendations. The Report of the Scientific Review Committee.* Ottawa: Supply and Services Canada.

Ho, G.P. Nolan, F.L., & Dodds, M.L. (1966). Adaptation to American dietary patterns by students from oriental countries. *Journal of American Dietetic Association, 58*, 277-80.

Hrboticky, N., & Krondl, M. (1984). Acculturation to Canadian foods by Chinese immigrant boys: Changes in the perceived flavour, health value and prestige of foods. *Appetite, 5*, 117-26.

— —. (1985). Dietary acculturation process of Chinese adolescent immigrants. *Nutrition Research, 5*, 1185-97.

Katona-Apte, J., & Apte, M.L. (1980). The role of food and food habits in the acculturation of Indians in the United States. In S. Parmamtma and E. Egmes (Eds.), *The New Ethnics: Asian Indians in the United States* (342-61). New York: Praeger.

Kelly, G.A. (1975). *The Psychology of Personal Constructs.* New York: Norton.

Krondl, M., & Coleman, P. (1986). Social and biological determinants of food selection. In R.K. Chandra (Ed.) Progress in Food and Nutrition Science, (vol. 10, 179-203). Elmsford, N.Y.: Pergamon Journals Ltd. USA.

Krondl, M., & Lau, D. (1978). Food habit modification as a public health measure. *Canadian Journal of Public Health, 69*, 39-45.

— —. (1982). Social determinants in human food selection. In L.M. Barker (Ed), *The Psychology of Human Food Selection* (139-52). Westport, CT; AVI Publishing.

Kumanyika, S. (1990). Diet and chronic disease issues for minority populations. *Journal of Nutrition Education, 22*(2), 89-96.

Lau, D. (1985). Nutrition Behaviour Analysis: Food Perceptions as Determinants of Food Use. Unpublished Ph.D. thesis, University of Toronto, Toronto.

— —. Krondl, M., & Coleman, P. (1984). Psychological factors affecting food selection. In J.R. Galler (Ed.), *Nutrition and Behaviour* (397-415). Vol. 5, *Human Nutrition: A Comprehensive Treatise*, R.B. Alfin-Slater & D. Kritchevsky (Eds.). New York: Plenum Press.

Ludman, E.K., & Newman, J.M. (1984). Yin and Yang in the health-related food practices of three Chinese groups. *Journal of Nutrition Education, 16*, 3-5.

Murray, T.K., & Beare-Rogers, J.L. (1990). Nutrition Recommendations, 1990. *Journal of Canadian Dietetic Association, 51*,(3), 391-93.

Neiwind, A.C., Krondl, M., & Van't Foort, t. (1986). Combinations of foods and their compatibility. *Ecology of Food and Nutrition, 19*, 131-c.39.

Olson, J.C. (1981). The importance of cognitive processes and existing knowledge structures for understanding food acceptance. In J. Solms and R.L. Hall (Eds.), *Criteria of Food Acceptance* (69-81). Zurich: Forster Publishing Ltd.

Parraga, I.M. (1990). Determinants of food consumption. *Journal of American Dietetic Association, 90*(5), 661-63.

Reaburn, J., Krondl, M., & Lau, D. (1979). Social determinants in food selection. *Journal of American Dietetic Association, 74*, 637-41.

Rozin, P., & Schiller, D. (1980). The nature and acquisition of a preference for chili pepper by humans. *Motivation and Emotion, 4*, 77-101.

Sanjur, D. (1982). Ethnicity and food habits. In *Social and Cultural Perspectives in Nutrition* (233-84). Englewood Cliffs, NJ: Prentice Hall.

Shepherd, R. (1988). Belief structure in relation to low-fat milk consumption. *Journal of Human Nutrition and Dietetics, 1*, 421-28.

Story, M., & Harris, L.J. (1989). Food habits and dietary changes of Southeast Asian refugees families living in the United States. *Journal of American Dietetic Association, 89*(6), 800-01.

Tillotson, J.I., Kato, H., Nichaman, M.Z., Miller, D.C., Gay, M.L., Johnson, K.G., & Rhodes, G.G. (1973). Epidemiology of coronary heart disease and stroke in Japanese men living in Japan, Hawaii and California: methodology for comparison of diet. *American Journal of Clinical Nutrition, 26*, 177-84.

Tong, A. (1986). Food habits of Vietnamese immigrants. *Family Economics Review, 2,* 28-32.

Unites States. Department of Health and Human Services. (1988). *The Surgeon General's Report on Nutrition and Health.* DHHS (PHS) Publication No: 88-50210. Washington DC: Superintendent of Documents, US Government Printing Office.

Wenkam, S.N. & Wolff, R.J. (1970). A half-century of changing food habits among Japanese in Hawaii. *Journal of American Dietetic Association, 57,* 29-32.

Yang, G.F., & Fox, H.M. (1979). Food habit changes of Chinese persons living in Lincoln, Nebraska. *Journal of American Dietetic Association, 75,* 29-32.

Yoshida, M. (1981). Trends in international and Japanese food consumption and desirable attributes of foods as assessed by Japanese consumers. In J. Solms and R.L. Hall (Eds.), Criteria of Food Acceptance (117-37). Zurich: Forster Publishing Ltd.

Ziegler, V.S., Sucher, I.P., & Downes, N.J. (1989). Southeast Asian renal exchange list. *Journal of American Dietetic Association, 89*(1), 85-92.

Zimmerman, S., & Krondl, M. (1986). Perceived intolerance of vegetables among the elderly. *Journal of American Dietetic Association, 86,* 1047-51.

- 13 -

Lay Health and Self-Care Beliefs and Practices: Responses of the Elderly to Illness in Four Cultural Settings in Canada and the United States

Amarjit Singh
Barry Kinsey

Human life everywhere is full of mystery and misfortune: various economic, political, social and cultural factors influence human conditions. Blumhagen rightly points out that "sickness is a ubiquitous human experience" (1980, 198). Health considerations are some of the most important factors contributing toward the general well-being of individuals; each society and culture provides its individuals with knowledge and experience to interpret the causes, management and anticipated outcomes of sickness and disease. In other words, each society creates its own definition of nosology (Illich, 1976) and also dictates how one should go about choosing ways and means to deal with associated health problems.

Medical sociologists, anthropologists and medical practitioners have been interested for many years in both modern medicine and traditional or "lay" health care beliefs. They have been particularly interested in the nature and assessment of the relationship between "lay" and "professional" belief systems. It has been generally assumed that "lay" and "professional" health care coexist in most societies. In this chapter, we review selected studies in this area, as well as selected changes that have recently taken place in the organization of the Canadian health care system.

In Canadian society, the publication of Lalonde's (1974) paper, *A New Perspective on the Health of Canadians*, emphasized the health risks associated with individual lifestyles and consumption patterns. He argued that "individual blame must be accepted by many of the deleterious effect on health of their respective lifestyles. Sedentary living, smoking, overeating, driving while impaired by alcohol, drug abuse and failure to wear seat belts are among the many contributors to physical or mental illness for which the individual must accept some responsibility and for which he should seek correction" (26). A recent policy paper by Epp (1986) focused attention on self-care and lifestyle. This approach to health care has become popular not only in Canada but also in other countries (Doyal & Pennel, 1979; Navarro, 1986; Waitzkin, 1983). Epp's policy paper points to three major challenges that are not adequately considered by current health policies and practices in Canada: (1) reducing inequalities in health and health care; (2) increasing the prevention effort; and (3) enhancing people's capacity to cope with chronic conditions, disabilities and mental health problems (Epp, 1986, 398-99). These challenges, the paper suggests, can be met through health promotion, which is defined as "the process of enabling people to increase control over, and to improve, their health" (ibid., 400). Self-care is offered as one of the intrinsic mechanisms to promote health, which "refers to the decisions taken and the practices adopted by an individual specifically for the preservation of his or her health ... simply put, encouraging self-care means encouraging healthy choices" (ibid., 401).

Epp's examples of self-care include eating a balanced diet and exercising daily. He considers mutual aid as a second intrinsic mechanism to promote health; this implies people working together, helping and supporting each other or forming self-help groups. A third mechanism to promote health is the creation of healthy environments. The paper acknowledged that "environmental change becomes by far the most complex and the most difficult of the three mechanisms or kinds of actions required for the promotion of health" (ibid., 403), but this mechanism, in fact, received very little attention in the policy paper. In his critical review of Epp's policy paper Bolaria (1988,

538) points out that "the policy paper tends to stress individual lifestyles, self-care, self-help groups, and other factors more in the individual's sphere of control than environmental factors which require social intervention." Bolaria contends that in this way both Lalonde's (1974) and Epp's (1986) policy papers "tend to downgrade the importance of the physical and social environment to the individual's health. The underlying assumption is that the basic cause of much ill health is the individual" (ibid., 538). We agree with Bolaria that a one-sided emphasis on lifestyles over social environment is an example of what Ryan (1971) called "blaming the victim." We also concede that in many situations individuals do not have any control over the social, economic and political relations that contribute to disease, injury, illness and death; and, therefore, social intervention is necessary to improve environmental factors.

The primary focus of this chapter, however, is on the self-care aspect of health care. In particular, we explore lay health care beliefs and practices among the elderly living in four different cultural communities in Canada and the United States. Self-care practices are rooted in culture, which means, as Ujimoto (1988) has pointed out, that perceptions of personal health and illness, and of the seriousness of the problem, responses to illness, health status, utilization of services, and coping responses and medications used to manage physical and psychological stress and illness are influenced by ethnic and cultural differences. He points out that "while there are several recent Canadian publications on aging and health, for example, Simmons-Tropea & Osborn (1987, 399), D'Arcy (1987, 424), Connidis (1987, 451), Marshall (1987, 473), Chappell (1987, 489), Schwenger (1987, 505), and Shapiro and Roos (1987, 520), cultural variation in Canadian society and its implications for the future health care provisions of aging ethnic minorities are not considered" (237). Similarly, Chappell, Strain and Blandford (1986) note that "the relevance of subculture (ethnic, minority and racial) for the elderly population and, in particular, for the provision of health care is an under-researched area in gerontology" (30). This situation is changing, however, and some studies are beginning to examine the relationship between aging and health by taking cultural interpretation into account (Rempel & Havens, 1986; Wong & Reker, 1985; Ujimoto, 1987; Hess, 1986).

The demographic profile of Canadian and American societies is changing. Both are becoming culturally and ethnically heterogeneous. Ujimoto (1988, 220-43) uses available Canadian and American data on the health statistics of ethnic minorities to illustrate some differences in health problems. We agree with his conclusion that "in order to understand the adjustment to aging by ethnic minorities and their attitudes and behaviour towards aging from a health care perspective, an understanding of what is meant by ethnicity is important" (240).

In any society, varieties of medical and health care systems and beliefs coexist. Such beliefs are rooted in the myth, magic and medicine of a given society. In many cultures it is almost impossible to separate medical practice and religion. Kleiman has pointed out: "Health care systems are symbolic systems built out of meanings, values, and behavioural norms. The health care system articulates illness as cultural idiom linking beliefs about disease causation, the experience of symptoms, specific patterns of illness behaviour, decisions concerning treatment alternative, actual therapeutic practices, and evaluations of therapeutic outcomes" (1978, 86). Medical sociologists and anthropologists have interpreted the emergence of these systems within the modernizing theory (Foster, 1976; King, 1962; Landy, 1974; Pfifferling, 1975; New, 1977; Blumhagan, 1980; Friedson, 1970; Rosengren, 1980; Saunders & Hewes, 1953; Cartwright & Martin, 1958; Gould, 1975; Bauer, 1969). Press points out the three most common meanings of the concept "folk medicine." These are "(1) any health system at variance with Western, scientific medicine; (2) any health system at variance with a codified, formal, and literate medical tradition (Western, scientific, ayurvedic, classical chinese, etc.), and (3) any system of health practice at variance with the official health practice of the community or nation" (1978, 72). The major thrust of these studies is that there is a constant two-way interchange between the two systems, that is "the two cannot be sharply differentiated since many elements are common to both" (Saunders & Hewes, 1953, 44). There is some evidence that the persistence of these models is related to both individual social characteristics and the type of illness. Other authors have identified groups among whom popular beliefs are more likely to be found. These include the elderly (Mabry, 1964); the poorly educated, lower classes (Watts, 1966; Koos, 1967; Davidson, 1970); ethnic minorities (Suchman, 1964; Snow, 1974); and rural residents (Mabry, 1964; Press, 1978). Finally, following modernization theory, it has been assumed that popular health belief systems will eventually disappear as medicalization of society further proceeds and deepens (Illich, 1976). However, "folk medicine is still being practised today in spite of high levels of medicalization (i.e., advances in medical knowledge, technology, increased availability of trained medical personnel, etc.) of Western societies" (Bauer, 1969, 42). Since North American society is increasingly becoming multicultural and heterogeneous, it is more likely that the interaction between popular health belief systems and modern medical health care systems will increase. Therefore, it is important to investigate the popular health beliefs of various cultural groups living in different communities. As Ujimoto (1988) contends, recognition of these beliefs will allow health care professionals and other providers of health care to avoid any "cultural misunderstandings." It is in the framework of this literature that we analyse "lay" conception of health and self-care responses by the elderly in four different communities in Canada and the United States.

LAY HEALTH CARE BELIEFS AND PRACTICES

Methodology and Data Collection

In collecting data for this study, several methodological and conceptual considerations were taken into account. These included (1) the perceived uniqueness of culture in Newfoundland, Canada; (2) the importance of understanding cultural factors in research in the area of a culture/ethnicity, aging and health; (3) the need to do more comparative studies; (4) the importance of having familiarity with the respondents' communities and culture; and (5) the difficulty of conceptualizing and operationalizing ethnicity and culture in the social sciences. Before elaborating on these issues, we will first briefly outline the procedures that were used to collect data.

The present study is part of a research project that focuses on the health and well-being of the elderly. A questionnaire was used to collect data on various aspects of health and well-being of older people living in four culturally diverse communities: (1) a small, transitional city in the southwestern United States; (2) a Philippine community in Toronto; (3) Newfoundland Community A, a group of small communities largely populated by descendants of Protestant immigrants from southwest Ireland and southeast England; and (4) Newfoundland Community B, a fishing village predominantly populated by Irish Catholic immigrants and their descendants. In addition, information pertaining to standard socio-demographical variables (such as age, sex, education and religion) and data relevant to health care beliefs and practices were collected. The primary purpose of the study was to contribute some data to the field of culture and health care by empirical exploration of the relationship between cultural factors and self-care. The focus was (1) to identify the nature of lay beliefs regarding the etiology, pathology and treatment of illness/disease; (2) to determine the nature and extent of lay self-care practices; and (3) to explore potential sources of cultural variation in these health care beliefs and practices.

The questionnaire was designed by the researchers at the Center for Aging, University of Manitoba, and was previously used by Chappell et. al (1984) and Segall (1987) to conduct various studies in that province. Data were collected from a total of 138 respondents, aged 65 and over. This included 30 respondents from Newfoundland Community A, 37 from Newfoundland Community B, 50 from Oklahoma and 21 from Toronto. The method used for selecting respondents could best be described as convenient sampling; however, steps were taken to determine the extent to which the respondents were representative of the larger population of elderly in the communities sampled. For example, the Canadian samples were not significantly different from Buehler's (1987) national survey of health status and activities of the aged in Canada.

In Oklahoma and Toronto we worked through local community agencies for the aged. We identified the most significant program for the aged in each community and asked the directors of these programs to assist us in distributing and collecting questionnaires and in recruiting respondents for interviews. In Oklahoma this was the director of the Senior Citizens Center, and in Toronto, the president of a senior citizens' club specifically organized to meet the needs of the Philippine elderly. In Newfoundland, data was collected in two ways. One set of data was collected in a single small community. There were 37 older people living in the community at the time and all were included in the study. This is referred to as the Newfoundland Community B sample. The second set of Newfoundland data was collected with the assistance of two community coordinators associated with the Red Cross. The coordinators had contacts with Red Cross workers who were in charge of various programs for the elderly in small communities scattered all over the province of Newfoundland. They provided a list of senior citizens over 65 who were living in these communities. The Newfoundland Community A sample (N = 30) was selected from this list so that respondents represented communities in different regions of the province.

Much of the research literature relevant to ethnicity, culture, aging and health tends to be somewhat confusing but does suggest that ethnic culture is important in explaining variation in health care (Ujimoto, 1988; Rosenthal, 1986). The confusion seems to result from difficulties in developing suitable and consistent conceptual and operational definitions of ethnicity and culture. To some extent, we believe that we have addressed this problem by collecting data from diverse but quite distinctive populations. Newfoundland Community B is a small community about 100 miles southwest of St. John's. Although it is situated on St. Mary's Bay, because of transportation and cultural links, the community has always been considered part of the "Cape Shore," a string of Irish communities on the eastern side of Placentia Bay near Cape St. Mary's. This community was originally settled about 1790 by three fishermen from Waterford in Ireland and today the population of approximately 650 people who live there are all descendants of these and other Irish, almost exclusively Roman Catholic, fishermen. While affected by change and a part of 20th-century Newfoundland, it remains very much what it always has been--primarily a fishing and farming community.

Most of the respondents in the other Newfoundland communities surveyed (Newfoundland Community A) were Protestants. In Newfoundland, religion is a good indicator of ethnic origin since most small communities were settled by fishermen "whose families were divided between Catholics from Southwest Ireland and Protestants from Southeast England" (McCann, 1988, 87).

As mentioned previously, the respondents from Toronto were immigrants from the Philippines, and the respondents from Oklahoma live in a small rural community that is gradually being transformed into a typical suburban bedroom city.

Past research had tended to use either subjective or objective definitions of ethnicity. In this study, both definitions were utilized. In selecting the four groups of respondents, the assumption was that they objectively lived in different cultures. For example, Canadian society has a cultural heritage that distinguishes it from American culture in many significant ways. Similarly, in her extensive survey of the literature of or about Newfoundland and Newfoundlanders, Drodge asserts that "there exists a popular and widely shared belief in the distinctiveness of Newfoundland and the character...of Newfoundlanders" (1982, 57). Newfoundlanders have distinctive "soul" (Poole, 1978). She further explains that in other parts of Canada the notion of "ethnicity" applies to immigrants, the Native peoples and others belonging to various religious and racial origins (Breton, 1964; Brettell, 1977; Briggs, 1971; Elliott, 1979; Isajiw, 1977; Porter 1965, 1975). Labels such as "Canadian" or "Albertan" are indicative of citizenship or region of birth or residence; they do not point to ethnicity. But "the designation 'Newfoundlander' like the term 'Québécois', is more of an ethnic label. It transcends the internal diversities of origin, dialect, religion, and the like, merging them into a common and distinctive identity. This appears to be so both in the objective and subjective senses, i.e., Newfoundlanders see themselves as unique and separate from the rest of Canada, and Canadians and other non-Newfoundlanders tend to perceive the people of this province as distinct" (Drodge, 1982, 60). Many authors have voiced such sentiments about the province and its people (England, 1924; Guy, 1976; Gwyn, 1968; Horwood, 1966; Moyles, 1975; O'Flaherty, 1979; Perlin, 1959; Smallwood, 1973; Smith, 1952). In the objective sense, the Philippine elderly also have roots in a very distinctive Asian culture.

Finally, ethnicity in this paper is also defined in terms of a subjective, social-psychological orientation. In this sense it refers to individuals expressing their own perceptions of distinctiveness of their culture through self-identification. It was operationalized by asking the respondents two questions: "Do you consider yourself a member of a particular ethnic group? If yes, which ethnic group?"

Major Independent Variables

Several cultural variables in the study were treated as independent variables, such as country of birth, membership in ethnic group, language spoken, bilingualism, religion, how long lived in the area and size of community. Other socio-demographic independent variables included gender, marital status (married, single, divorced, widowed or separated), years of schooling, major occupation in life and satisfaction with current income and assets. Two other independent variables, self-assessed health status and medical care contact, were also included. The literature suggests that these two variables are correlates of age and potential determinants of self-care behaviour. Several different indicators were used to measure self-assessed health status and medical care contact. Health status was measured by three questions: (1) "For your age, would you say, in general, your health is excellent, good, fair or poor?" (2) "About how many days have you spent in a hospital during the last twelve months?" (3) "About how many days during the past twelve months have you been in bed at home all or most of the day?"

In the literature several behavioural and attitudinal components are identified that may influence medical care contact and self-care. Respondents were asked only one question about their utilization of physician services: "Do you have a regular doctor?" (Yes/No). Finally, several dimensions of medical skepticism were identified. Among these two main dimensions were (1) a skeptical attitude about the things that doctors say; (2) a skeptical attitude about the things that doctors do. Both these subscales of medical skepticism were included in the analysis as measures of respondents' attitude towards physicians because in the literature, medical skepticism is seen as a factor that has influence on self-care.

Major Dependent Variables

Two health maintenance beliefs and two self-care practices were investigated. First, to measure health maintenance beliefs, respondents were presented with a list of types of things individuals do to stay healthy (i.e., maintain his/her health) and were asked "How frequently do you do those things?" (Often/Sometimes/Occasionally/Never).

Each respondent was assigned a scale score on the basis of the number of these activities identified that he/she did often for health maintenance. Following are some of examples of the types of things included: eat balanced diet, take vitamins, exercise, avoid stress, get routine medical check-ups, get together with friends, pray, avoid smoking, use car seat belts, get enough sleep, do self-examination and get immunized.

Secondly, "popular" beliefs about health as a measure of health maintenance were investigated. These beliefs are rooted in the cultural context, and therefore, are part of the collective wisdom of individuals living in that culture. That is why they are characterized "popular." As cited in the literature, these "popular" beliefs constitute health systems that are different from the professional health care system. Thus "popular" health belief systems exist alongside the professional health system and provide individuals with wide varieties of alternate knowledge and experience to interpret the causes, management and anticipated outcome of sickness and disease. Thus these beliefs are seen as important factors that may influence the decision to engage in self-care behaviour. Respondents were presented with a list of nine "popular beliefs" about health (such as "eating carrots improves your vision") and were asked to indicate which ones they believed to be correct. Each respondent was assigned a scale score on the basis of the number of these beliefs accepted as correct.

The two self-care beliefs that were considered in this study were self-help responses to symptoms of illness and the use of home remedies. The measurement of response to symptoms of illness (symptomatic response) involved presenting the respondents with a list of eleven conditions and asking in each case whether they had experienced any of these conditions during the past year, and what was their first response. The conditions were a feeling of dizziness, bowel irregularity, constant tiredness, frequent headaches, rash or itch, shortness of breath, difficulty sleeping at night, loss of appetite, stomach upset, indigestion and greater than usual happiness or depression, for a considerable length of time. The response categories were "self treatment" (a person should try to take care of it him/herself) and "expert advice" (a person should see a doctor about it right away). Each respondent was assigned a scale score on the basis of the number of these symptomatic conditions that he/she would handle by self-care.

Finally, we asked the respondents about their familiarity with home remedies. This aspect of self-care behaviour was explored by asking the respondents to respond to the question: "Are you familiar with any home remedies that you believe are effective and would recommend others to use?" (Yes/No). If the response was positive, respondents were given an opportunity to explain each home remedy (in an open-ended format). Scale scores were assigned on the basis of the number of home remedies cited.

Data Analysis

The statistical analysis of data was done at the Institute for Research and Development in Education, Memorial University. The first concern was to compile a socio-demographic profile of the respondents in four communities. Second, differences in responses of the elderly in four communities to dependent variables were investigated. For this purpose a cross-tabulation analysis was carried out. Further, to investigate the significance of variance in the responses of the elderly in the four communities, the data was subjected to ANOVA analysis of variance procedures. Finally, a multivariate analysis of the data using stepwise multiple regression was carried out.

For this latter procedure, the four health beliefs and self-care practices were treated as dependent variables and all others as independent variables. Cultural factors were allowed to "compete" with the other independent factors to assess their predictive ability. This was done to evaluate the relative explanatory power of cultural variables compared to other socio-demographic attributes, health status and medical care contact, in order to account for variance in lay health beliefs and self-care practices. The main intention was to identify the best set of predictors of self-care behaviour.

A Socio-Demographic Profile of the Respondents

No significant differences exist among the four cultural groups in terms of age, sex, marital status and use of community agencies. However, differences were seen with respect to other socio-demographic characteristics. The Philippine elderly tended to have more than 12 years of schooling whereas the elderly in Oklahoma and Newfoundland communities were more likely to have 9 to 12 years of schooling. The Philippine elderly in Toronto tended to be first generation immigrants (95% of Philippine elderly in the sample were born in the Philippines). Immigration selection policies often favour those with more education. The majority of older people in Oklahoma (96%) were born in the United States and 97% of the people in Newfoundland were born in the same province. Significant differences among the four groups also emerged with respect to occupation. Fewer Philippine elderly tended to report being housewives. Among all the groups (except for Newfoundland Community B), higher percentages of Philippine elderly reported having professional occupations. The fact that respondents in Newfoundland Community B were more likely to have different levels of occupation than the respondents from Newfoundland Community A is indicative of the diversity that seems to exist among various communities in the province. Newfoundland culture and communities were not homogeneous. Further, in terms of religion, most elderly from the Philippines were likely to be Roman Catholic. This was also true for the respondents from Newfoundland Community B. In Oklahoma and Newfoundland Community A, higher percentages of respondents were Protestants. Historically, the population in Newfoundland had its roots either in Ireland or in the British Isles. Thus, ethnically and culturally some groups identified themselves as Irish and others as "Anglo" or of British ancestry. Understandably, everybody in Oklahoma and Newfoundland spoke English at home, while most Philippine elderly were likely to be bilingual. Although bilingual, the majority of Philippine respondents, like others, usually spoke English at home. Significant differences also emerged with respect to ethnic identification, participation in social activities, volunteer time spent with community agencies or groups, number of years living within 30 miles of the city of the town in which the respondents were currently living, size of the place the respondents lived before moving to their current place of residence and duration of stay in the current neighborhood or site in the town or city.

Cultural Factors, Health Status and Utilization of Medical Care

Three measures of health status were used: self-reported health at present, days spent in a hospital during the last 12 months and days spent being sick in the bed at home during the past 12 months. In addition to these indicators of health status, the study also included an attitudinal measure of medical skepticism. The majority of the respondents described their present health in very positive terms; most (90.6%) said they were either in "excellent" or in "good" health. In addition many respondents reported they did not spend much time either in hospital or being sick in bed at home during the past 12 months. For the last 12 months the mean number of days spent by the respondents in a hospital was 3.31 and the mean for days being sick in bed at home was 2.50.

However, statistically significant differences were found in the responses of the elderly in four communities to self-rated health status. More respondents from Oklahoma (27%) reported being in "excellent" health as compared to 24% of Philippine elderly and 17% of elderly in Newfoundland Community B (except for 38% in Community A) who reported being in "excellent" health. On the other hand more respondents from Newfoundland Community B (69%) and 40% in Community A said their health was "good" as compared to 33% and 24% respondents in Oklahoma and Toronto. The majority of the Philippine elderly (48%) reported their health was fair; only 25% of the respondents in Oklahoma and 23% in Newfoundland Community A and 8% in Community B said their health was fair. ANOVA results for health status variables by community type are presented in Table 1.

Cultural differences, while not statistically significant, were also found when the focus was shifted to the analysis of the second indicator of health status, the number of days spent in hospital during the last 12 months. More elderly in Oklahoma (84%) and Newfoundland (82%) spent zero days in hospital; only 60% of the Philippine elderly spent zero days in the hospital. It appears that the elderly in this sample were not heavy users of health services, although it is generally "well known that the elderly are disproportionately heavy users of health services" (Wolinsky et. al., 1983, 325).

The relationship between cultural background and health services utilization pattern has also been subjected to considerable research (Wong and Reker, 1985, 33; Rempel and Havens, 1986, 9; Ujimoto, 1987, 117). Research indicates that the non-white ethnic groups under-utilize health care services. In this study, however, more Philippine elderly (40%) spent more days in hospital than either the Oklahoma or Newfoundland elderly. How can these utilization data be reconciled with the hypothesis that the elderly, in general, and non-white elderly in particular, are more skeptical of physicians and are reluctant to use their services? In order to answer this question for the elderly in general, as Segall points out, "requires empirical evidence which clearly distinguishes between physician and patient initiated contact. Mean number of physician visits per year may be more accurately a reflection of the medicalization of aging, than help-seeking behaviour on the part of the elderly. Furthermore, since increasing age is often accompanied by a greater incidence of chronic illness and frequent medical check-ups, these utilization

data may be more valid indicators of medically defined treatment patterns for the chronically ill, than demand for services by
the elderly. Perhaps medical skepticism among older persons is
the outcome of, rather than determinant of, frequent use of
medical services" (1987, 55). The Philippine elderly, as new
immigrants, find themselves in a new societal setting and perhaps in the beginning are more prone to help-seeking behaviour.
But once they experience physician-patient interaction, their
help-seeking behaviour, utilization of medical services and
medical skepticism perhaps can best be explained within the
framework of the medicalization of aging in North America.

Further suggestion is often made in literature "that the elderly may lack confidence in professional health care and have a
negative image of physicians" (Nuttbrock and Kosberg, 1980).
Two main subscales of medical skepticism were developed to
collect responses about the things that doctors say and do. Three
items were included to record responses of the elderly's
skepticism about the things that doctors say: (1) "I have my
doubts about some things doctors say they can do for you"; (2)
"Doctors often tell you there's nothing wrong with you, when
you know there is"; and (3) "I believe in trying out different
doctors to find out which one I think will give me the best care."
Statistically significant difference was found among four cultural groups only in regard to the last two questions. More
Philippine elderly said (81%) they believed in trying out different doctors as compared to 21% in Oklahoma, 29% in Newfoundland Community A and 14% in Newfoundland Community B.

The second subscale of medical skepticism (skepticism about
the things that doctors do) had three items: (1) "If you wait long
enough, you can get over most sickness without going to the
doctor"; (2) "Some home remedies are still better than prescribed drugs for curing sickness"; and (3) "A person under-
stands his/her own state of health better than most doctors."
Some differences (statistically insignificant) were found among
four groups in their responses to these questions. For example,
in the case of the last question, more elderly (67%) in Oklahoma
agreed with the statement. Only 56% of the Philippine elderly
agreed with the statement. In Newfoundland Community A,
31% agreed and in Newfoundland Community B, 46%. On the
whole, medical skepticism was not prevalent among the elderly
in this sample in any major way and statistically significant
cultural differences were found only in some areas. ANOVA
results for medical skepticism variables by community type are
presented in Table 2.

Table 1
ANOVA Results for health status variables by community types

Dependent Variables	Sources	SS	DF	Mean Square	F	Sig. P
Self-assessed health status	1	.575	3	.191	2.654	.051*
	2	9.535	132	.0722		
Days of Hospitalization	1	801.180	3	267.060	2.135	.098
	2	16632.323	133	125.055		
Days sick in bed	1	92.010	3	30.670	.350	.788
	2	11379.489	130	87.534		

Note: * $p \leq .05$, 1 = between groups; 2 = within groups; SS = sum of squares; DF = degrees of freedom.

Table 2
ANOVA results for medical skepticism variables by community type

Dependent Variables	Source	SS	DF	Mean Square	F	Sig. P
Whenever I get sick, it is because of something I have done or not done.	1	3.492	3	1.164	.925	.430
	2	156.007	124	1.258		
When I fell ill, I know it is because I have not been getting the proper exercise or eating right.	1	12.189	3	4.063	3.508	.017**
	2	145.933	126	1.158		
When I think I am getting sick, I find it difficult to talk to others about it.	1	7.836	3	2.612	1.869	.138
	2	176.040	126	1.397		

Table 2 continued

Dependent Variables	Source	SS	DF	Mean Square	F	Sig. P
The trouble with being ill is that you have to depend on other people.	1	35.701	3	11.900	14.463	.0000***
	2	104.497	127	.822		
I have my doubts about some things doctors say they can do for you.	1	3.254	3	1.084	.764	.515
	2	178.776	126	1.418		
I believe in trying out doctors to find out which one I think will give me the best care.	1	18.110	3	6.036	3.579	.015**
	2	210.789	125	1.686		
If you wait long enough, you can get over most sicknesses without going to the doctor.	1	7.887	3	2.629	1.842	.142
	2	178.360	125	1.426		
Some home remedies are still better than prescribed drugs for curing sickness.	1	3.430	3	1.143	.914	.436
	2	158.889	127	1.251		
A person understands his/her own state of health better than most doctors.	1	3.242	3	1.080	.839	.474
	2	163.460	127	1.287		
Doctors often tell you there's nothing wrong with you, when you know there is.	1	14.686	3	4.895	3.205	.025**
	2	193.939	127	1.527		

Note: *p≤.01; ***p≤.001; 1 = between groups; 2 = within groups; SS = sum of squares; DF = degrees of freedom.

Cultural Factors, Health Beliefs and Self-Care Practices

The analysis in this section is presented in steps. First, the ANOVA results for health maintenance and popular health beliefs are presented. The purpose of doing this is to highlight variance in elderly's health beliefs and self-care practices in four cultural settings. Following this, a correlational and multiple regression analysis was performed to answer the questions: How effectively can socio-demographic, sociomedical and cultural factors predict lay health beliefs and self-care behaviour? What is the relative explanatory power of cultural factors for variance in health beliefs and self-care practices? The results of the ANOVA are discussed first.

The respondents were asked how frequently they did (or do) the following things to stay healthy or to maintain their health: eat a balanced diet, take vitamins, exercise, avoid smoking, use car seat belts, avoid stress, get enough sleep, get routine medical check-ups, do self-examination, get immunized, get together with close friends, pray, or do some other things. Analysis of the data reveal significant differences among the groups in seven areas: take vitamins, avoid smoking, get enough sleep, do self-examination, get immunized, get together with close friends and get routine medical check-up. For example, a high percentage of Newfoundlanders - 69% in Community A and 62% in Community B - never take vitamins to maintain their health as compared to 17% of the elderly in Toronto and 35% in Oklahoma. ANOVA results for health maintenance variables by community type are presented in Table 3.

Now we shift our focus to the relationship between cultural factors and the "popular" health beliefs investigated in this study. Significant differences seem to exist among the four groups in their responses to the six out of nine "popular" health beliefs investigated in this study. The differences related to their beliefs about wet feet, eating carrots, eating garlic, bowel movements, eating licorice, and feeding a cold. For example, more elderly in Newfoundland Community B (65%) believed that wet feet would cause a cold as compared to only 55% in Toronto, 40% in Newfoundland Community A and 14% in Oklahoma. More Philippine elderly in Toronto (81%) as compared to 47% in Newfoundland Community A, 46% in Newfoundland Community B and only 30% in Oklahoma believed that eating carrots would improve their vision. In Newfoundland Community B, 38% did not know whether this was true or not. In

Table 3
ANOVA results for health maintenance variables by community type

Dependent Variables	Source	SS	DF	Mean Square	F	Sig. P
Eat a balanced diet.	1	1.477	3	.492	1.725	.165
	2	36.823	129	.2855		
Take vitamins.	1	25.356	3	8.452	5.977	.0008***
	2	180.977	128	1.413		
Exercise.	1	12.735	3	4.245	3.543	.016**
	2	153.348	128	1.198		
Avoid smoking.	1	28.398	3	9.466	5.017	.002***
	2	235.988	125	1.887		
Use care seat belts.	1	8.020	3	2.673	2.104	.102
	2	168.986	133	1.270		
Avoid stress.	1	5.740	3	1.913	2.029	.113
	2	115.976	123	.942		
Get enough sleep.	1	12.629	3	4.209	9.272	.001***
	2	59.929	132	.454		
Get routine medical check-up.	1	11.360	3	3.786	3.786	.012**
	2	133.004	133	1.000		
Do self examination.	1	30.744	3	10.248	10.084	.001***
	2	119.919	118	1.016		

Table 3 continued

Dependent Variables	Source	SS	DF	Mean Square	F	Sig. P
Get immunized.	1	29.146	3	9.715	9.482	.001***
	2	132.162	129	1.024		
Get together with close friends.	1	5.878	3	1.959	2.575	.056*
	2	101.186	133	.760		
Pray.	1	.215	3	.071	.250	.861
	2	38.222	133	.287		

Note: *p≤.05; **p≤.01; *** p≤.001; 1 = between groups; 2 = within groups; SS = sum of squares; DF = degrees of freedom.

Oklahoma, 6% said it was not true. Again, 76% of the Philippine elderly in Toronto believed that eating garlic was good for their health as compared to 42% in Oklahoma and 30% in Newfoundland Community A. In Newfoundland Community B, 83% did not know whether this was true or not. Except in the case of the elderly in Oklahoma (26%), a large number of elderly believed that bowels should move every day in order to be healthy (81% in Toronto, 70% in Newfoundland Community B and 66% in Newfoundland Community A. What is good for your digestive system? How can you beat your fever? Except in Newfoundland Community B, a relatively high percentage of the elderly believed eating licorice was not good for digestive problems (65% in Oklahoma, 55% in Toronto, 50% in Newfoundland Community A and only 14% in Newfoundland Community B said no). The majority of elderly in Newfoundland Community B (54%) said they did not know whether eating licorice was good or not for digestive problems. Some elderly did believe in this kind of cure (35% in Toronto, 32% in Newfoundland Community B, 13% in Oklahoma and 10% in Newfoundland Community A). And finally, most elderly in each community, except in Toronto, believed feeding a cold would get rid of a fever (59% in Oklahoma, 60% in Newfoundland Community A, 43% in Newfoundland Community B and only 20% in Toronto). It may be interesting to note the responses of the Philippine elderly in this study in regard to eating garlic and carrots. Most of these elderly believed that eating them was good for maintaining their health. That these elderly would have such a belief is understandable because, like most people in Asia, the Philippine elderly are "vegetarian," that is, they are used to eating varieties of vegetables with their meals. In contrast, eating a sufficient quantity of varieties of vegetables with daily meals is rare in Newfoundland and among many groups in North America. For example, very few people in North America eat garlic or ginger daily.

Congruent with the modernization theory, North Americans are seen as modern and the Philippine elderly as traditional, and traditional people are seen as having popular beliefs. We may conclude the analysis of the relationship between cultural factors and popular beliefs by stating that data in this study show that the elderly do subscribe to "popular" beliefs about health and that significant differences exist in several areas in the responses of the elderly living in different cultural settings. Segall reported that significant age differences exist in the popular health beliefs, implying that those 60 and over more often subscribed to these beliefs, and that these beliefs "are most prevalent among the elderly with lower levels of formal education" (1987, 56-57). In this study most respondents were over 60 years of age and significant differences were found in the educational levels of the respondents, but no statistically significant correlation was found between education and "popular" beliefs. ANOVA results for popular health beliefs variables by community type are presented in Table 4.

No significant differences were found in the symptomatic responses (self-care) of the elderly in four communities. Few respondents would define the conditions presented as unimportant and simply ignore them. The majority of respondents in Oklahoma, Toronto and Newfoundland would see a doctor without delay if they experienced "dizziness" (82%), "bowel irregularity" (73%), "constant tiredness" (92%), "frequent headaches" (70%), and "rash or itch" (71%). ANOVA results for self-treatment responses to symptoms of illness by community type are presented in Table 5.

Finally, significant variation was found in the use of home remedies by the elderly in four communities. For example, 65% of the Philippine elderly and 61% of the elderly in Newfoundland Community B knew home remedies. In contrast, only 9% of the elderly in Oklahoma and 41% of the elderly in Newfoundland Community A knew home remedies.

On the whole, in this study 61% of the elderly indicated that they were not familiar with any home remedy, while 39% said they were. It is also interesting to note that most respondents in Oklahoma (98%) and Newfoundland Community A (90%) were Protestant and most respondents in Toronto (62%) and Newfoundland Community B (97%) were Roman Catholic. Similarly, most participants in this study equated their ethnic identity with their nationalities; in Oklahoma 100% said they were American; in Toronto, 71% said they were "Filipinos," while 29% identified themselves as Asian or Oceanic; in Newfoundland Community A, 88% said they were Canadians, while 68% in Newfoundland Community B identified themselves as "Newfoundlanders," and only 30% as Canadian and 3% as British. ANOVA results for home remedies by community are presented in Table 6.

Table 4
ANOVA results for poplar health belief variables by community type

Dependent Variables	Source	SS	DF	Mean Square	F	Sig. P
Gargling with aspirin relieves a sore throat.	1	1.621	3	.540	2.341	.077
	2	25.396	110	.230		
If your feet get wet, you will get a cold.	1	5.111	3	1.703	8.058	.001***
	2	25.372	120	.211		
Eating garlic is good for your heart.	1	3.284	3	1.094	4.939	.003***
	2	18.393	83	.221		
Eating carrots improves your vision.	1	4.432	3	1.477	6.841	.003***
	2	23.752	110	.215		
Bowels should move everyday without fail.	1	5.559	3	1.853	8.922	.0000***
	2	26.171	126	.207		
Sleeping with the window open will cause headcolds.	1	.094	3	.031	.154	.926
	2	25.409	125	.203		
Eating licorice is good for digestive problems.	1	3.883	3	1.294	7.188	.0002***
	2	15.307	85	.180		
Feed a cold, and starve a fever.	1	2.737	3	.912	4.247	.007***
	2	21.913	102	.214		
You should put butter on a burn.	1	.776	3	.258	1.415	.241
	2	20.465	112	.182		

Note: *p≤.001; 1 = between groups; 2 = within groups; SS = sum of squares; DF = degrees of freedom.

Table 5: ANOVA results for self-treatment responses to symptoms of illness by community type

Dependent Variables	Source	SS	DF	Mean Square	F	Sig. P
Feeling of dizziness	1	.583	3	.194	.777	.530
	2	2.750	11	.250		
Bowel irregularity	1	.696	3	.232	2.104	.137
	2	1.875	17	.110		
Constant tiredness	1	.250	3	.083	.470	.711
	2	1.416	8	.177		
Frequent headaches	1	.250	2	.125	1.687	.238
	2	.666	9	.074		
Rash or itch	1	.300	3	.1000	.2000	.888
	2	.500	1	.5000		
Shortness of breath	1	.348	3	.116	1.064	.397
	2	1.416	13	.109		
Difficulty sleeping at night	1	.508	3	.169	.695	.572
	2	2.928	12	.244		

Note: 1 = between groups; 2 = within groups; SS = sum of squares; DF = degrees of freedom.

Table 6: ANOVA results for home remedies by community type

Dependent Variables	Source	SS	DF	Mean Square	F	Sig. P
Number of home remedies recommended.	1	7.054	3	2.351	12.434	.0000***
	2	23.260	123	.189		

Note: ***p ≤ .001; 1 = between groups; 2 = within groups; SS = sum of squares; DF = degrees of freedom.

Correlational coefficients were calculated for cultural factors and health maintenance and popular health beliefs. Zero-order correlation coefficients for the relationship between socio-demographic attributes, health status, medical care contact, health beliefs and self-care practices are shown in Table 7. Looking at these results it is clear that several cultural factors (country of birth, membership in ethnic group, identification with specific ethnic group, number of years lived in the area, size of community and bilingualism, i.e., language spoken other than English and religion) were found to be correlates of health beliefs and self-care practices.

Multiple Regression

The main objectives of data analysis at this stage were (1) to identify the set of factors that would best predict lay health beliefs and self-treatment practices (self-care practices); (2) to find out how much of the variance is explained by the selected socio-demographic and socio-medical factors; and (3) to determine the relative explanatory value of cultural factors. The result of the regression analysis are summarized in Table 8. In examining the data in Table 8, it is important to note that independent variables which did not meet the minimum significance level for entry into the model were excluded automatically following the stepwise multiple regression procedure.

It is clear from Table 8 that some of the independent cultural factors (size of the community, bilingualism, English spoken and religion did meet the minimum level of statistical significance and thus appeared as good predictors in three of the four models by the stepwise multiple regression procedure (health maintenance beliefs, "popular health beliefs") and the use of home remedies. For self-help responses to symptoms of illness (symptomatic responses), none of the cultural factors met the minimum level of significance for entry into the model. In other words, even when other factors were controlled, none of the cultural factors were found to be significantly related to self-help responses to symptoms of illness.

Of the other **socio-demographic attributes**, only occupation is included among the best predictor in one model ("popular health beliefs"). Age, sex, marital status, education and income were not among the best predictors for any of the four models (for the four lay health beliefs and self-care practices investigated in this study).

Table 7
ZERO-order correlation coefficients for the relationship between sociodemographic attributes, health status, medical care contact, health beliefs and self-care practices

	Health Maintenance Belief	Popular Health	Symptomatic Responses	Home Remedies
Country born	.059	.006	.180	.196**
Member of ethnic group	.206**	.064	.180	.018
What ethnic group	.137	-.023	.211	-.297***
How long lived in the area	.173*	.135	-.092	-.011
Size of community	.321**	.052	-.420*	-.150
English language spoken	.022	.187**	-.098	-.124
What other languages spoken	.193	.911***	1.00***	-.271
Religion	.121	.140*	.143	-.290***
Christian	-.328*	.061	.103	-.108
Male/widowed	.641*	-.057	-.209	-.065
Occupation	-.036	.221***	-.043	.046
Skepticism about what doctors say	-.041	.164*	-.335**	-.060
Skepticism about what doctors do	-.221*	.129	-.317*	-.175*
Present status of health	-.179*	-.041	.452***	.143*
Number of days spent in hospital	-.244*	.207***	.502***	-.082
Number of days spent in bed	-.207*	.160*	.761***	-.157*
Income	-.139	.067	.041	-.163*
Education	.161	-.040	.085	-.115
Age	-.081	.033	.054	-.039

Note: *p≤.05; **p≤.01; ***p≤.001

Table 8
Stepwise multiple regression analysis of the relationship between sociodemographic attributes, health status, medical care contact and health beliefs and self-care practices

Health Beliefs and Practices	Independent Variables in Model	Standardized Regression Coefficients (Beta)
Health Maintenance	Skepticism about what doctors do	-.192
	Number of days spent in hospital	-.224
	Size of the community	.232
	Self-assessed health status	-.173
	$R^2 = .153$, Adjusted $R^2 = .127$, F = 6.013, P .0002	
Popular Health Beliefs	What other language spoken (Bilingual)	.235
	Number of days spent in hospital	.203
	English spoken	.209
	Occupation	.200
	$R^2 = .175$, Adjusted $R^2 = .150$, F = 7.080, P .0000	
Symptomatic Responses	Number of days spent in hospital	.415
	Self-assessed health status	.287
	Skepticism about what doctors say	-.176
	$R^2 = .284$, Adjusted $R^2 = .268$, F = 17.740, P .0000	
Home Remedies	Skepticism about what doctors do	-.175
	Religion	-.286
	$R^2 = .110$, Adjusted $R^2 = .097$, F = 8.409, P .0004	

Of the **socio-medical indicators**, number of days spent in hospital appears to be the best predictor of the three of the four health beliefs and practices investigated (health maintenance beliefs, "popular health beliefs" and self-help responses to symptoms of illness).

Self-assessed health over the past 12 months as an indicator of health status appears to be a good predictor of two models (self-help responses to symptoms of illness and health maintenance beliefs).

On the whole, none of the socio-medical factors (self-assessed health status, number of days spent in hospital and number of days spent in bed at home) appear to be connected to use of home remedies as a self-care practice. In contrast, the attitudinal dimension explored (medical skepticism) proved to be an important predictor. In particular, skepticism about the things that doctors do was one of the best predictors of not only for the use of home remedies but also for the health maintenance beliefs. Skepticism about the things that doctor say was one the best predictors for symptomatic responses.

Turning to the explanatory power of these indicators, cultural factors alone explained little of the variance in health beliefs and practices. When cultural factors were combined with all other independent variables (socio-demographic indicators, health status and attitudes toward doctors), a moderate proportion of the variance was explained. This varied from a low of 9% for the use of home remedies (adjusted R^2), 12% for the health maintenance beliefs, to a high of 15% for the popular health beliefs. In case of self-help responses to symptoms of illness, cultural attributes didn't meet the regression criteria and were thus excluded from the model. In contrast, health status indicators and medical skepticism explained 26% of the variance for the symptomatic responses. Thus more explanations are needed about the nature of lay health beliefs and self-care behavior to fully understand these factors.

CONCLUSION

This study is based on data obtained from four culturally diverse communities: (1) a small, transitional city in the southwestern United States; (2) a Philippine community in Toronto; (3) Newfoundland Community A, small communities largely populated by descendants of Protestant immigrants from south-west Ireland and Southeast England; and (4) Newfoundland Community B, a fishing village populated mostly by Irish Roman Catholic immigrants and their descendants.

It explores the health care beliefs and practices among the elderly living in these four communities. Statistical analysis is used to assess the hypothesized relationships between cultural/ethnic factors and lay health care beliefs and practices, and to evaluate the explanatory power of cultural/ethnic factors when compared to other socio-demographic factors, self-reported health status and medical care contacts. The results presented in this study clearly suggest that lay health care beliefs and behaviors do exist and that cultural/ethnic factors do have some explanatory power. The findings also suggest that the relationship between cultural factors and health maintenance and health self-care behavior is complex. More cross-cultural studies need to be carried out in this area using similar instruments and methodologies. Also variations in health care responses among different "Anglo" groups living in various community settings need to be studied. More studies of lay populations of different ethnic and cultural backgrounds are needed to provide useful information and insight into self-care behaviors. It should be recognized that lay persons are not only consumers of professional care, but are actively involved in the process of providing primary health care. It is also clear that self-care behaviours coexist with professional health care, and that they are not mutually exclusive. Therefore, special attention should be paid to this insight in conceptualizing health care in multicultural Canadian society to avoid cultural misunderstandings and to improve the well-being of different cultural groups in Canadian society.

REFERENCES

Bauer, F. (1969). *Potions, remedies and old wives tales.* New York: Doubleday & Co.

Blumhagen, D. (1980). Hyper-tension: A folk illness with a medical name. *Culture, Medicine and Psychiatry, 1,* 197-227.

Bolaria, B.S. (1988). The politics and ideology of self-care and lifestyles. In B.S. Bolaria and H.D. Dickinson (Eds.). *Sociology of health care in Canada* (537-49). Toronto: Harcourt Brace Javanovich.

Breton, R. (1964). Institutional completeness of ethnic communities and the personal relations of immigrants. *American Journal of Sociology, 70,* 193-205.

Brettell, C.B. (1977). Ethnicity and entrepreneurs: Portuguese immigrants in a Canadian city. In G. Hicks and P. Leis, (Eds.), *Ethnic encounters* (169-80). Belmont, CA: Wadsworth Publishing.

Briggs, J. (1971). Strategies of perception in the management of ethnic identity. In R. Paine (Ed.), *Patrons and brokers in the East Arctic* (55-73). St. John's: Memorial University of Newfoundland, Institute of Social and Economic Research.

Buehler, S.K. (1987). *The active health report: The health promotion survey in Newfoundland.* Department of Health, Government of Newfoundland and Labrador.

Cartwright, A., & Martin, F.M. (1958). Some popular beliefs concerning the causes of cancer. *British Medical Journal, 2,* 592-94.

Chappell, N. (1987). Canadian income and health care policy: Implications for the elderly. In V.W. Marshall (Ed.), *Aging in Canada* (489-504). Toronto: Fitzhenry and Whiteside, Ltd.

Chappell, N.L., & Penning, M.J. (1984). Informal social supports: Examining ethnic variation. Paper presented at the annual meeting of the Gerontological Society of America, San Antonio, Texas.

Chappell, N., Strain, L.A., & Blandford, A.A. (1986). *Aging and health care.* Toronto: Rinehart and Winston.

Connidis, I. (1987). Life in older age: The view from the top. In V.W. Marshall (Ed.), *Aging in Canada* (451-72). Toronto: Fitzhenry and Whiteside, Ltd.

D'Arcy, C. (1987). Aging and mental health. In V.W. Marshall (Ed.), *Aging in Canada* (424-50). Toronto: Fitzhenry and Whiteside, Ltd.

Davidson, K.R. (1970). Conceptions of illness and health practices in a Nova Scotia community. *Canadian Journal of Public Health, 61,* 232-42.

Doyal, Lesley, and Pennell, R. (1979). *The political economy of health.* London: Pluto Press.

Drodge, J.A. (1982). *A heritage portrayed: Nationalist theatre in Newfoundland 1972-82.* Unpublished master's thesis, Department of Anthropology, Memorial University of Newfoundland, St. John's, Nfld.

Elliott, J.L. (Ed.) (1979). *Two nations, many cultures: Ethnic groups in Canada.* Scarborough, Ontario: Prentice-Hall Canada.

England, G.A. (1924). *The greatest hunt in the world.* Montreal: Tundra Books.

Epp, J. (1986). Achieving health for all: A framework for health promotion. *Canadian Journal of Public Health, 77* (6), 394-407.

Foster, G. (1976). Disease aetiologies in non-Western medical systems. *American Anthropologist, 78,* 773-82.

Freidson, E. (1970). *Profession of medicine.* New York: Dodd, Mead & Col.

Gould, H.A. (1975). The implications of technological change for folk and scientific medicine. *American Anthropologist, 59,* 507-16.

Guy, R. (1976). *That far greater bay.* Portugal Cove, Newfoundland: Breakwater Books.

Gwyn, R. (1968). *Smallwood: The unlikely revolutionary.* Toronto: McClelland and Stewart.

Hess, P. (1986). Chinese and Hispanic elders and OTC drugs. *Geriatric Nursing, American Journal of Care for the Aging, 7,* 314-18.

Horwood, H. (1966). *Tomorrow will be Sunday.* Garden City, NY: Doubleday.

Illich, I. (1976). *Limits to medicine: Medical neurosis, the expropriation of health.* New York: Pantheon.

Isajiw, W.W. (1977). *Identities: The impact of ethnicity on Canadian society.* Toronto: Peter Martin Associates.

King, S. (1962). *Perceptions of illness and medical practice.* New York: Russell Sage Foundation.

Kleiman, A. (1978). Concepts and a model for the comparison of medical system as cultural system. In C. Leslie (Ed.) *Science and Medicine,* Vol. 12, No. 1B (85-92). New York: Pergamon Press.

Koos, E.L. (1967). *The health of Regionville.* New York: Hafner Publishing.

Lalonde, M. (1974). *A new perspective on the health of Canadians.* Ottawa: Information Canada.

Landy, D. (1974). Role adaptation: Traditional cures under the impact of Western medicine. *American Ethnologist, 1,* 102-103.

Mabry, J. (1964). Lay conceptions of etiology. *Journal of Chronic Diseases, 17,* 371-86.

Marshall, V.W. (Ed.) (1987). *Aging in Canada.* Toronto: Fitzhenry and Whiteside Ltd.

McCann, P. (1988). Culture, state formation and the invention of tradition: Newfoundland 1832-1855. *Journal of Canadian Studies, 23,* 86-103.

Moyles, R.G. (1975). *Complaints is many and various but the odd devil likes it: Nineteenth century view of Newfoundland.* Toronto: Peter Martin Associates.

Navarro, V. (1986). *Crisis, health, and Medicine.* New York Tavistock Publications.

New, P. (1977). Traditional and modern health care: An appraisal of complementarity. *International Social Science Journal, 29,* 483-95.

O'Flaherty, P. (1979). *The rock observed: Studies in the literature of Newfoundland.* Toronto: University of Toronto Press.

Perlin, A.B. (1959). *The story of Newfoundland.* St. John's: Creative Printers and Publishers.

Pfifferling, J.H. (1975). Some issues in the consideration of non-Western and Western folk practices as epidemiologic data. *Social Science and Medicine, 9,* 655-58.

Poole, C.F. (1978). The soul of a Newfoundlander. *The Newfoundland Quarterly, 9,* 19-24.

Porter, J. (1965). *The vertical mosaic.* Toronto: University of Toronto Press.

— —. (1975). Ethnic pluralism in Canadian perspective. In N. Glazer and D.P. Moynihand (Eds.), *Ethnicity: Theory and experience* (267-304). Cambridge, Massachusetts: Harvard University Press.

Press, I. (1978). Urban folk medicine: A functional overview. *American Anthropologist, 80,* 71-84.

— —. (1980). Problems in the definition and classification of medical systems. *Social Science and Medicine, 14B,* 45-57.

Rempel, J.D., & Havens, B. (1986). Aged health experiences as interpreted through culture. Paper presented at the Canadian Sociology and Anthropology Association Annual Meeting, Winnipeg, Man.

Rosengren, W.R. (1980). *Sociology of medicine.* New York: Harper and Row.

Rosenthal, C. (1986). Family support in later life: Does ethnicity make a difference? *Gerontology, 26*(1), 19-24.

Ryan, W. (1971). *Blaming the victim.* New York: Vintage Books.

Saunders, L., & G. Hewes (1953). Folk medicine and medical practice. *Journal of Medical Education, 28,* 43-46.

Schwenger, C.W. (1987). Formal health care for the elderly in Canada. In V.W. Marshall (ed.), *Aging in Canada* (505-19). Toronto: Fitzhenry and Whiteside Ltd.

Segall, A. (1987). Age differences in lay conceptions of health and self-care responses to illness. *Canadian Journal on Aging, 6* (1), 47-65.

Shapiro, E., & Roos, N.P. (1987). Predictors, patterns and consequences of nursing-home use in one Canadian province. In V.W. Marshall (Ed.), *Aging in Canada* (520-37). Toronto: Fitzhenry and Whiteside Ltd.

Simmons-Tropea, D., & Osborn, R. (1987). Diseases, survival and death: The health status of Canada's elderly. In V.W. Marshall (Ed.), *Aging in Canada.* (395-423).Toronto: Fitzhenry and Whiteside Ltd.

Smallwood, J.R. (1973). *I chose Canada.* Toronto: MacMillan of Canada.

Smith, J.H. (1952). *Newfoundland holiday.* Toronto: Ryerson Press.

Snow, L. (1974). Folk medical beliefs and their implications for cure of patients. *Annals of Internal Medicine, 81,* 82-96.

Suchman, E.A. (1964). Sociomedical variations among ethnic groups. *American Journal of Sociology, 70,* 319-331.

Ujimoto, K.V. (1987). The ethnic dimension of aging in Canada. In V.W. Marshall (Ed.), *Aging in Canada* (111-37). Toronto: Fitzhenry and Whiteside Ltd.

—— . (1988). Aging, ethnicity, and health. In Bolaria, B.S., & Dickinson, H.D. (Eds.), *Sociology of health care in Canada,* (220-43). Toronto: Harcourt Brace Jovanovich, Canada.

Waitzkin, H. (1983). *The second sickness.* New York: Free Press.

Watts, D. (1966). Factors related to the acceptance of modern medicine. *American Journal of Public Health, 56,* 1205-12.

Wolinsky, F.D., Coe, R.M., Miller, D.K., Prenergast, J.M., Creel, M.J., & Chávez, M.N. (1983). Health services utilization among the non-institutionalized elderly, *Journal of Health and Social Behavior, 24,* 325-337.

Wong, P.T.P., & Reker, G.T. (1985). Stress, coping, and well-being in Anglo and Chinese elderly. *Canadian Journal on Aging, 4,* 29-37.

- 14 -

Cultural Factors Affecting Self-Assessment of Health Satisfaction of Asian Canadian Elderly

K. Victor Ujimoto
Harry K. Nishio
Paul T.P. Wong
Lawrence Lam

There is an increasing awareness of the multicultural nature of our aging population. Recent publications by Tseng and Wu (1985), England (1986), Rosenthal (1986), Chappel et al. (1986), Driedger and Chappell (1987), Disman (1987), and Ujimoto (1987a, 1987b, 1988) have all noted the salience of ethnicity in aging and health studies. With reference to aging and health, however, very few studies have examined the cross-cultural variations in self-reported well-being concerning health. Furthermore, the meaning of health satisfaction from different cultural perspectives is yet to be explored in Canada. As a small step towards addressing this issue, we have been engaged in a study of aged Chinese, Japanese, and Korean Canadians for the past several years. Although our research had several related objectives, only those aspects related to cultural variations and the self-assessment of health satisfaction will be discussed here.

STUDY OF ASIAN CANADIAN ELDERLY

Characteristics of the Asian Canadian Elderly

The Asian Canadian elderly selected for our study consisted of Chinese, Japanese and Korean Canadians sixty-five years of age or older who resided mostly in urban areas. Our respondents had several distinguishing characteristics that must be noted prior to any comparative analyses of the data on self-assessed well-being concerning health. First, the Japanese Canadian elderly in our sample had been in Canada longer than the other two groups. Of those who had immigrated to Canada, 93.8 percent had migrated prior to World War II, as compared with only 11 percent of the Chinese elderly. In our sample, all of the Korean respondents had arrived in Canada after the Korean War. In contrast, only 6.2 percent of the Japanese Canadian elderly and a very high proportion of the Chinese, 88.1 percent, had come to Canada during the postwar period. This means that there were individual differences in terms of level of education, occupation and expectations which will impact on their adjustment to Canadian society and their current appraisal of health satisfaction.

A second factor to note concerning our Asian Canadian sample is that the longer the duration of residence in Canada, the older the second generation. Therefore, while 62.7 percent of the Japanese elderly were of the first generation, 94.3 percent of the Chinese and 100 percent of the Korean elderly were of the first generation. In contrast, 29.9 percent of the Japanese elderly and 5.7 percent of the Chinese elderly were Canadian-born. For the Japanese, there is another group of elderly known as the *kika-nisei*. The *kika-nisei* refers to those who were born in Canada, but who were exiled to Japan during or after World War II. They constituted 7.5 percent of our sample.

A final factor to keep in mind as we examine our data on aged Asian Canadians is their prior socialization. Depending on whether the respondents were socialized in Canada or elsewhere during their most formative years, there may be differences in their outlook on life in general, and on health care in particular. The retention of certain cultural values may facilitate or hinder day-to-day social interaction or communications.

Methodology

In order to establish the general size and socio-demographic characteristics of our subjects, we utilized the 1981 Census to obtain the necessary information on sex, marital status, age and general immigration statistics. This was done in order to compare our overall community data to some established data base to ascertain the general representativeness of our sample. We obtained the names of elderly Chinese, Japanese and Korean Canadians through various community services. The Asian communities had maintained good records of their members. Although there were duplicates in some membership lists, a simple computer program successfully deleted these and we were able to establish a fairly accurate universe from which to make a random selection of respondents.

Our survey instruments consisted of a questionnaire to obtain the standard information on education, age, marital status, occupational changes and other socio-demographic factors; the Michalos Life Satisfaction Instrument (MLSI), and Time-Budget forms to record daily activities for a whole week. The MLSI provided life satisfaction data in terms of several dimensions such as health, financial security, family relations, housing, residential area, recreational activity, religion, self-esteem, transportation and government services. The respondents were asked to indicate how they considered their daily life "as it is now" by checking one of the categories marked "terrible," "very dissatisfying," "dissatisfying," "mixed," "satisfying," "very satisfying," "delightful" or "no opinion." The respondents were requested to fill in the MLSI at their leisure after the initial questionnaire interview had taken place. Similarly, the respondents were provided with time-budget forms to record their daily activities in sequential order commencing with activity at midnight. Respondents were asked to fill in their forms at frequent intervals in order to obtain an accurate record of their activities, with whom these activities took place, and the location of the activities. Time-budget methodology is described elsewhere by Ujimoto (1987b, 1990).

Data and Discussion

The self-reported data on health satisfaction of our elderly Asian Canadians are shown in Table 1 below. Generally, a high proportion of respondents were satisfied with their health. The Chinese respondents appeared to be the most satisfied, followed by the Japanese, but the Japanese elderly tended to have the highest mixed feelings about their health compared to the Chinese and Korean elderly. Of those respondents who were dissatisfied with their present health status, the Koreans were the most dissatisfied.

Table 1
Health satisfaction of aged Asian Canadians by ethnic group (n=774)

Health Satisfaction	Chinese (%)	Japanese (%)	Korean (%)
Dissatisfied	15.7	10.2	21.9
Mixed	8.1	20.1	10.1
Satisfied	76.2	69.7	68.0
	100.0	100.0	100.0
	(223)	(373)	(178)

The relatively high percentage of Korean elderly who were dissatisfied with their own self-assessment of health appears to be in contrast to earlier studies, which indicated that Koreans were well adjusted. In a study by Kim and Berry (1986) that assessed the mental health of Korean immigrants who resided in Toronto, they found that the Koreans scored low on the Cawte Stress Scale and also on the Mann Marginality Scale when compared to other groups undergoing acculturation in Canada. Kim (1987) argues that these findings are consistent with several other studies. He notes that several factors may account for the successful adaptation of Korean immigrants. First, Kim states that since the Koreans were voluntary immigrants, their mental health status would be better than for others who were involuntary, such as refugees. Second, Kim notes that the Koreans have developed better coping skills to deal with stressful life events. A third factor is that the Canadian government selection criteria are such that only those who are highly educated or who have occupational skills are chosen to immigrate.

Finally, both the relatively high degree of established Korean community institutions and the policy of multiculturalism encourage Korean immigrants in Canada to retain their cultural identity. How then can we account for the relatively high degree of dissatisfaction reported by the Korean elderly?

In terms of possible contradiction between our data and the previously reported findings, caution must be exercised in interpreting and comparing data. By utilizing the standard stress and marginality instruments, it is conceivable that fairly consistent results can be obtained. However, a much different picture emerges if we attempt to seek health information from the Korean health professionals themselves. Kim's (1987) intensive interviews with medical and social support staff revealed that the Koreans tended to internalize their feelings, thus making it difficult for health care personnel to assess the real problem.

Kim (1987) reports that the Koreans do not want to admit that they are sick, or to show any signs of weakness; they tend to somatize their illnesses because of the stigma attached to psychological illnesses. Korean doctors have reported to Kim that many of the Korean illnesses are psychological and stem from loneliness, depression and anxiety. These, in turn, further aggravate the existing somatic problems. These illness characteristics and behaviour are not limited to the Korean elderly, but are very often manifested by other Asian Canadian elderly, particularly the first generation. Indeed, Liu (1986) notes that "somatization is culturally sanctioned in Chinese society, it is an adaptive coping response that allows the person to escape stigmatization." Our data in Table 2 below indicate that the highest degree of self-reported health dissatisfaction is by the first generation and the most satisfied are the second generation and *kika-nisei*.

Table 2
Health satisfaction by generation (n=774)

Health Satisfaction	First Generation (%)	Second Generation (%)	Kika- Nisei (%)
Dissatisfied	16.3	8.0	3.6
Mixed	13.8	16.8	14.3
Satisfied	69.9	75.2	82.1
	100.0	100.0	100.0
	(621)	(125)	(28)

Further insight regarding the relatively high percentage of Korean elderly reporting dissatisfaction with their health can be obtained from our time-budget data. Koreans as a group are extremely devoted to hard and long hours of work. More time devoted to work means less time for family and leisure activities, and eventually, this has an impact on a person's health. Kim (1987) reports that about half of the Korean households in Toronto operate a small business; many of them are open from 14 to 16 hours a day. A few are open 24 hours a day.

Gender differences in self-reported health satisfaction are shown in Table 3 below. It will be noted that both Chinese and Korean elderly women reported a higher degree of dissatisfaction with their health compared to the Japanese elderly women. While both Japanese men and women expressed similar degrees of mixed feelings, both Chinese and Korean elderly men reported higher degrees of health satisfaction. The dissatisfaction expressed by the elderly Korean and Chinese women may stem from the fact that both Chinese and Korean women immigrated to Canada as "captive immigrants," a term used by Kim (1987) to describe Korean parents or grandparents who came to Canada because of their sense of responsibility toward their family. In Korean households that operate a small business or have dual-income earners, the baby-sitting role is most often provided by the parents or grandparents. This appears to be the only role given to the elderly Koreans, thus compounding their sense of anxiety and depression. Such a limited role does not provide the elderly with the opportunity to become fully integrated into Canadian society. Kim notes that the Korean elderly are totally dependent on their children or grandchildren and that "they do not have the cognitive and social skills to participate in the larger society and their adjustment is limited to the ethnic pockets."

CULTURAL FACTORS AND AGING

One of the key cultural variables that requires examination is the degree of obligation that is perceived by the children toward their parents. The concept of filial piety has its roots in Confucianism and involves several types of obligations. According to Osako and Liu (1986, 130), the child must obey his or her parents, support them in old age and must succeed in a career to bring honour to parents and ancestors. What happens then, when

Table 3
Health satisfaction by ethnic group and gender (n=774)

Health Satisfaction	Chinese M (%)	Chinese F (%)	Japanese M (%)	Japanese F (%)	Korean M (%)	Korean F (%)
Dissatisfied	9.2	20.8	11.4	8.6	12.8	29.0
Mixed	6.1	9.6	19.9	20.4	9.0	11.0
Satisfied	84.7	69.6	68.7	71.0	78.2	60.0
	100.0	100.0	100.0	100.0	100.0	100.0
	(98)	(125)	(211)	(162)	(78)	(100)

children do not fulfil the filial roles as expected by their parents? As a partial response to this question, it is suggested that intergenerational conflict is one possible outcome, and in those situations where conflict appears to be minimal, it is the parents who internalize their feelings and suffer the consequences in silence. This tends to be more true for elderly immigrants who are recent arrivals than for those who have become acculturated to Canadian societal norms.

Table 4 illustrates the variations in responses to the question "What aspects of your cultural heritage do you feel have enabled you to grow old successfully?" It can be seen from Table 4 that 25.5 percent of the Korean elderly indicated that filial piety was the key cultural variable for successful aging. This contrasts with the Chinese and Japanese elderly respondents of whom 12.2 percent and 7.1 percent respectively indicated filial piety. The Korean elderly also indicated that pride in their cultural heritage was important. It should be observed here, however, that the Koreans were the most recent immigrants to Canada among the Asian elderly studied here. This means that most of the socialization had taken place in Korea and it can thus be argued that there is a relatively strong attachment to traditional Korean values. The Chinese tend to fall between the Korean and Japanese responses.

From Table 4 it can be seen that an extremely high percentage of Japanese elderly indicated that discipline and perseverance were important cultural factors that contributed to their successful aging. The Japanese term *gaman* was most frequently cited. According to Kobata (1979), *gaman* is literally translated as "self-control." The outward manifestation of this is the tendency to suppress emotions whether they be positive or negative. In traditional Japanese society, *gaman* was seen as virtuous and Kobata argues that "the tendency to suffer in silence with a great deal of forbearance provides some insights into the nature of the family as the source for dealing with problems rather than the outside service providers." It is not surprising, therefore, to note in Table 1 that the Japanese elderly have the highest percentage of mixed feelings regarding their own evaluation of health. Both dissatisfaction and satisfaction appear to be suppressed in comparison to the Korean and Chinese elderly.

Associated with the concept of *gaman* or self-control is *enryo*. According to Kobata (1979), "the norm of *enryo* includes, but is not limited to, reserve, reticence, self-effacement, deference, humility, hesitation, and denigration of one's self and possessions." Because of the plethora of terms that can be associated with *enryo*, it is extremely difficult to assess the well-being of the Japanese elderly. As Kobata notes, "the concept had its origin in the cultural norm of knowing one's position in relation to another when interacting with others perceived as 'inferior' or 'superior' to oneself." Thus, in interactions with authority figures, for example doctors, the Japanese elderly very often do not volunteer their true feelings. How can researchers differentiate

Table 4
Cultural factors considered important for successful aging by ethnic group (n=632)

Cultural Factors	Chinese (%)	Japanese (%)	Korean (%)
Discipline, diligence	0.6	18.4	1.9
Patience, tolerance	3.3	20.1	2.5
Filial piety	12.2	7.1	25.5
Group loyalty	1.7	2.7	1.9
Sense of duty	3.3	3.7	3.8
Thriftiness	1.7	1.0	—
Moral obligations	0.6	3.4	8.3
Emphasis on education	17.7	3.1	5.3
Pride in culture, tradition	24.6	8.2	10.8
Honesty, courtesy, manners	—	10.6	0.6
Religious teachings	2.8	2.7	3.8
Traditional family emphasis	1.7	3.7	—
Fatalism	2.2	0.3	—
Deferred gratification	—	1.4	0.6
Martial and traditional arts	—	2.0	—
Modesty	0.6	2.4	—
Self-reliance	6.6	2.4	0.6
Optimism	7.7	—	—
Nothing in particular	12.7	6.8	34.4
	100.0	100.0	100.0
Total Numbers	(181)	(294)	(157)

empirically whether it is *gaman* or *enryo* or both that are operating in order to account for the lack of interaction? This is an extremely crucial aspect to understand if health care providers are to provide effective care. Our data revealed that 15.7 percent of the Japanese elderly respondents and 6.1 percent of the Korean respondents indicated that *enryo* or reserve was a negative aspect of their culture that impacted on their well-being. This is particularly true in health care settings in which those who are able to complain the loudest very often receive the most care.

DISCUSSION AND CONCLUSION

Although we have not discussed all of the cultural factors noted in Table 4, the significance of understanding various cultural factors must be underscored in providing effective health care. As noted by Kreps and Thornton (1984, 191), culture is particularly important in effective communication between health care personnel and their clients. Furthermore, as noted above, the influence of traditional cultural values may impact on a person's social interaction pattern and thus create a situation in which the elderly may feel powerless. The lack of effective communication may also result in low self-esteem which, in turn, as Dreher (1987, 69) has argued, will have a negative effect on the health of individuals.

The extent to which various cultural values are retained by the Chinese, Japanese and Korean Canadian elderly is related to the socialization process experienced earlier, whether in Canada or in the country of emigration. As Sugiman and Nishio (1983, 20) have indicated, the retention of cultural norms is also a function of the immigrant's attitudes towards acculturation. In the case of Japanese Canadians, the immigrant or first generation group appears to have supported the idea of acculturation. Consequently, Sugiman and Nishio argue that the *Issei* made only modest demands on their children to fulfil filial obligations. This view appears to be supported even in contemporary Japan today. The *Japan Times* (1987) reports that the elderly in Japan look less to their children to look after them and prefer to be taken care of by their spouse.

Another important point to consider when examining the extent to which traditional values are retained concerns the supportive or non-supportive environment in which one's traditional culture can survive. Clearly, the lack of institutional support for the transmission of Japanese culture and language during the time of their internment cannot be compared to today's multicultural environment, which encourages the retention of traditional cultural heritage. Thus, it is expected that the Chinese and Korean Canadian elderly manifest a higher degree of cultural retention compared to the elderly Japanese Canadians. Indeed, our data in Table 4 indicate that the Chinese and Korean elderly consider filial piety and pride in one's traditional culture to be very important.

Although we have not been able to explore all of the cultural variables that have their roots in the Confucian ethic, our examination of a few selected variables suggests that an understanding of cultural traditionals of aged ethnic minorities are important if effective health care services are to be provided. As we have illustrated, reference to data obtained through accepted social science methodology may not provide the same information that the health care professionals who are members of a given ethnic group can obtain because of their understanding of the psychological make-up of the particular ethnic group. Therefore, as a subsequent step in our endeavour to bridge the cultural gaps in the provision of health care, we are in the process of establishing a data bank consisting of transcultural health information (Ujimoto, 1987c). When the project is completed, it is hoped that a simple multivariate display of information will be readily available. Advances in information technology have made this possible and as empirical data becomes avail, refinements can be made to our traditional data information system.

REFERENCES

Canada. *1981 Census*. Population, Ethnic Origin. Statistics Canada. Cat. 92-911 Vol. 1 - National Series. Ottawa: Ministry of Supply & Service

Chappell, N.L., Strain, L.A., & Blandford, A. (1986). *Aging and Health Care, A Social Perspective*. Toronto: Holt, Rinehart and Winston.

Disman, M. (1987). Explorations in Ethnic Identity, Oldness and Continuity. In D.E. Gelfand and C.M. Barresi (Eds.), *Ethnic Dimensions of Aging* (64-74). New York: Springer Publishing Co.

Driedger, L. & Chappell, N. (1987). *Aging and Ethnicity, Toward an Interface*. Toronto: Butterworths.

Dreher, B.B. (1987). *Communication Skills for Workings with Elders*. New York: Springer Publishing Co.

England, J. (1986). Cross-Cultural Health Care. *Canada's Mental Health*, 34(4), 13-15.

Japan Times Weekly Overseas. (1987). Elderly Look Less to Children for Care. October 3.

Kim, U. & Berry, J.W. (1986). Predictors of Acculturative Stress: Korean Immigrants in Toronto, Canada. In L.H. Ekstrand (Ed.), *Ethnic Minorities and Immigrants in Cross Cultural Perspectives*. Lisse: Swets and Zeitlinger.

Kim, U. (1987). Illness Behaviour Patterns of Korean Immigrants in Toronto: What are the Hidden Costs? In K. Victor Ujimoto and Josephine Naidoo (Eds.), *Asian Canadians: Contemporary Issues* (194-219). Guelph: University of Guelph.

Kobata, F. (1979). The Influence of Culture on Family Relations: The Asian American Experience. In P.K. Ragan (Ed.), *Aging Parents* (94-106). Los Angeles: University of Southern California Press.

Kreps, G.L. & Thornton, B.C. (1984). *Health Communications, Theory and Practice*. New York: Longman.

Levkoff, S.E., Cleary, P.D., and Wetle, T. (1987). Differences in the Appraisal of Health Between Aged and Middle-Aged Adults. *Journal of Gerontology, 42*(1), 114-20.

Liu, W.T. (1986). Culture and Social Support. *Research on Aging, 8*, 57-83.

Masi, R. (1986). *Partnerships in Health in a Multicultural Society*. Downsview, Ont. Multicultural Health Coalition.

Osako, M.M., and Liu, W.T. (1986). Intergenerational Relations and the Aged Among Japanese Americans. *Research on Aging, 8*, 128-55.

Rosenthal, C. (1986). Family Supports in Life: Does Ethnicity Make a Difference? *The Gerontologist, 26*(1), 19-24.

Sugiman, P. and Nishio, H.K. (1983). Socialization and Cultural Duality Among Aging Japanese Canadians. *Canadian Ethnic Studies, 15*, 17-35.

Hayami-Steven, J. Kadota, C. and Ujimoto, K.V. (1990). *The Best Years: The First Japanese Canadian Conference on Aging*. Winnipeg: The National Association of Japanese Canadians.

Tseng, W. and Wu, Y.H. (1985). *Chinese Culture and Mental Health*. Don Mills: Academic Press.

Ujimoto, K.V. (1987a). The Ethnic Dimensions of Aging in Canada. In V.W. Marshall (Ed.), *Aging in Canada: Social Perspectives*, (2nd Edition, 111-37). Toronto: Fitzhenry and Whiteside.

— —. (1987b). Organizational Activities, Cultural Factors, and Well-Being of Aged Japanese Canadians. In D.E. Gelfand and C.M. Barresi (Eds.), *Ethnic Dimensions of Aging*. New York: Springer Publishing.

— —. (1987c). Aging, Health, and Information Technology in a Multicultural Society. Submission prepared for the Standing Committee on Multiculturalism, Toronto, Ont. 7 December.

— —. (1988). Aging, Ethnicity, and Health. In B.S. Bolaria and H.D. Dickenson (Eds.), *Sociology of Health Care in Canada*. Don Mills: Harcourt Brace Jovanovich Canada.

— —. (1990). Time-Budget Methodology for Research on Aging. *Social Indicators Research*, 23, 381-93.

Waxler-Morrison, N., Anderson, J. and Richardson, E. (1990). *Cross-Cultural Caring: A Handbook for Health Professionals in Western Canada*. Vancouver: University of British Columbia Press.

- 15 -

The Semiotic Representation of "Health" and "Disease"

Marcel Danesi

It is a widely known fact that the mind can influence the body. But it is not commonly known that the science of semiotics grew out of attempts by the first physicians of the Western world to understand how this mind/body interaction operates within specific cultural domains. Indeed, in its oldest usage (Nöth 1990, 12-14), the term *semiotics* was applied to the study of the observable pattern of physiological symptoms induced by particular diseases. Hippocrates (460?-377? B.C.)—the founder of medical science—viewed the semiotic ways in which a culture would portray the symptomatology associated with a disease as the basis upon which to carry out an appropriate diagnosis and then to formulate a culturally suitable prognosis. As Fisch (1978, 41) has pointed out, it was soon after Hippocrates's utilization of the term *semiosis* to refer to the cultural representation of symptomatic signs that it came to mean—by the time of Aristotle (384-322 B.C.—the "action" of a sign itself, or the correlative act of sign interpretation.

So, from the dawn of civilization to the present age of high-technology health care, it has always been recognized, at least implicitly, that there is an intrinsic connection between physical health and the semiotic codes that human beings create to represent and think about physical health. Rarely, however, have medical practitioners ventured to give serious consideration to the possibility that these codes may not only help to define a disease in cultural terms, but also to actually affect its etiology and medical treatment. These are the semiotic themes explored in this essay. On the basis of the relevant insights derived from the field of semiotics, the case will be argued that the definition of health and the successful treatment of disease are dependent to a large extent upon cultural perceptions and models of "health" and "disease." Needless to say, in multicultural societies this constitutes a particularly pertinent mode of medical inquiry. Specifically, this essay will discuss the ways in which cultures encode (refer to) health features and disease symptoms. It will then consider the implications such cultural encoding systems have for the administration of health care in multicultural societies.

SEMIOTICS AND REALITY

Before examining the case that health and the culturally specific semiotic codes used to represent it are cognitively interdependent, it is useful to describe briefly the analytical tools that semiotics makes available for the study of so-called "reality." The raison d'etre of semiotics is, arguably, to investigate whether or not reality can exist independently of the cultural codes that human beings create to represent and think about it. Is the physical universe a great machine operating according to natural laws that may be discovered by human reason? Or, on the other hand, is everything "out there" no more than a construction of the human mind projecting itself onto the world of sensations and perceptions? Although an answer to this fundamental question will clearly never be possible, one of the important offshoots of the search for an answer has been a systematic form of inquiry into how the mind's symbolic products and the body's natural processes are interrelated (Sebeok, 1976, 1979).

Semiotics is the term commonly used to refer to the study of the innate capacity of human beings to produce and understand signs of all kinds (from those belonging to simple physiological signalling systems to those that reveal a highly complex symbolic structure). The etymology of the term is traceable to the Greek word *sema* meaning "mark" or "sign," which is also the root of the related term *semantics* "the study of meaning." In the theoretical semiotic literature, the term *semiosis* is used to refer to the actual comprehension and production of signs.

In all the main conceptualizations of semiosis, the primary components of this mental process are seen to be the *sign* (a representative image or icon, a word, etc.), the *object* referred to (which can be either concrete or abstract) and the *meaning* that results when the sign and the object are linked together by association. It would appear that the human cognitive system operates on the basis of this triadic nexus. Indeed, many semioticians now would claim that it underlies the very structure of the mind. Thus, for instance, the word *cat* is a verbal sign that can be seen to relate the animal (its object) to the meaning "cat" (the domesticated carnivorous mammal with retractile claws, which kills mice and rats, etc.). Similarly, the use of the index finger to point to an object in a room creates a concrete existential meaning relation between the so-called indexical sign (the pointing finger) and the object. Following Charles Sanders Peirce (1931-58), most semioticians now add the notion of *interpretant* to the process of semiosis. This is Peirce's term for the individual's particular interpretation of the triadic relationship that inheres in semiosis: "A sign addresses somebody, that is, creates in the mind of that person an equivalent sign, or perhaps a more developed sign. The sign which it creates I call the *interpretant* of the first sign (ibid., vol. 2, 228.).

There are various theories on the phylogenesis of the semiotic capacity, but perhaps the most plausible one traces it to the mind's innate ability to transform sense impressions into memorable experiences through the formation of images (see Danesi (1990a) for a detailed discussion of this hypothesis). Although all species participate by instinct in the experiential universe, only humans are endowed with the capacity to model their sense impressions in the form of mental images. It is when these transformations of our bodily experiences are codified into signs and sign systems that they become permanently transportable in the form of cognitive units, phenomenologically free from their physiological units of occurrence. Indeed, the work on semiosis has made it possible to relate the world of sensorial experience to the world of abstraction and thought, by showing the latter to be a kind of evolutionary "outgrowth" of the former.

In the area of health, the following semiotic hypothesis can now be formulated. "Health" can be posited as constituting a culturally specific code whose meaning, or semantic range, is delimited by the particular signs in the code used to represent bodily processes (the object). As in the case of any semiotic code (e.g., food, clothing, etc.), the semantic relations among its signs are maintained by a psychological dichotomy—"healthy" vs. "non-healthy." So the ways in which health is spoken about, the ways in which a healthy complexion or bodily state is visualized form the signs of the code that define "health," and its converse. This "health code" is, in other words, a cognitive strategy for organizing and rationalizing the flux of changes that the body is perceived to undergo.

The hypothesis upon which most of Western medicine has conventionally operated is, on the contrary, the one that claims that bodily health is a knowable phenomenon to all physicians in all cultures in exactly the same cognitive ways. However, the reliance on the traditional scientific arguments to support such an objectivist perspective has been weakened in this century by the intriguing theoretical debates in physics. The great 20th century physicist Werner Heisenberg (e.g., 1949) was, in fact, the first to debunk the notion that science was capable of discovering so-called "objective reality." His uncertainty, or indeterminacy, principle, for which he won the Nobel Prize in 1931, has come to have a profound influence on scientific thinking in the latter part of this century. In essence, Heisenberg showed that the idea of an objectively knowable universe that is independent of our culturally shaped modes of observation is just that—a human idea. Heisenberg argued that the construct of "objective reality" had to be replaced by the one of "observer-dependent reality." His uncertainty principle, whose repercussions are being felt in all the sciences (including the medical ones) lends substantial credibility to the argument that conceptualizations of health and disease are dependent in large part upon the ways in which cultures represent them semiotically.

THE SEMIOTIC REPRESENTATION OF "HEALTH" AND "DISEASE"

What, if any, are the specific implications of the foregoing discussion for the scientific study of health and the medical treatment of disease? Basically, it suggests that these concepts are constrained by the cultural contexts in which they appear. What is considered to be healthy in one culture may not coincide with what it is to be healthy in another. Health, like all the phenomena codified by scientists, cannot be defined ahistorically, aculturally or in purely absolutist terms. As a corollary, it is obvious that for any treatment of a disease to be meaningful (and consequently effective), it will have to be grounded in cultural reality.

This semiotic perspective does not deny the existence of events and states in the body that will lead it to malfunctioning. All organisms have an innate warning system that alerts them to dangerous changes in bodily states. But only in the case of the human organism are fluctuations in bodily functions codified semiotically and thus made available to reflective consciousness. Once a specific pattern of fluctuation has been selected and codified as "healthy," then its absence or its converse becomes an immediate sign of "disease." Problems in interpreting this sign as indicative of a "disease state" emerge when an individual comes from a culture that has not codified the bodily fluctuations in question in similar ways.

At this point an illustrative analogy is in order. The world of flora and fauna is classified semiotically by all cultures into a dichotomy of "edible" and "non-edible" categories. However, the inclusion of an item in one or the other category is a culture-specific decision. Rabbits, many kinds of flowers and silkworms, for instance, would be classified by and large as "non-edible" by North American culture. However, Europeans regularly cook rabbit meat and various types of flowers, and Mexicans eat cooked silkworms with no adverse physical reactions whatsoever. But if such substances were to be presented to North Americans in a prepared culinary form, chances are, given the semiotic valence they have in their own culture, that they would suffer an adverse reaction if told what they were eating. This example shows, in an intuitively obvious way, how culture can influence our physical responses.

Perhaps the best way to approach the mind/body interaction in the domain of health care is to enlist the ideas of Giambattista Vico, the great 18th century Neapolitan philosopher whose 1725 book, *The New Science* (Bergin and Fisch, 1984), offers some truly remarkable insights into how to understand this interaction. In his penetrating analysis of the human mind, Vico posits the existence of two cognitive layers—a deep layer and a surface layer (Danesi, 1990b). At the deep level human sense impressions are registered and organized into categories which schematize the physiological and affective responses to the stimuli and signals present in the environment in the form of images. Although all species participate in the universe of experience, only humans are endowed with the capacity to transform sense impressions into memorable images. This is the primordial function of the human imagination, and it is at this deep level that one can talk of "universals" (e.g., Verene, 1981).

It is only when these mental images of bodily experiences are codified, especially by language, that a surface form of cognition crystallizes. The particular characteristics of this form will, clearly, vary from person to person and from culture to culture. Surface-level signs eventually become independent from their imagistic origins and generate highly abstract systems of thought that subsequently guide the mind's efforts to understand the world of reality. These efforts produce our institutions, scientific theories and ultimately our cultures.

Vico's insights on the nature of mind suggest that there is an objective reality to which the human organism responds in universal ways. At this deep level, the mind transforms sensorial input into image schemas. But only those schemas codified semiotically (e.g., by language) become subsequently retrievable as units of recurring and meaningful pattern. Therefore, problems in understanding health conceptually can be seen to emerge at the culturally shaped surface level of cognition. The semiotic categories that make up this level (e.g., the words used to describe a healthy state) eventually develop into culturally specific models of health and disease.

The question now becomes: How do we come to conceptualize health in culturally specific ways? Even a superficial consideration of this question will suggest that we do so through the template of the surface-level signs that cultures utilize to represent health and its converse. Thus, for instance, in some cultures a "healthy body" is considered to be one that is lean and muscular. Conversely, in others it might be conceptualized as being one that is plump and rotund. A "healthy lifestyle" might be seen by some cultures to inhere in rigorous physical activity, while in others it might be envisaged as inhering in a more leisurely and sedentary form of behaviour.

But perhaps the "semiotic key" that allows us best to access the conceptualization of health in a culture is the language used to refer to "healthy" and "unhealthy" states. Consider, for example, the following common metaphorical portrayals of health by our own North American culture (see also Lakoff & Johnson, 1980, 15, 50):

1. You're at the *peak* of your health
2. My health is *down*.
3. You're in *top* shape.
4. My body is in perfect *working order*.
5. My body is *breaking down*.
6. My health is going *down the drain*.

7. His pain *went away*.
8. I'm going to *flush out* my cold.

The first three sentences represent health in terms of an orientation analogy: i.e. the state of being healthy is depicted as being oriented in an upwards direction, while the opposite state is portrayed as being oriented in a downward direction. This is probably because in this culture, as Lakoff and Johnson point out, serious "illness forces us to lie down physically" (ibid., 15). Sentences (4) and (5) compare health, and its converse, to a machine. And in the last three sentences health and its converse are envisaged as being entities within a person. This is why they can *go away*, they can be *flushed out*, and so on.

The study of metaphorical formulas such as these (e.g., Johnson, 1987; Lakoff, 1987; Lakoff & Johnson, 1980; Lakoff & Turner, 1989) reveals that they underlie the representation of most of our concepts. Since 1977 the increase in the number of psychologically oriented studies on metaphor has been rather dramatic. That was the year in which Pollio and his associates (1977) presented data that demonstrated how pervasive figurative language was at all levels of communication and conceptualization. Such research found that most speakers of English uttered about 3,000 novel metaphors and 7,000 idiomatic expressions per week. It became immediately apparent to the scientific community at large that metaphor was hardly to be considered a rhetorical ornament or frill. And, indeed, in the last decade or so, cognitive scientists have been coming more and more to the realization that metaphor plays a key role in everyday concepts (see Danesi 1989 for a review of the relevant literature). The gist of most of the research in this area has been that metaphor structures the ways in which we perceive, think and act.

It is interesting to note that even before the current wave of fascination with metaphor within cognitive science, the writer Susan Sontag wrote a compelling book, *Illness as metaphor* (1978), that has become a classic study of how metaphor shapes our conceptualizations of disease. A decade later, after the advent of AIDS, Sontag (1989) followed this up with a sequel study on the metaphors commonly used to portray AIDS. The main point made by Sontag in these two books was that illness is not a metaphor, but that cultures invariably think of diseases in metaphorical ways. Using the example of cancer, Sontag pointed out that in the not too distant past the very word *cancer* was said to have killed some patients who would not have necessarily succumbed to the malignancy from which they suffered: "As long as a particular disease is treated as an evil, invincible predator, not just a disease, most people with cancer will indeed be demoralized by learning what disease they have" (1979, 7). Sontag's point that people suffer more from conceptualizing about their disease than from the disease itself is, indeed, a well-taken and instructive one.

It is also interesting to note that medical practitioners can easily come under the spell of health and body symbolism. As Averill (1990) has recently argued, cultural shaping of health and disease concepts probably takes its origins from the fact that the functioning of the human body is of utmost importance to both the individual and society. As he eloquently puts it: "From a psychological point of view, our body is as much symbol as substance" (1990, 117). However, it is to be noted that the semiotic transformation of the body can have serious consequences for the practice of medicine. To quote just one example, Hudson (1972) found that medical specialists trained in private British schools were more likely to achieve distinction and prominence by working on the head as opposed to the lower part of the body, on the surface as opposed to the inside of the body and on the male as opposed to the female body. Hudson correctly suggested that the only way to interpret such behaviours was in cultural terms: that is, parts of the body, evidently, possessed a symbolic significance that influenced the decisions taken by medical students: "students from an upper-middle-class background are more likely than those from a lower-middle-class background to find their way into specialties that are seen for symbolic reasons as desirable" (ibid., 282). Examples such as this highlight the intrinsic interconnection that exists between medical practice and the cultural context in which it takes place.

IMPLICATIONS FOR HEALTH CARE IN MULTICULTURAL SOCIETIES

I would like to suggest that there are two main implications that health care practitioners working in multicultural societies can distil from the foregoing semiotic discussion. The first is that the human body, as the anthropologist Mary Douglas (1973, 98) has phrased it, is generally "treated as an image of society." And as Danziger (1990, 349) has similarly remarked, the "structure of the body, or the mind, confirms the consonant structure of the social order and vice versa." The awareness that the body, health and disease are conceptualized differently by various cultures will in itself assist those involved in administering health care in multicultural contexts. Understanding how individuals from different cultural backgrounds conceptualize body image, health and disease will help practitioners to program an intervention strategy for clients that is more suitable and effective. The main lesson would seem to be that a successful health care strategy is, in large part, dependent upon it being synchronized with the client's cultural codes and expectations. A health care professional should, therefore, attempt to be particularly sensitive to cultural differences and to learn as much as he/she can about them.

To see how this sensitivity to cultural differences can be helpful to the practitioner, consider the recent research on the experience of pain. This area of medical inquiry has long been shaped by a strictly physical view: namely that pain "is a specific sensation subserved by a straight-through transmission system from skin to brain, and that intensity of pain is proportional to the extent of tissue damage" (Melzack, 1988, 288). But recent research has shown that pain thresholds are also influenced by non-physical factors, such as the unique past history of the individual and his/her cognitive experiences (Melzack & Wall, 1982). This suggests that culturally specific conceptual models of pain can affect the patient's response and threshold patterns. As a specific example, consider the experience of childbirth. As Melzack (1972, 223) observes, in North American culture "childbirth is widely regarded as a painful experience." However, anthropologists have documented "cultures in which the women show virtually no distress during childbirth." Melzack, a psychologist, goes on to provide what is, remarkably, a semiotic explanation of such a behavioral discrepancy:

> Can this mean that all women in our culture are making up their pain? Not at all. It happens to be part of our culture to recognize childbirth as possibly endangering the life of the mother, and young girls learn to fear it in the course of growing up. Books on "natural childbirth" ("childbirth without fear") stress the extent to which fear increases the amount of pain felt during labour and birth and point how difficult it is to dispel it. (ibid., 223)

A health care professional who does not take into account such culturally shaped response patterns to childbirth will generally tend to ascribe them to individual threshold levels. Clearly, such an approach would have missed the point completely and could potentially lead to undesirable results.

The second main implication to be drawn from a semiotic consideration of health and disease follows directly from the first one: namely that training in semiotic analysis should probably be made an intrinsic part of the practitioner's education, so as to improve his/her knowledge and skills in serving a multicultural clientele. As pointed out at the beginning of this essay, this certainly would not constitute an improper suggestion, given that in its oldest usage semiotics referred to a branch of medicine. For example, the physician Galen of Pergamum (C.130-200 A.D.) referred to diagnosis as a process of semiosis (Nöth, 1990, 13). In Italy, the term *semeiotica* continues, to this day, to be used in medical science to refer to the study of symptoms.

By way of conclusion, it is instructive, and germane to the theme of this essay, to consider the point made by John Morreall (1983) on the vital role that humour often plays in medical practice. Morreall suggests that humour creates an important "distancing effect" that is used by doctors in operation and emergency rooms as a strategy for coping with stressful and life-threatening situations (ibid., 104-105). It can be suggested that a semiotic knowledge of the patient's cultural conceptualizations of health and disease will also create a distancing effect that will put the practitioner into a much better position to understand how and why certain patients in multicultural societies respond to treatment and care in the way that they do. This is one of the ways that will allow medical practitioners to become more capable of coping effectively with those individual response patterns that arise, not from the body, but from the domain of culture. After all, as Harris et al. emphasize in their classic textbook on medical practice, the physician becomes an effective healer only when he/she views the patient not as a collection of symptoms, disordered functions, damaged organs and disturbed emotions, but as a human being in his/her individual and cultural totality: treatment of a patient consists in more than the dispassionate confrontation of a disease. It embodies also the exercise of warmth, compassion, and understanding. In the now famous words of Peabody, "one of the essential qualities of the clinician is interest in humanity, for the secret of the care of the patient is in caring for the patient" (1966, 9).

REFERENCES

Averill, J.R. (1990). Inner feelings, works of the flesh, the beast within, diseases of the mind, driving force, and putting on a show: Six metaphors of emotion and their theoretical extensions. In D.E. Leary (Ed.), *Metaphors in the history of psychology* (104-32). Cambridge: Cambridge University Press.

Bergin, T.G., & Fisch, M.H. (1984). *The new science of Giambattista Vica.* Ithaca: Cornell University Press.

Danesi, M. (1989). The role of metaphor in cognition. *Semiotica, 77,* 521-31.

— —. (1990a). Thinking is seeing: Visual metaphors and the nature of abstract thought. *Semiotica, 80,* 221-37.

— —. (1990b). Semiosis, cognition, and reality: A Vichian commentary on Krausz's anthology on relativism. *New Vico Studies, 8,* 71 - 78.

Danziger, K. (1990). Generative metaphor and the history of psychological discourse. In D.E. Leary (Ed.), *Metaphors in the history of psychology* (331-56). Cambridge: Cambridge University Press.

Douglas, M. (1973). *Natural symbols.* Harmondsworth: Penguin.

Fisch, Max H. (1978). Peirce's General Theory of Signs. In T.A. Sebeok (Ed.), *Sight, sound, and sense* (31-70). Bloomington: Indiana University Press.

Harris, T.R., Adams, R.D., Bennett, I.L., Resnick, W.H., thorn, G.W., Wintrobe, M.M. (1966). *Principles of internal medicine.* New York: McGraw-Hill.

Heisenberg, W. (1949). *The physical principles of the quantum theory.* New York: Dover.

Hudson, L. (1972). *The cult of the fact.* New York: Harper and Row.

Johnson, M. (1987). *The body in the mind: The bodily basis of meaning, imagination, and reason.* Chicago: University of Chicago Press.

Lakoff, G. (1987). *Women, fire and dangerous things: What categories reveal about the mind.* Chicago: University of Chicago Press.

Lakoff, G., & Johnson, M. (1980). *Metaphors we live by.* Chicago: University of Chicago Press.

Lakoff, G., & Turner, M. (1989). *More than cool reason: A field guide to poetic metaphor.* Chicago: University of Chicago Press.

Melzack, R. (1972). The perception of pain. In R.F. Thompson
(Ed.), *Physiological psychology* (223-31). San Francisco: Free-
man.
— —. (1988). Pain. In J. Kuper (Ed.), *A lexicon of psychology,
psychiatry and psychoanalysis* (288-91). London: Routledge.
Melzack, R. & Wall, P. D. (1982). *The challenge of pain.*
Harmondsworth: Penguin.
Morreall, J. (1983). *Taking laughter seriously.* Albany: State Uni-
versity of New York Press.
Nöth, Winfred. (1990). *Handbook of semiotics.* Bloomington: Indi-
ana University Press.
Peirce, C.S. (1931-58). *Collected papers.* Vols. 1-6. Cambridge,
Mass.: Harvard University Press.
Pollio, H., Barlow, J., fine, H., & Pollio, M. (1977). *The poetics of
growth: Figurative language in psychology, psychotherapy,
and education.* Hillsdale, N.J.: Lawrence Erlbaum Associ-
ates.
Sebeok, T.A. (1976). *Contributions to the doctrine of signs.* Lanham,
Maryland: University Press of America.
— —. (1979). *The sign and its masters.* Austin: University of Texas
Press.
Sontag, S. (1978). *Illness as metaphor.* New York: Farrar, Straus &
Giroux.
— —. (1989). *AIDS and its metaphors.* New York: Farrar, Straus &
Giroux.
Verene, D.P. (1981). *Vico's science of the imagination.* Ithaca:
Cornell University Press.

- 16 -

Ethics in Cross-Cultural Health

When future historians describe the last two decades of the 20th century, they may well use the term "the ethics era." We are witnessing an explosion of interest in the ethical dimensions of various aspects of society, including business, politics, the environment, war and peace and health care. This interest is reflected through reports in the media, the activities of citizens' groups and professional associations, and government initiatives such as royal commissions dealing with particular ethical issues. Such activities are bound to increase, as ever more areas of public life are subjected to ethical analysis.

The field in which this wave of interest in ethics originated and where the most work has been done is that of health care. However, there are many areas of health care where ethical analysis has hardly begun, including the one that is the subject of this book. In this chapter I will attempt to remedy this deficiency by identifying some of the major ethical problems that arise in the provision of health care in a multicultural setting and by suggesting how they can be resolved. The chapter will first explore the relation of ethics and culture; second, describe the role of ethics in health care; third, discuss the requirements of ethics in cross-cultural health care; and finally, make some suggestions for the education of health care workers in cross-cultural ethics.

ETHICS AND CULTURE

Ethics is the study of morality, of the good and the bad, the right and the wrong in human decision making and behaviour. Morality is and always has been an essential feature of humanity. In the words of the social anthropologist Lionel Tiger, "Ethical behaviour is a primitive behaviour. Even though it calls us all to the highest standards and lays claim to the most generous of human purposes, it is as basic a business as suckling or stalking. It involves ancient social responses which we share with other creatures" (1987, 22).

Although morality most probably originated in the earliest human family and clan groupings, its formulation into rules and codes of conduct followed upon the establishment of pastoral and agriculturally based civilizations beginning approximately 10,000 years ago: "An important force which helped produce the ethical codifications accompanying agriculture and pastoralism was precisely the one that could adjust a species with a certain behavioral grammar to a new set of requirements arising out of new and more crowded conditions of social life" (ibid., 38). The development of these more systematic codes of conduct gave rise in some cultures to a new branch of intellectual inquiry— ethics. In the majority of cultures, ethics was and is an integral part of the study of religion, since moral rules are justified by reference to religious myths, scriptures and authorities. In the cultures from which Western civilization originated, however, namely the Greek and Roman cultures, a rival to the religious monopoly in ethics emerged and developed. That rival was philosophy, and its founding fathers were the well-known Athenians, Socrates, Plato and Aristotle.

Ethics, whether religious or philosophical, is a major academic field, with many competing schools, an enormous literature, and a very interested public. In most Western countries, debates about public morality are usually decided according to philosophical rather than religious standards. The dominant Western culture is rationalist and secular, and religion is widely perceived as irrational and potentially divisive in pluralist societies. Individuals are free to abide by the prescriptions of religious morality in their private and family lives, but these rules are considered to be inappropriate for regulating the relations between social groups such as governments, businesses, labour unions and professional associations.

This attempt to circumscribe religious morality is widely contested by many groups in the Western countries (Williams, 1984; Brown and Brown, 1989). In other parts of the world, similar attempts have met with outright rejection (Iran is one notable example; the former Soviet Union is another) or else have succeeded to a very limited degree (e.g., India). All attempts to construct a transcultural ethics, based on reason alone, have been failures, and must necessarily be so, given the cultural specificity and religious diversity of moral beliefs and practices.

As long as a cultural group keeps to itself, its ethics may function in a relatively unproblematic fashion. However, as soon as the group, or some of its members, encounter another culture with different ethics, problems occur. This chapter will consider such situations. It will attempt to formulate an approach to health care ethics which is *cross-cultural*, in that the problems it examines arise from the fact that members of one cultural group find themselves in a health care system that is based on the values of a quite different culture. The approach of this chapter is also *multicultural*, since it argues that the health care system should recognize that its clientele is made up of members of many different cultural groups, and it is *intercultural*, because the resolution of problems in this context depends to a large extent on the interaction and cooperation of different cultural groups, not just on the representatives of the dominant culture. This approach should not, however, be described as *transcultural*, simply because it is impossible to transcend culture, and any claim to do so is in reality an attempt to impose one culture on all others.

ETHICS IN HEALTH CARE

Of all the fields of professional activity, the one which has probably been most subject to ethical analysis throughout history, at least in the Western world, is medicine. In the West there has been an unbroken tradition of medical ethics since the time of the Greek physician Hippocrates (5th century B.C.E.). For most of this period medical ethics was concerned primarily, if not exclusively, with the decision making and behaviour of *physicians*. There was very little attention paid to the rights and duties of other health care workers or of patients. This is not to say that physicians were the only ones who engaged in medical ethics. Many theologians and philosophers devoted themselves to the study of medical morality by applying the teachings of religion and the insights of human reason to problems encountered in medical practice. However, they had little more to say about the behaviour of patients and other health care workers than did the physician-ethicists.

This virtual identification of medical ethics with the concerns of physicians began to dissolve in the 1960s, because of certain important developments in medical science and practice and other social changes. The explosive growth of modern medical science and technology during the past 30 years has raised many new issues for scientists, health care professionals, public policy officials, jurists and the general public. The harmful effects of many scientific discoveries (e.g., thalidomide), the shortage of certain life-saving technologies (e.g., dialysis machines), and the need to redefine such fundamental concepts as death (in order to permit the removal of cadaver organs for transplantation) served to convince all those involved in the health care field that a new approach was required to deal with moral problems in medical science and practice.

The contentious nature of these scientific and technological developments is compounded by other major changes in society since the 1960s. Three of these are of particular relevance for medical ethics: the triumph of moral pluralism in many Western countries, as evidenced by the removal of legal barriers to sexual practices such as contraception, abortion and homosexual relations; a great increase in concern for the protection of human rights, including the right to decide about one's medical care; and the overcoming of the taboo against discussing death, which has led to an upsurge of interest in the conditions for the withdrawal of life-support systems for seriously ill patients and in the pros and cons of active euthanasia.

In response to these developments, a new field of study and practice has emerged during the past 25 years. It is referred to as bioethics, biomedical ethics or health care ethics. Medical ethics is just one subset of this field, as are nursing, dental and health administration ethics. Activities in bioethics include research and publication, courses in medical, nursing, dental and health administration programs and philosophy and religious studies departments, conferences and workshops, consultations on difficult patient cases, the development of hospital policies on a wide range of ethical topics and the study of contentious ethical issues by public groups such as the Law Reform Commission of Canada and the Royal Commission on New Reproductive Technologies.

The primary role of bioethics is to identify and describe the often hidden presuppositions and prejudices about values which influence decisions regarding appropriate medical care. For example, whether a senior citizen in the early stages of Alzheimer's disease should be operated on for a hip replacement raises questions about the desires of the patient, the attitudes of care-givers and the best use of scarce medical resources. Once the sources of value conflicts are brought to light, bioethics can help to balance conflicting values or at least to determine what to do when compromise is impossible. In situations where agreement cannot be reached at the patient's bedside, many institutions have developed mechanisms for resolution of conflicts, such as a clinical ethics committee or consultation service. Finally, over and above its value for particular medical cases and policies, bioethics has an important educational function for health care professionals, policy makers and the general public. This function is exercised in a wide variety of ways, including formal courses, lectures and conferences, books and articles and radio and television programs.

As its name indicates, bioethics is an interdisciplinary field which requires the participation of experts in both ethics and biomedicine. The latter include medical and life scientists; physicians, nurses and other clinicians; and health care administrators and public policy officials. Other participants in the field include members of the legal profession, social scientists, representatives of citizens groups, and perhaps the most important category of all, patients and their family members. The interaction of this expertise and experience takes many different forms, such as a solitary author reading the works of experts in the field and using them to formulate a new position on some problem, or an hospital ethics committee discussing a problematic case from many different perspectives and coming to a consensus about what should be done.

As a relatively new field, bioethics is characterized by a great diversity of opinion on almost every issue. Those who look to ethics for the definitive word on whether a proposed action is right or wrong are disappointed by this diversity. Other regard it as a sign of vitality, in that practitioners in this field are keenly interested in developing and testing new approaches. Another major challenge for bioethics arises out of the vast extent and complexity of modern health care. Bioethicists have responded to this challenge in part by moving beyond their preoccupation with certain stock issues (abortion, euthanasia, informed consent, confidentiality, etc.) to explore many other problems in clinical practice, experimentation on human subjects and animals, and the development and implementation of health policies at the institutional, provincial, national and international levels.

Much of this work has just begun, and there are other areas which bioethics has hardly touched. Furthermore, most of the recent work in this field has been conducted with little awareness of the cultural diversity of the participants in the health care field, especially patients. The remainder of this chapter will describe the ill effects of bioethics' neglect of multiculturalism and will show how they can be overcome.

ETHICS IN CROSS-CULTURAL HEALTH

Thanks to the rapid diffusion of modern medical technology, high-quality health care is available in almost every country, at least to those who can afford it. The ethical problems which follow from the use of this technology have provided the substance of bioethical reflection and action in North America, Europe and, to a lesser extent, in certain other countries. Up to now, most of this work has reflected a monocultural perspective on both health care and ethics. If bioethics is to be of service to members of different cultural groups, it will have to develop a much greater sensitivity to the realities of cross-cultural health.

The origin of bioethics' monoculturalism is relatively easy to explain. Bioethics began in the United States, the home of the "melting pot" ideology. Although many of the pioneers in the field during the 1960s and 1970s were religious scholars who were well aware of different value systems (Walters, 1985), bioethics soon became dominated by secular philosophers who favoured a uniform, rational approach to the subject, one in which cultural and religious variations have no validity (Toulmin, 1982). The competent, rational, individual adult became the norm for ethical decision making, and all were expected to fulfil this norm or else be subject to other, equally rational, procedures (such as court orders).

In recent years there has been a growing recognition that this approach to bioethics is inadequate. Philosophers such as Alasdair MacIntyre (1984, 1988) have argued that secular liberalism is just one culture among others, and not what it proclaims itself to be—the universal, rational foundation of all cultures. Speakers at a conference on "Transcultural Dimensions of Medical Ethics" in Washington, DC (26-27 April, 1990) demonstrated that the dominant North American approach to bioethics, especially its emphasis on the autonomous individual in medical decision making, is actually a minority position within the global community (see also Fox and Swazey 1984; Veatch 1988, 1989). Even in North America, the dominant position, despite being incorporated into medical practice and the law, does not do justice to the cultural values of minority groups: the First Nations, Afro-Americans and more recent groups of immigrants.

The importance of cultural factors for bioethics can be seen from a brief examination of three of the major recurrent ethical issues in contemporary health care: informed consent, telling the truth to terminally ill patients and withholding/withdrawing life-sustaining treatment.

Informed Consent

In Canada and the United States there has developed over the past 20 years a legal and ethical consensus on the right of individuals to make decisions about their medical treatment (Faden and Beauchamp 1986). The traditional approach of medical "paternalism," whereby physicians made all such decisions and often did not tell patients what was being done to them, has been thoroughly discredited. The ethical principle which paternalism was supposed to reflect, namely "beneficence" (acting in the best interests of the patient) is now subordinated to the principle of "autonomy," which entails the right of individuals to make their own medical decisions, based on all available information about different treatment options.

This doctrine of informed consent is based on an understanding of human beings as competent, rational and autonomous decision-makers. For those patients who do not meet these criteria, such as infants, those who suffer from serious mental illness and unconscious and severely demented patients, other procedures for medical decision making must be implemented. But even for normal adults the ideal of informed consent may be difficult to achieve. It is not surprising, then, that this doctrine encounters particular difficulty in cross-cultural health care.

We need to be very careful when making general statements about different cultures. Nevertheless, it can safely be said that many cultures are less individualistic than the one which prevails in North American. The family, the clan or the nation count for more than the individual, and decision-making authority about such matters as one's medical treatment may well be someone else's prerogative—a parent, spouse, elder or health professional. In many cultures medical paternalism is the morally correct way to make treatment decisions, and other approaches are simply wrong.

These different concepts of medical decision making can give rise to clashes throughout the health care system. Just one example will have to suffice here. In a major Canadian city with a large immigrant population, both public and private family planning programs have a policy of distributing contraceptives to all clients who seek them, regardless of age or marital status. Neither program inquires whether married women using the clinics have the consent of their husbands. Some ethnic leaders charge that this practice is, in their society, an open invitation to infidelity. They believe that there has in fact been a notable rise in adultery since the programs were initiated. They want the clinics to require spousal consent before dispensing contraceptives. Spokespersons for both programs defend their policies on the grounds that it is their task to prevent unwanted births, and that they are not moral police officers. They also point out that the World Population Plan of Action states that individuals have the right to the means for determining the number of, and spacing of, their children. The question which this case raises is to what extent is informed consent (in this instance, freedom of contraceptive choice) a higher priority value than ethnic social and religious traditions and beliefs with respect to sexual behaviour.[1]

Telling the Truth to Terminally Ill Patients

In order for informed consent to be operative, subjects must have access to all the necessary information to make appropriate health care decisions. In practice this means that their

---

[1]This case is adapted from Levine and Veatch (1982).

physicians must tell them the truth about their diagnosis and prognosis. In the same way as the patient's decision making prerogative was traditionally overridden by medical paternalism, the patient's right to be told the truth has generally been subject to the physician's "therapeutic privilege." This expression refers to the legal doctrine that physicians may justifiably withhold information from patients if they reasonably believe this information would not be in the patients' best interests or would interfere with treatment and care.

Although therapeutic privilege is still practised today in countries such as Canada (for example, in giving placebos to hypochondriacs), its scope is far more limited than in previous times. Until quite recently it was unusual for patients to be told by a physician that they were suffering from a terminal illness such as cancer (Oken, 1961). It was felt that such knowledge would spoil the remaining days of the patients and might even cause them to commit suicide.

Another reason for physicians to withhold information from patients, one which is still operative in certain cultures, is the desire to preserve the traditional physician-patient relationship. It is felt that the therapeutic bond between these two parties depends in large measure on the confidence the patient has in the physician's knowledge and ability. If physicians were to admit that they do not know the best treatment for the patient, or worse still, that they can do nothing more to help the patient, it is likely that the patient's hope for recovery would be destroyed.

What should a nurse or doctor in a Canadian hospital say to a Chinese or Japanese patient who is dying from cancer? Ethics, law and hospital policy may all require that patients be fully informed about their condition, and that others be told only with the patient's permission. However, the patient's family may insist that the truth not be revealed, since it would have a terrible effect on the physical and mental well-being of the patient. For members of the dominant North American culture, who have come to expect the truth about their condition, no matter how negative, such family pleadings can generally be disregarded. Is it right to do so for other cultural groups?

Withholding/Withdrawing Life-Sustaining Treatment

For most of medical history, neither physicians nor patients had very much control over the duration of life. Medical, surgical and other forms of treatment were relatively limited, both in quantity and in efficacy. Life expectancy was short, and infectious diseases were often fatal.

All this has changed in the 20th century. With the development of antibiotics and other "wonder" drugs, and advances in surgical techniques and medical technology, both the quantity and the quality of life has been greatly enhanced. However, the application of these life-preserving measures is not always an unqualified good. Many individuals whose lives have been saved by these innovations wish that they had been allowed to die, and others attempt to ensure that when the time comes, they will not be kept alive at what they consider to be an unacceptable quality of life.

In the Western medical tradition, physicians have had an almost absolute duty to preserve life. At first, modern medical technology and drugs seemed to be a great help in achieving this goal. However, when physicians saw that the extra days, months and years of numerous severely deformed newborns and demented elderly persons resulted only in prolonging suffering, they began to rethink this commitment to life at all costs. At the same time, a powerful "right to die" movement used the doctrine of informed consent to enable individuals to refuse life-sustaining treatment either directly or through devices such as the "living will."

At present, Canadian and American law generally recognize the right of competent persons to refuse life-sustaining treatment, and most jurisdictions have procedures which allow such treatment to be withheld or withdrawn from incompetent patients. When to exercise this prerogative is, however, a major issue for bioethics. A considerable literature has developed on the difference between "killing" and "letting die," the appropriate use of "do not resuscitate" orders and other related topics.

The acceptability of withholding or withdrawing life-sustaining medical treatment differs from one culture to another. In the Jewish tradition there is a very strong commitment to preserving life as long as possible, no matter what its quality. According to this view, it is wrong to refuse any treatment which has a good possibility of extending life. Other religious groups not only do not require all such treatments, but actually forbid some of them. Jehovah's Witnesses, for example, are required to refuse blood transfusion even if death will be the result. Needless to say, a knowledge of the patient's views on this matter is of decisive importance when life and death decisions have to be made.

FINDING SOLUTIONS

Apart from the case of Jehovah's Witnesses, which has been the subject of much legal and ethical discussion during the past 20 years, the above-mentioned ethical problems in cross-cultural health care have no clear-cut solutions. To date bioethics has not developed a sensitivity to the cultural dimensions of the issues which it treats. Given the multicultural reality of Canadian society, however, especially in the larger cities, it is high time to develop a cross-cultural bioethics. This will require the contributions of the academic disciplines which deal with cultural matters, especially medical and cultural anthropology and religious studies.

Anthropology

The ultimate aim of bioethics is to determine what ought to be done for patients. One important factor in this process is their physical and/or mental condition. There are some significant biological variations among races which need to be known when determining treatment options (Masi, 1989, 69-71). However, by far the greater source of variation among patients is due to cultural factors. For knowledge of these factors, we turn to medical and cultural anthropology.

Masi (1988, 1989) has provided a useful overview of the principal cultural elements in health and illness. These include beliefs about the natural environment, the relation of human beings to the environment (e.g., good health as a balance of hot and cold or Yin and Yang properties), and the interrelation of physical, mental and spiritual aspects of the human person; interpretations of symptoms of ill health; and appropriate remedies for various types of sickness. Specific examples of these factors will be found in other chapters of this book.

A cross-cultural bioethics must incorporate an understanding of the cultural diversity of patients and must tailor health care policies and practices to the specific requirements of a multicultural clientele. A basic requirement for such understanding is adequate communication between patients and caregivers, which will in many cases depend on greatly improved translation services. Respect for the patient entails as well the maintenance of confidentiality and the provision of the same level of health care services as is available to all other individuals.

Religious Studies

In Western scientific-technological culture, religion has been marginalized. Health and illness are explained in a purely naturalistic and materialistic fashion; the only important question is **how** disease operates and can be overcome, not **why** it happens. The latter is a matter for inconclusive speculation, and can be safely left to religion.

In most other cultures, religion deals as much with the how as with the why of health and illness (Numbers & Amundsen, 1986; Sullivan, 1989). Disease is likely to be caused by offending against a god or supernatural spirit, another person or animal, or the tribe. It may also result from the malevolent intentions of another, for example by means of voodoo or the "evil eye." Preservation and restoration of good health often requires the services of religious authorities, the invocation of a god or spirit and a change in behaviour.

Although anthropologists deal with religion as part of their cultural studies, their work needs to be supplemented by that of religious specialists. The latter delve into all aspects of the teachings and practices of religions in areas such as health: their history, scriptures, organizational structures, rituals and ethics. Together, these people provide a comprehensive view of how and why members of different religious groups act as they do.

One branch of religious studies is particularly important for the development of a cross-cultural health care ethics, namely comparative religious ethics. Since the publication of *Comparative Religious Ethics* by Little and Twiss in 1978, this field of study has undergone considerable advancement in its methodology and its application to numerous topics in ethical foundations and in personal and social ethics. Like bioethics, it is an interdisciplinary endeavour. Two of its leading exponents explain its components and *modus operandi* thus: "Anthropologists, cultural historians, and historians of religion make a tradition available for comparative study by detailing the modes in which its moral beliefs may be expressed (legal codes, wisdom literature, ritual actions, etc.), relating these modes of expression to other aspects of the tradition's view of the world and identifying the typical moves by which problems of choice and action are resolved in the context of the whole system of factual and moral beliefs" (Lovin & Reynolds, 1985, 4). As so described, the work of religious ethicists constitutes a useful, even essential, element of cross-cultural bioethics.

SKILLS DEVELOPMENT

This chapter has argued the need to develop a cross-cultural bioethics and has indicated some of the features which it should incorporate. However, those involved in cross-cultural health care delivery cannot wait for bioethics to complete this work; they face major ethical problems right now. They need to know how they can equip themselves to deal with such issues.

The basic features of cross-cultural health education are dealt with elsewhere in this book. What follow are suggestions for incorporating ethical concerns in this education, and for ensuring that cross-cultural concerns are included in the teaching of bioethics. Due to space limitations, these suggestions will be of a general nature, applicable to all health professions.

Basic Formation

For several years now, training in ethics has been an integral part of the undergraduate educational programs of all health professions, although not in every school or faculty (Williams, 1986). Students are introduced to this subject in a variety of ways: full courses in ethics; some ethics instruction as part of a more comprehensive course (e.g., "Medicine and Society" or "Issues in Professional Nursing and Health Care") and special lectures or rounds.

Due to timetable, personnel and other restraints, this ethics instruction seldom provides students with more than a minimal exposure to the field. Thus it may seem utopian to expect that the cross-cultural dimensions of health care be addressed along with everything else. However, if it is realised that cross-cultural bioethics does not treat any additional problems but rather the same problems in different (cultural) contexts, then the challenge of including this dimension within the current ethics programs becomes much less formidable. Another way of promoting cross-cultural ethics in the curriculum is to ensure that ethical concerns are introduced into the programs of cross-cultural education, training and communication.

The means to be employed in incorporating cultural factors into bioethics instruction include the following: selection of issues and examples which illustrate cultural concerns in health care (such as those listed above), incorporation of anthropological and religious studies titles in course readings and bibliographies, and encouragement of students and professors to discuss the influence of their culture on their approach to health care. As the student body and professorate become more multicultural, health care education, including ethics, should naturally develop a more cross-cultural character.

Post-graduate Training

Whereas undergraduate programs should provide a basic exposure to cross-cultural bioethics, there is a further need for advanced training in this field to prepare educators, administrators and policy makers to recognize and deal with the specific ethical problems of cultural communities. Unfortunately, there are very few graduate programs in bioethics in Canada, especially in the health professional faculties. Likewise, there are few, if any, graduate programs in cross-cultural health care which include a focus on ethics. Those who wish to specialize in bioethics generally have recourse to advanced degree programs in philosophy or religious studies or else turn to more professionally oriented programs in other countries.

A cross-cultural bioethics degree program, were it to be established, would require expertise in medical and cultural anthropology and religious studies along with the usual components of bioethics: the health sciences, law and ethics. Such a program could serve as an important link between the fields of cross-cultural health care and bioethics, to the mutual enrichment of both.

Continuing Education

Continuing education programs, such as conferences and workshops, offer the best opportunity for practising health professionals to become skilled in dealing with cross-cultural bioethical problems. They can be organized much more easily than formal courses and degree programs, and they require considerably less time and effort from participants.

The ideal type of conference or workshop for this purpose is one devoted exclusively to cross-cultural health care ethics. Examples of this approach are the aforementioned Washington conference on "Transcultural Dimensions of Medical Ethics" and a November 1989 workshop entitled "Between Two Worlds" Ethical Issues in Intercultural Health Care," organized by the Center for Bioethics, Clinical Research Institute of Montreal. Another way of dealing with this topic is to include a discussion of ethical issues as part of a program on cross-cultural health care; this approach was followed at the "Multicultural Health Symposium" in Richmond, British Columbia in February 1989 and at a conference on "Health Care and Multiculturalism" in Toronto the following month.

Finally, cultural issues in health care can and should be discussed in conferences and workshops on bioethics.

CONCLUSION

Despite the growing awareness of ethical issues in health care and the necessity of a systematic approach for dealing with these issues, the field of bioethics is still struggling for its place in the health care system. All too often, technological, economic and bureaucratic considerations prevail when decisions have to be made about the care of individual patients, hospital policies, or government priorities in health care. The situation of bioethics in this regard is similar to that of cross-cultural health, which likewise has an active and growing constituency but is still somewhat marginal to the main concerns of the system.

This mutual lack of status can be overcome to a certain extent by greater cooperation between the bioethics and the cross-cultural health communities. This chapter has argued that these two groups have much in common, and indeed the work of each is incomplete without the other. By combining their efforts whenever possible, they may ensure that the concerns of each group will find the recognition and support which they need and deserve.

REFERENCES

Brown, R.M., & Brown, S.T. (Eds.). (1989). *A Cry for Justice*: The Churches and Synagogues Speak. New York: Paulist Press.

Faden, R., & Beauchamp, T. (1986). *A History and Theory of Informed Consent*. New York: Oxford University Press.

Fox, R.C., & J.P. Swazey. (1984). Medical Morality is not Bioethics-Medical Ethics in China and the United States. *Perspectives in Biology and Medicine, 27*(3), 336-60.

Levine, C., & Veatch, R.M. (Eds.). (1982). *Cases in Bioethics*. Hastings-on-Hudson, New York: The Hastings Center.

Little, D., & Twiss, S.B. (1978). *Comparative Religious Ethics*. New York: Harper & Row.

Lovin, R.W., & Reynolds, F.E. (Eds.). (1985). *Cosmogony and Ethical Order: New Studies in Comparative Ethics*. Chicago: University of Chicago Press.

MacIntyre, A. (1984). *After Virtue*. Notre Dame, Indiana: University of Notre Dame Press.

— —. (1988). *Whose Justice? Which Rationality?* Notre Dame, Indiana: University of Notre Dame Press.

Masi, R. (1988). Multiculturalism, Medicine and Health Parts I-III. *Canadian Family Physician, 34*, 2173-8; 2429-34; 2649-53.

— —. (1989). Multiculturalism, Medicine and Health Parts IV-VI. *Canadian Family Physician, 35*, 69-73; 251-4; 537-9.

Numbers, R.L., & Amundsen, D.W. (Eds.). (1986). *Caring and Curing: Health and Medicine in the Western Religious Traditions*. New York: Macmillan.

Oken, D. (1961). What to Tell Cancer Patients: A Study of Medical Attitudes. *Journal of the American Medical Association, 175*, 1, 120-28.

Sullivan, L.E. (Ed.). (1989). *Healing and Restoring: Health and Medicine in the World's Religious Traditions*. New York: Macmillan.

Tiger, L. (1987). *The Manufacture of Evil: Ethics, Evolution and the Industrial System*. New York: Harper & Row.

Toulmin, S. (1982). How Medicine Saved the Life of Ethics. *Perspectives in Biology and Medicine, 25*(4), 736-50.

Veatch, R.M. (Ed.). (1988). Comparative Medical Ethics. *The Journal of Medicine and Philosophy, 13*(3).

— —. (1989). *Cross Cultural Perspectives in Medical Ethics: Readings*. Boston: Jones and Bartlett.

Walters, L. (1985). Religion and the Renaissance of Medical Ethics in the United States: 1965-1975. In E.E. Shelp (Ed.) *Theology and Bioethics: Exploring the Foundations and Frontiers* (3-16). Dordrecht/Boston/Lancaster/Tokyo: D. Reidel.

Williams, J.R. (Ed.). (1984). *Canadian Churches and Social Justice*. Toronto: Anglican Book Centre and James Lorimer.

Williams, J.R. (1986). *Biomedical Ethics in Canada*. Queenston, Ontario: Edwin Mellen.

- 17 -

Cancer and Cultural Attitudes

Marion Poliakoff

Unless it has been displaced by AIDS, cancer is probably today's most feared disease. People often fear the word itself and try to avoid it. In *Illness As Metaphor*, Susan Sontag (1978) maintains that, like tuberculosis (TB) before it, cancer has taken on metaphorical attributes. She points out that because it is not understood, cancer is feared, and given its own mythology, which is expressed in the history of many cultures. Sontag relates how we project feelings of evil onto cancer and use such punitive words to describe it as a "killer disease" and "shameful" illness (ibid., 57).

Educational efforts by cancer agencies in Canada, the United States and other countries to counter such beliefs have made some progress. However, reports by health professionals indicate negligible impact on many cancer patients and families, particularly those from non-Western backgrounds. Because of this extra dimension or emotional overlay that exists with cancer, it is particularly important for health professionals and other involved in the care of cancer patients to be familiar with the emotions and beliefs that can influence the treatment compliance and coping skills of patients with varying ethnocultural origins.

How many people are we talking about? The most recent figures from the Canadian Cancer Society (National Cancer Institute of Canada, 1990) tell us that the incidence of all cancer in males is increasing at a rate of just over 1 percent per year, and just under that in females. In 1992 there were expected to be 115,000 Canadians faced with the diagnosis of cancer, bringing the total number of Canadians receiving medical care for cancer to approximately 315,000. Mortality from many types of cancer is declining, but the disease is still the second leading cause of death in Canada and the United States.

There are no figures available that identify cancer patients throughout Canada by ethnic background. We do know from Statistics Canada, however, that there are more than 100 distinct ethnic and cultural communities in this nation (Statistics Canada, 1989b, 35). We also know that the pattern of immigration has been changing, with an increasing proportion of new Canadians arriving from Asian rather than from European countries. We also have more immigrants with Caribbean and African origins (ibid, 7).

With these trends in mind, we can make some estimates based on an attempt at data collection by the British Columbia Cancer Agency (BCCA) - Vancouver Clinic. Of new patients identifying their ethnic group in 1986, about 3 percent were Chinese and an additional three percent were from other Asian backgrounds (Japanese, Indo-Pakistani, Vietnamese, Filipino). Because of changing immigration patterns, we can estimate that approximately nine percent of new cancer patients in Vancouver in 1992 had non-European backgrounds and that number will continue to increase in future years. Another group with European roots is likely to be influenced by attitudes and beliefs prevalent in their countries of origin. How will all these patients and their families react to this dread diagnosis?

Although we are learning more and more about cultural attitudes and beliefs related to disease and illness in general, there is little in the literature on the particular subject of cancer. It is possible to develop a worthwhile body of knowledge, nevertheless, by extrapolating from general writings on multicultural health to key elements of cancer care. In addition, the material included here is based on information from interviews with cancer patients and health professionals over the past several years, particularly at the BCCA in Vancouver. The areas we will explore include disclosure of the diagnosis and prognosis, use of interpreters, pain reactions, food beliefs, blood tests, beliefs about contagion, attitudes toward death and bereavement, and prevention and compliance.

DISCLOSURE OF DIAGNOSIS

Whatever their cultural background, most people who go for medical help expect to get a diagnosis that explains why they are feeling ill. They also hope that a treatment program will be prescribed that will bring them relief. When the diagnosis is cancer, however, there seems to be a common practice outside of North America to conceal that information. The long-held belief that cancer is inevitably fatal contributes to this conspiracy of silence between physicians, patients and their families.

"You have a tumour and we will try to get rid of it," is one of the euphemisms often used. Patients will lose hope and may even refuse treatment if they are told they have cancer, some doctors fear. An example is given of a chief surgeon in the former Soviet Union who developed lung cancer. In keeping with the Soviet practice of not telling patients their diagnosis when it is cancer, the colleagues of this surgeon kept two patient histories—a false one to give to the surgeon when he asked to see his records, and an accurate one for the hospital. When the surgeon asked to see his chest x-rays, he was given someone else's!

Most North American cancer specialists, on the other hand, are convinced that it is better to tell the true diagnosis to the patient. One doctor who had originally been an oncologist in an Eastern European country spoke about the difficulty that he had had in sharing the cancer diagnosis with patients when he first came to Canada. Now he is one of the many cancer specialists who believe in full disclosure, so that all concerned can mobilize their energies to fight the disease.

This attitude is born out by slowly changing attitudes in France. The head nurse in an oncology unit of a French hospital writes that "the majority of physicians and surgeons refuse to disclose the truth, sometimes even to the patient's family, and it follows that they never recommend relevant postoperative treatment which could, in any case, change the prognostic outlook" (Adonis, 1978, 113). She adds that her medical team is moving increasingly toward disclosure in the belief that "patients who know what they are fighting for have a better chance of being successful thanks to modern therapeutic advances" (ibid.).

In the Chinese culture, as well as in others, the family members may be concerned about more than the loss of hope. Many Chinese as well as those from other cultures, believe that cancer is a punishment for some "sin" or evil act committed by the patient, or even by a member of the patient's family. A cancer diagnosis could bring shame or ridicule to the family, or they could be ostracized by their entire community.

In a recent study of the needs of ethnic Chinese cancer patients in Vancouver (Ho, 1990), 14 family doctors of Chinese origin were interviewed. They agreed that a major problem for them was that family members of elderly patients often requested that the doctor not inform the patient of the diagnosis. "The doctors would normally comply but the families would be explained the pros and cons of so doing and the rights of the patients and let them decide what to do," (ibid., 37).

In the Ho study, one elderly male patient reported that he suspected that he was not getting all the information about his disease or treatment, but he could not ask. When he was referred to the BCCA, "the doctor pushed his grandchild (who was acting as interpreter) to disclose the information to him." The report states that the patient appreciated the protectiveness of his family, but wanted to know the prognosis "so that he could plan to live out the rest of his life. He was grateful to the doctor who asked his grandchild to let him know about his disease." (ibid., 40)

The Ho study also revealed the frustrations of doctors at the BCCA who believed that the patients should have the right to know their disease and make decisions about their treatment plans. The doctors were also concerned that if the patients did not know the details of their disease and proposed treatment, they could not really give informed consent, which created an ethical dilemma. In addition to the possible impact on treatment, practical disadvantages can result from concealing a cancer diagnosis, as the following case illustrates.

Mrs. L. was a thirty-two-year-old woman of Chinese origin with a recurrence of breast cancer. The social worker informed Mrs. L. that she was eligible for Unemployment Insurance sick benefits because she was unable to work during the course of her treatments, but the patient stated that she was "ashamed" to let her employer or co-workers know why she could not work. She and her husband also did not want the children's school nurse informed of the diagnosis. Continual understanding support for the family by the "Anglo" social worker, plus the efforts of a Chinese-speaking male Home Care nurse who was able to increase the husband's acceptance of the situation, eventually resulted in a successful resolution of the problems. The patient expressed her surprise at how supportive her employer and co-workers were.

Another example is that of a thirty-three-year-old East Indian male, born in Uganda, whose leukemia had been in remission for some time. For several years Mr. P. would not join the medical and dental plans at his work place because of his feelings of shame and disgrace. When he eventually did share his medical history with his employer, he also expressed to the social worker his surprise and pleasure at the understanding and sympathy he received.

This same social worker was not as successful in convincing a forty-six-year-old woman from the Philippines to share her breast cancer diagnosis with the female tenants in her basement suite who could have provided babysitting when Mrs. A. went for treatments. She also would not accept rides in a patient services van because the name of the cancer agency was on it. In this instance, the social worker supported the patient's concerns by arranging for her treatment at times when her husband had finished work and could take her to the clinic and care for the children.

Francis (1986) emphasizes the added stress on families when they are told that a loved one is dying, but either choose or are asked by the doctor not to share the information with the patient. Her study and others found that concealing information created a barrier between the patient and the family because communications had to be so guarded.

These examples, and many like them, have a common denominator: lack of education about cancer increases the likelihood that cultural myths and biases will interfere with the best medical care and the benefits of other supports. Nevertheless, these are deeply held beliefs and it seems incumbent on doctors and other health professionals to deal with them as sensitively and constructively as possible.

INTERPRETER PROBLEMS

Many studies emphasize the difficulties that medical personnel and patients encounter because they do not speak the same language. Although this is a general concern, cultural biases about cancer can deepen the problem. They can also place a heavy emotional burden on the person doing the interpreting.

In the Ho study, staff members at the BCCA who were used frequently to interpret for Chinese patients talked about their discomfort in passing on "bad news" to the patient or family. (Ho, 1990, 33) They were also unhappy about the time pressures when they were called away from their own professional responsibilities. The dilemma is that in many hospitals and treatment centres, doctors prefer to use medically trained staff members as interpreters, rather than family members or even interpreters from a community agency. Doctors are concerned that when family members are involved, they cannot clearly pass on vital information because of lack of familiarity with medical terminology. In addition, they may "screen" the information in a desire to "protect" the patient.

In research for her MSW thesis, for example, Lai (1990) learned from three breast cancer patients about their dissatisfaction with the translations provided by their husbands. They felt that since what the husbands told them was so much briefer than the doctor's remarks, a significant part of the information must have been left out. This increased their anxiety (ibid., 53).

Even experienced interpreters from community agencies have difficulty explaining the reasons for the many tests that cancer patients may require, let alone the pros and cons of radiation, chemotherapy and surgery. Confidentiality is something else that bothers medical staff, as well as patients and their families. Even though interpreters may be well trained, families may be reluctant to use community interpreters because of the worry that the information will reach the broader community.

"Culturally my people are not ready to share. They know there can be a lot of gossip," commented a psychologist of Greek background (personal communication, September, 1988). This concern about "community gossip" was also expressed to researchers in a study at the University of British Columbia School of Nursing (Anderson & Lynam, 1988). There can also be political, religious or class divisions within an ethnic group that make using community interpreters a delicate business.

This problem is illustrated by the experience of a San Diego research group. When they used a bicultural, bilingual psychologist "who happened to be from a relatively well-to-do Mexican family" to interview families who had come from Mexico for cancer treatment, people were ill at ease. When they switched to using an interviewer who was an older woman with little education and who had lost a husband and a son to cancer, the discussion of feelings and concerns was much more open (Spinetta, 1984, 2330).

With so many factors to consider, the provision of suitable interpreter services for cancer patients and their families has no simple solution. Most institutions would find it too costly to employ a team of trained interpreters. Some of the options recommended in the Ho study could have application beyond the target group of that study, such as making sure that only those staff members at ease with interpreting are on the volunteer interpreter list, rather than including everyone with special language capabilities; and providing training about cancer and medical terminology to interpreters from community agencies. Also, professional organizations of translators and interpreters could be enlisted to help find appropriate solutions to overcoming language barriers to effective treatment of cancer patients.

COPING WITH PAIN

We know that severe pain can accompany certain stages of cancer. In fact, it is fear of such pain that contributes to cancer being such a dreaded disease. We need to pay special attention, therefore, to how patients of different cultural backgrounds are likely to respond to pain. Granted, even members of the same family can have different pain thresholds. However, many studies verify that different ethnic groups apparently have dissimilar patterns of response to pain.

In a classic study, Zborowski (1952) found that persons of Italian and Jewish backgrounds displayed greater sensitivity to pain and expressed it more openly than "old Americans" (i.e., those of English background). The latter's chief concern was that they would be pitied, which helped motivate them to keep that "stiff upper lip." Another study in the United States that compared persons of Italian and Irish origins with the same illness found that the Irish denied pain more while the Italians coped by dramatizing their pain (Spector, 1979).

A study in a Hawaiian nursing facility compared patients of Caucasian, Chinese, Filipino, Hawaiian and Japanese backgrounds. A much smaller percentage of the Chinese, Japanese and Filipinos made demands on the staff, cried or requested medication than did the Caucasians and Hawaiians (Lister, 1977, 220).

Health professionals in Canada report that Native Indian, as well as Chinese, Vietnamese and Japanese cancer patients tend to be stoical about pain. In fact, hospital nurses writing about cancer often stress the importance of paying special attention to

the need for pain control for patients with these cultural backgrounds, as the need may be there but not be apparent (Francis,
1986). Others have pointed to the pressure to be a "good patient," especially when there is a language barrier and a hospital
patient may already feel "at the mercy" of the nurses and doctors
(Phung Pham in Wong, 1989). As well, when a patient's greatest
desire is to go home from the hospital, he or she may be less
likely to communicate pain (Stevenson in Victoria Cancer Clinic,
1990).

Another problem is the reluctance within some cultural groups
to use pain medications. The Chinese are one such group.
According to Chinese-Canadian professionals, there are two
reasons for this: a fear of being out of control; and a belief that
pain killers cause a person to sweat and that this loss of body
fluid induces weakness.

Patients of the Hindu faith who know that they are facing
death also prefer to be clear-headed rather than sedated
(Swerdlow and Stjernsward, 1982). Although they make a strong
case for better management of cancer pain with all the modern
remedies available, these authors also stress the importance of
traditional cultural and religious supports for some patients.
"We must be careful not to remove this support, but instead
supplement it with effective analgesic therapy when such native
healing is inadequate," they state (ibid., 327).

Francis (1986) emphasizes the advantages of determining the
cancer patient's religious and cultural beliefs. In a series of
interviews she carried out with Hindu patients in New Delhi,
she found a "quiet acceptance of pain" that she associated with
their belief in karma, that is, that all experience results from
previous actions and that illness and disease is a result of
negative behaviour in this or a past life. However, Francis
reasons, since the philosophy of karma encourages the pursuit
of a better life, "the relief of pain is not in contradiction to the
belief in karma" (ibid., 169).

Obviously it takes much time and patience to bridge the gap
between traditional beliefs and modern medicine but efforts of
this kind are surely worthwhile because of their potential to
bring substantial relief to suffering cancer patients. At the same
time, hospital staff need to be sensitive to the fact that outcries
of some patients can be as much a cultural expression, as a
reflection of the degree of discomfort that they are experiencing.
A typical example was the case of the East Indian woman in the
BCCA hospital unit in Vancouver who was constantly moaning

and unduly disturbing other patients. When the nurses learned in a case conference that she was expressing her distress as custom demanded, they were able to enlist the help of appropriate family members in modifying her behaviour.

BELIEFS ABOUT FOOD

The healing qualities of chicken soup as extolled by traditional Jewish women have attained near mythic proportions. Such a product is actually sold in at least one major treatment centre in New York City! While this may be "tongue in cheek," it is an example of how strong folklore about food can become in relation to health and illness.

For cancer patients with roots in Asian and Hispanic cultures in particular, beliefs related to food can have a major impact. The basis of these beliefs is the concepts that the forces of yin (negative) and yang (positive) in the human body must be in harmonious balance to maintain health. Foods are classified as "hot" or "cold," and are used to contribute to that balance (Lai & Yue, 1990, 78). In other words, if a disease is thought of as "yin" or "hot," it would be deemed essential to use "yang" or "cold" foods to ensure a change from illness to good health.

There does not seem to be one universal classification system, but the consensus seems to be that gallbladder, stomach, intestine, bladder and lymph systems are considered "yang" or "hot," while the liver, heart, spleen, lungs and kidney are "yin" or "cold" (Spector, 1979). It is also important to understand that "hot" and "cold" does not refer to the temperature of the food, but to the traditional classification in a particular culture. This can vary even within the same country. Here is one description from a community in India. "Most foods with a pungent, acidic or salty taste were considered 'hot,' and foods with a sweet, astringent or bitter taste were 'cold,' (Storer, 1997 in Sampson, 1982, 28). In the Iranian culture, foods such as honey, sugar and nuts are considered "hot," while yogurt, berries and watermelon are considered "cold," (Behjati-Sabet, 1990, 105). The Vietnamese consider meat, fish sauce, sweets, coffee, spices, garlic, ginger and onion to be "hot" foods, while most vegetables, fruit, potatoes, fish and duck are "cold" (ibid., 209). While dieticians and other health professionals need not have detailed knowledge about these varying classifications and their application, they should be familiar enough with the basic principles so they can take them into account when they are making recommendations for a patient who is not eating well.

A seventy-eight-year-old Chinese matriarch in an Ontario hospital refused to eat the Western food she was given. There was uncertainty about her medical diagnosis. Once it was established that she had lymphoma, the family could have her disease classified as "hot" or "cold" by a traditional herbalist and ensure that her food "fit" the desired balance.

It is also important to be aware that these same yin/yang-hot/cold principles apply to medications. Because most Western medications are considered "hot," for example, a patient with an illness that is considered "hot" may not follow through on the prescribed treatment, or may reduce the dosage. There can be other reasons for noncompliance (the medication or treatment might be stopped prematurely because the symptoms have abated), but the principles discussed above are often behind the decisions of patients or the family members responsible for them.

There are also practical ways in which a health professional sensitive to such beliefs can help to remedy a serious situation. A case in point concerned a sixty-two-year-old refugee from Nicaragua who had been diagnosed with lymphoma. Mrs. M. and her two daughters were living in a one-room apartment and could not afford the "cold" foods that they considered appropriate to her illness, such as papayas. The BCCA social worker and dietician became aware of the problem and wrote the necessary letters so that the family could receive additional income for "dietary extras."

SIGNIFICANCE OF BLOOD

Frequent blood tests are often necessary for cancer patients in order to monitor the course of their disease and/or the effect of chemotherapy and other treatments. While the average patient may simply regard this as an uncomfortable nuisance, in some cultures the removal of even a small amount of blood is much more threatening.

The Vietnamese, for instance, "may fear and resist blood tests that require even small samples of blood, mainly because they believe that the body has a finite, irreplaceable amount of blood. Some may attribute symptoms such as headaches or weakness to the loss of blood during blood tests, even single tests done several years earlier" (Dinh et al, 1990, 203).

As well, patients of Cambodian, Laotian and Chinese background may refuse blood tests because they believe the loss of blood will weaken their bodies and even be life threatening (Richardson, 1990, 27; Lai & Yue, 1990, 84). In the Chinese culture, the loss of blood would be connected with the loss of "chi," which is thought of as a finite vital substance within the body that contains blood.

When such resistance to blood tests is encountered, careful explanations should be given and tests should be kept to a minimum. Sometimes a little "subterfuge" may be a useful compromise, particularly with elderly, uneducated patients. One doctor, for example, knowing that his elderly Chinese patient would not accept a physiological explanation, told him that he was very ill and that withdrawing some of the "bad blood" would help him get better. Some patients may be reassured if they are given a liquid to drink after a blood test, and a red drink such as cranberry juice might be particularly strengthening—to the spirit if not the body! (A.K.H.Ho, personal communication, January, 1991).

CONCERNS ABOUT CONTAGION

Patients and their families from varying backgrounds (including fifth-generation Canadians!) sometimes need reassurance that cancer is not contagious. Fear of contagion has become relatively uncommon because of the education programs of the Canadian Cancer Society. There is also increasing evidence that certain food patterns, lifestyles and environmental factors and/or gene patterns might explain why a particular family appears to be predisposed to cancer. Nevertheless, it seems more difficult to dispel the fear of contagion among members of some ethnic groups than among others, particularly the Chinese. In the Ho study (1990), 12 percent of those interviewed thought cancer was contagious.

Why should this be? One doctor of Asian descent speculated that it might stem from a confusion in the "old country" between TB, which is contagious, and lung cancer which is not, but exhibits some of the same symptoms. The importance of countering such beliefs, which can occur even with persons from a more educated background, is pointed up by this case related by a Vancouver doctor of Chinese origin (Dr. W.H.L., personal communication, 1983):

Mrs. L. was an elderly widow who came from Hong Kong to join her five children, all of whom had gone to university in Canada and were married. She had a cough when she came, but waited the three months for her medical card before going to a doctor. What she feared might be TB turned out to be lung cancer. Although she managed her surgery and chemotherapy well and the disease was in check, she remained severely depressed, attempted suicide and eventually starved herself to death. The problem was that her daughter-in-law with whom she lived believed her cancer was contagious and insisted on isolating her. She could no longer have contact with her grandchildren. She did not want to make trouble between her son and his wife or go to an extended care facility, and chose another solution.

While this may be an extreme case, there are many other cases where sexual relationships are ended between husband and wife because of fear of contagion, or a patient is no longer welcome at family social activities. In this latter instance, it is not necessarily the cancer per se that is feared, but that the "sick" person (who has probably not been told that he/she has cancer) will spread "bad luck" to other members of the family. The need to prevent such social isolation is self-evident. The challenge is to find effective ways to educate all the generations in a family. The Canadian Cancer Society, B.C. and Yukon Division, has made a commendable start through its Chinese Canadian Education Committee by providing brochures, pamphlets and videotapes on cancer and related issues.

DEATH AND BEREAVEMENT

While the mortality rate for many types of cancers is declining, the ratio of deaths to new cases in Canada was estimated at 51 percent in 1992, and the ratio was much higher for lung, stomach, brain, pancreas, ovary and leukemia (National Cancer

Institute, 1992). Obviously, health professionals working with cancer patients should be familiar with strongly held beliefs of their clients about death and bereavement. These often have a religious base.

Several publications provide detailed descriptions of the relevant beliefs of many cultural groups and religions, including Bradley et al, *Caring Across Cultures* (1988); sections on Death and Drying in each chapter of Waxler-Morrison (1990); and Henley (1979, 1983a, 1983b).

One attitude that stands out as being very different among ethnocultural groups is the choice of where to die. Doctors are frequently confronted with decisions about sending terminal cancer patients home to die, transferring them to a hospice or palliative-care bed, or keeping them in an acute-care hospital. It is important that health professionals understand the cultural reasons behind the request of patients and their families.

In the Chinese culture, for example, many people would consider it bad luck to have someone die at home. More specifically, there is the fear that a "yin" or negative spirit will remain to haunt the house, interfering with daily living. While the terminal patient of Chinese background may be reluctant to be admitted to a hospital, which would be considered almost synonymous with a "death sentence," the family may feel that such a move is essential. The sensitive doctor, visiting nurse or social worker involved in the case will have to assess which is the correct decision for the good of the patient, as well as being supportive of the family.

In contrast, older people of Vietnamese background believe it will bring bad luck to their children and grandchildren if they die away from home. They believe the soul "may get lost on the way home or on its journey to Nirvana" (Dinh et al., 1990, 201).

Indo-Canadians from various South Asian origins share a similar desire to die peacefully at home, attended by family members. One reason for this is that most of these people have religious rituals and actions that are prescribed for just before and just after death. For example, when the patient who is dying is Muslim, the patient is supposed to be turned on his or her side with the head slightly raised, and if possible, should face in the direction of the Central Mosque in Mecca (Bradley et al., 1988, 26). Muslims, Hindus and Sikhs all have rituals related to washing the body, and family members rather than staff should be allowed to do this if the patient dies in the hospital.

A belief that the wandering spirit of a dead person may cause difficulties for the living may be common among West Indians. They are more fearful of spirits when the death has been untimely, and a cancer death is often in this category. Family members may exhibit considerable grief at the death of a cancer patient, because they are more worried about the soul of that person than when there is a natural death, such as from old age (Glasgow & Adaskin, 1990, 241).

North American Native people are among those who may be more stoical and accepting in the face of death. Perhaps because of their traditional closeness to nature and their hunting and fishing background (Spector, 1979, 278), they may have experienced death in many forms at close range.

The examples used here merely highlight the variety of beliefs and behaviours that come into play at a most distressing time for patients and their families. Such examples are an indication of the need for anyone working with cancer patients, particularly in hospitals and palliative care centres, to become informed about the specific background of the client in order to provide appropriate support.

PREVENTION AND COMPLIANCE

In the 1990's, the concept of "prevention" in health care may finally be coming into its own. Rising health care costs are making it at least a topic of discussion in governmental financing circles. In cancer control it has long been a major focus, and a sizeable portion of the funds collected by the Canadian Cancer Society goes for public education. The evidence has been in for a long time that the incidence of some cancers can be radically reduced by changes in lifestyle such as cutting out smoking to reduce lung cancer—the number one cause of cancer deaths for men and the second leading cause for women. Equally important, many cancers can be cured if detected early enough.

This becomes an enormous challenge when discussing the relationship between cancer and cultural attitudes. It is those very attitudes that often result in patients seeking medical attention only when their cancers are already well advanced. Jones writes: "Disparities in knowledge, attitudes, and practices between minorities and non-minorities may explain the longer delay in seeking diagnosis and treatment among minorities, and thus the greater prevalence of more advanced cancers, and poorer survival" (1989, 4). The studies in this book deal with the four main racial/ethnic groups in the United States—Blacks, Hispanics, Asian/Pacific Islanders and Native Americans. One study by the American Cancer Society in 1985 found that Hispanics were less familiar with the warning signs of cancer than were persons in the general population; they were also less aware of available cancer-screening tests, less convinced of the effectiveness of cancer treatments.

Several other studies in Jones (1989) look at the higher overall age-adjusted incidence rates of cancer in Blacks as compared to Whites. Blacks tend to be less knowledgeable about cancer, underestimate its prevalence and the significance of the common warning signs, less aware of the benefits of screening and self-examination methods, and more fatalistic. "These pessimistic attitudes...influence medical care-seeking behaviour and could account in part for the delays of 3 to 6 months (Natarajan et al., 1985) in seeking diagnosis and treatment" according to Baquet, Clayton and Robinson (Jones, 1989, 71). A community-based preventive effort of Blacks in Nashville, Tennessee is described, aimed at decreasing cancer risks related to dietary and nutrition factors. This educational effort took the form of health fairs in four churches, and included materials related to hypertension and cardiovascular disease as well as cancer. This comprehensive approach, as well as the location of the fairs, was selected after careful study of how best to reach the target audience in view of the tendency of Blacks to avoid cancer-related programs (Hargreaves, 1989, 77ff).

A low level of compliance in relation to medication instructions has been a concern of health practitioners in general, and cancer health workers more specifically. Esparza writes that Hispanics who do not comply often believe that they are not capable of changing their destinies; moreover, they do not believe in the efficacy of the treatments (1989, 279-81). She also points out that some patients will stop taking medications in the mistaken belief that they are cured if symptoms are not present.

Villejo (in Jones, 1989, 295-300) describes the efforts of the Bilingual Information and Education Advisory Group at the M.D. Anderson Cancer Center, University of Texas, to meet the special needs of Spanish-speaking patients and family members. This group, formed in 1983, includes physicians, social workers, nurses, dietitians, interpreters, volunteer coordinators, and public and patient education specialists. Their task has been to evaluate and promote Spanish-language patient education activities and improved communication between health professionals and patients and their families. They have developed and conducted patient education classes in chemotherapy and central venous catheter care in Spanish, published dozens of printed and audiovisual materials in Spanish, helped select materials for a Health Information Center, established a Spanish-language student internship at a local university, and constructed Spanish-language bulletin boards in clinics and in the hospital to advertise the availability of Spanish-language resources. Follow-up evaluation with patients indicated that these efforts were well received and made them more confident about required self-care. In addition, these activities have encouraged the hospital administration to meet the special needs of the Spanish-speaking patients.

The information and efforts described above certainly have application in Canada. An example of a Canadian effort at prevention and improved compliance has followed from the Ho (1990) study, which documented the need for improved educational efforts aimed at the Chinese population in the Vancouver area. As a result an ethnic Chinese social worker was employed by the Canadian Cancer Society to work with a volunteer committee to develop more educational materials and programs in Chinese on the prevention and treatment of cancer. There is also liaison with Chinese community agencies to provide educational programs, as well as to recruit and train Chinese-speaking volunteers. Some of these volunteers have been trained to provide support visits to Chinese cancer patients; others answer the phones and respond to queries on a Chinese Cancer Information Line that operates out of the Canadian Cancer Society headquarters. It is to be hoped that such efforts will be duplicated by various other ethnic groups in many Canadian communities, since prevention, early detection and treatment compliance are all crucial in preventing cancer deaths.

CONCLUSIONS

A diagnosis of cancer is devastating for anyone. Medical explanations of the type of cancer, prognosis and treatment options may be complex. Treatment may involve uncomfortable tests, disfiguring surgery and/or debilitating chemotherapy and radiation. Understanding what is involved, as well as what hope exists for recovery or remission can make a great deal of difference in the coping abilities of patients and their families.

We have discussed some of the elements that prevent that kind of understanding and hope, especially when the normal practices of Western medicine conflict with ethnocultural beliefs and practices about health and illness. While these conflicts can and often do interfere with the effectiveness of health care programs in general, we have tried to indicate that they can be especially dangerous when the illness is cancer. Late detection, lack of treatment compliance because of language barriers or varying belief systems, misinformation about factors such as contagion can all be deadly. In addition, there can be unnecessary stress for patients and families when health professionals do not understand cultural attitudes related to such things as blood tests, pain, food preferences, family decision-making patterns and fear of community stigma.

The knowledge base is available, as evidenced by the wealth of information in this publication, on ways to deal successfully with cultural conflicts in health services. We need to put that knowledge to work, both within the ethnic communities where we are aware that such conflicts exist, and within the health professions where work must be done with cancer patients and their families. Nor must health providers in this field spend years in cross-cultural training in order to provide culturally sensitive care. We need to acknowledge the importance of such an approach, look for ways to share our convictions and successful models with colleagues, and press for the necessary support systems in our workplaces and the community. Otherwise, despite the encouraging technological advances in the cancer field, we can fail to achieve the earlier detection, appropriate care and treatment compliance needed to improve survival rates for cancer patients from all ethnocultural backgrounds.

REFERENCES

Adonis, C. (1978). French cultural attitudes toward cancer. *Cancer Nursing, 1*(2), 113-13.

Anderson, J.M., & Lynman, M.J. (1988). Immigrant women: issues in health care. *Multicultural Health Bulletin, 4*(3), 3-5.

Baquet, C.R., Clayton, L.A., & Robinson, R.G. (1989). Cancer Prevention and Control. In L.A. Jones (Ed.), *Minorities and Cancer*. Verlag, N.Y.: Springer.

Behjati-Sabet, A. (1990). The Iranians. In N. Waxler-Morrison et al. (Eds.), *Cross-Cultural Caring: A Handbook for Professionals in Western Canada* (91-115). Vancouver: University of British Columbia Press.

Bradley, H.A., Leishman, M., Lemmon, B.E., Lundy, M.J., Mildon, B.L., Snape, H.A., & Wiggan, C.G. (1988). *Caring Across Cultures: Multicultural Considerations in Palliative Care.* Don Mills, Ont.: Saint Elizabeth Visiting Nurses' Association of Ontario.

Canada. Statistics Canada (1989a). *Dimensions, 1986 Census Data, Profile of Ethnic Groups.* Ottawa: Minister of Supply and Services Canada.

———. (1989b). *Focus on Canada, 1986 Census Data. Ethnic Diversity in Canada.* Ottawa: Minister of Supply and Services Canada.

Canadian Cancer Society. (1991). *1991: The Facts.* Toronto: Canadian Cancer Society.

Copeland, D.R., Silberberg, Y., & Pfefferbaum, B. (1983). Attitudes and practices of families of children in treatment for cancer, a cross-cultural study. *American Journal of Pediatric Hematology & Oncology, 5*(1), 65-71.

Dinh, D.K., Ganesan, S., & Waxler-Morrison, N. (1990). The Vietnamese. In N. Waxler-Morrison et al. (Eds.), *Cross-Cultural Caring: A Handbook for Professionals in Western Canada* (181-213). Vancouver: University of British Columbia Press.

Esparza, Q.M. (1989). Ethnic patient values and cancer nursing. In L.A. Jones (Ed.), *Minorities and Cancer* (279-81). Verlay, N.Y.: Springer.

Francis, M.R. (1986). Concerns of terminally ill adult Hindu cancer patients. *Cancer Nursing, 9*(4), 164-71.

Glasgow, J.H., & Adaskin, E.J. (1990). The West Indians. In N. Waxler-Morrison et al. (Eds.) *Cross-Cultural Caring: A Handbook for Professionals in Western Canada* (214-44). Vancouver: University of British Columbia Press.

Greenwald, H.P., & Nevitt, M.C. (1982). Physician attitudes toward communication with cancer patients. *Social Science Medicine, (16)*, 591-94.

Hargreaves, M.K., Ahmed, O.I., Semenja, K.A., Pearson, L., Sheth, N., Hardy, R.E., & Bernard, Louis J. (1989). Nutrition and Cancer Risk: Assessment and Preventive Program Strategies for Black Americans. In L.A. Jones (Ed.), *Minorities and Cancer* (77-94). Verlay, N.Y.: Springer.

Henley, A. (1979). *Asian patients in hospital and at home*. London: King's Fund Publishing Office.

————. (1982). *Caring for Muslims and their families: religious aspects of care*. Cambridge: National Extension College.

————. (1983a). *Caring for Hindus and their families: religious aspects of care*. Cambridge: National Extension College.

————. (1983b). *Caring for Sikhs and their families: religious aspects of care*. Cambridge: National Extension College.

Ho, A.K.H. (1990). Report on the study assessing the needs of ethnic Chinese cancer patients in Vancouver. Vancouver: Canadian Cancer Society, B.C. & Yukon Division.

Jones, L.A. (Ed.). (1989). *Minorities and Cancer*. Verlag, N.Y.: Springer.

Jussawalla, D.J., Yeole, B.B., Natekar, M.V., & Rajagopalan, T.R. (1985). Cancer in Indian Moslems. *Cancer, 55*, 1149-58.

Kesselring, A., Dodd, M.J., Lindsey, A.M., & Strauss, A.L. (1986). Attitudes of patients living in Switzerland about cancer and its treatment. *Cancer Nursing, 9*(2), 77-85.

Lai, M.C. & Yue, K.M.K. (1990). The Chinese. In N. Waxler-Morrison et al. (Eds.), *Cross-Cultural Caring: A Handbook for Professionals in Western Canada*, (68-90). Vancouver: University of British Columbia Press.

Lai, L.P.C. (1990). Understanding and caring for the Chinese-Canadian Cancer Patient: the perspective of a social worker. MSW thesis, University of British Columbia.

Lister, Larry. (1977). Cultural perspectives on death as viewed from within a skilled nursing facility. In E.R. Prichard et al. (Eds.), *Social Work with the Dying Patient and the Family* (216-29). New York: Columbia University Press.

National Cancer Institute of Canada. (1992). *Canadian Cancer Statistics 1992*. Toronto: The Institute.

Richardson, E. The Cambodians and Laotians. In N. Waxler-Morrison et al. (Eds.), *Cross-Cultural Caring: A Handbook for Professionals in Western Canada* (11-35). Vancouver: University of British Columbia Press.

Schriever, S.H. (1990). Comparison of beliefs and practices of ethnic Viet and Lao Hmong concerning illness, healing, death and mourning: implications for hospice care with refugees in Canada. *Journal of Palliative Care, 6*(1), 42-49.

Sontag, S. (1978). *Illness As Metaphor*. Toronto: McGraw-Hill Ryerson.

Spector, R.E. (1979). *Cultural Diversity in Health and Illness*. New York: Appleton-Century Croft.

Spinetta, J.J. (1984). Measurement of family function, communication, and cultural effects. *Cancer. 53*(Suppl.), 2330-37.

Storer, J. (1977). "Hot" and "Cold" food beliefs in an Indian community and their significance. In A.C.M. Sampson (Ed.), *The Neglected Ethic*. London: McGraw-Hill Book Co. (UK) Ltd.

Swerdlow, M., & Stjernsward, J. (1982). Cancer pain relief—an urgent problem. *World Health Forum, 3*(3), 325-30.

Victoria Cancer Clinic. (1990). *Cultural beliefs and its impact on patients' acceptance of medical diagnosis and treatment* (videocassette.). Victoria, B.C.

Villejo, L.A. (1989). Patient Education for Hispanic Cancer Patients. In L.A. Jones (Ed.), *Minorities and Cancer*. Verlag, N.Y.: Springer.

Walker-Morrison, N., Anderson, J., & Richardson, E. (1990). *Cross-Cultural Caring: A Handbook for Health Professionals in Western Canada*. Vancouver: University of British Columbia Press.

Wong, H. (1989). Cross-cultural perspective on health care, (videocassette). Victoria, B.C. Cancer Clinic.

Wood, M.R. (1983). Indo-Canadian behaviour and belief related to serious illness in the family. *The Lines: Newsletter of Canadian Association for Enterostomal Therapy, 1*, 11-12.

Zborowski, M. (1952). Cultural Components in Responses to Pain. *Journal of Social Issues, 8*, 16-30.

RESOURCES

I appreciate very much the assistance of the following:

Dr. Soma Ganesan

Mary Frey

Alfred K.H. Ho

Lorraine Kaszor

Azmina Lakhani

Speare H. Lee

Dr. W. H. L.

David Noble

Mahie Resnick, M.A.

Dr. Kenneth Swenerton

Marisa Tuzi

M.R. Wood

- 18 -

Seniors, Culture and Institutionalization

Milada Disman
Miroslav Disman

The Canadian research on ethnicity and aging is in its infancy. Only in the last few years has the issue of the relationship between health, culture and long-term care facilities come into focus in Canada. Consequently, very little information is available on the institutionalization of our culturally and racially diverse geriatric population.

There has been a growing recognition in social gerontology that the elderly are a heterogenous category of individuals. Generally this heterogeneity has been acknowledged to be the result of diversified life experiences within the "Anglo" stream. Most existing Canadian research is based on the assumption that the Anglo perspective and values are generally applicable to the elderly in Canada. This situation is beginning to change thanks to various initiatives of federal and provincial governments and of the Canadian Council on Multicultural Health. Nevertheless, there is still a paucity of literature on the long-term care facilities in culturally and racially diverse Canadian society.

In this chapter, first, meeting cultural needs of seniors in existing types long-term care facilities will be addressed to promote an understanding of the principles of cross-cultural health care that are applicable to long-term care. Second, the current perspective on institutionalized living will be challenged and a different framework will be offered. Third, findings from a survey on attitudes toward institutionalization among elderly persons of Canadian, Italian and Portuguese origin will be presented.

CULTURAL NEEDS OF SENIORS IN LONG-TERM CARE FACILITIES

It is self-evident that all seniors have cultural needs. The purpose of current multicultural initiatives is to meet cultural needs of every person in Canada through the health and social services system. However, we are concerned here with those seniors whose needs may not be met—those from ethnic groups other than English and French.

In order to create culturally sensitive environments in long-term care facilities, Snyder advocates creating "environments which are compatible with the residents' former lifestyles" (1982,22). Since residents have various perceptions of the outdoors, space allocation and indoor furnishings, Snyder emphasizes the importance of the staff being aware of "the usual lifestyle and general background of the people for whom they are providing care (ibid., 24). Specific points given by Snyder to be considered in meeting cultural needs of seniors in regard to the design of facilities include accessibility, the type of landscaping, arrangements of gardens, types of plant furnishings and special decorations. For example, for some people the garden means lush green plants, for others it means ornamental gardens.

Research among the foreign-born elderly has shown that the issue of continuity appeared to them more important than ethnicity. For example, an elderly Jewish woman, who had spent some years in Italy and lived in an Italian neighbourhood in Toronto, refused to move to Baycrest, a home for the Jewish elderly. After being accepted in an Italian home, she happily spent her remaining years there.

In contrast, however, a Dutch couple, strongly linked to the Dutch community in Toronto, could not imagine themselves living in a home for the elderly that was not Dutch (Disman, 1987b).

Meeting cultural needs of seniors in daily activities may focus on such considerations as styles of dress, frequency of bathing and their preferences in the use of time spent on culturally compatible activities (Snyder, 1982,926). Other concerns include cultural preferences in foods and cultural factors in the types of relationships formed "with relatives, friends, neighbours and care-givers" (ibid., 24). The expectations that seniors have of appropriate behaviour for themselves and others are shaped by their cultural backgrounds. "Formality, intimacy, sharing of personal information, physical contact, expressions of emotions, and dependency or boldness" with authority figures affect daily interactions in an institution (ibid., 24-25). Recognizing culturally influenced beliefs about health, illness, appropriate remedies and treatments may provide a basis for communication between staff and residents (ibid., 14).

A note of caution must be sounded, however, since cultural needs may vary, not only among different cultural backgrounds, but also among seniors of a single background. Thus inter-ethnic as well as intra-ethnic variations must be recognized. One major reason for diversity of needs among ethnic seniors is their age at the time of immigration and their subsequent experiences, in Canada.

What about the cultural needs of the future seniors? The pilot research (Disman, 1986) among second-generation Italians who were born in Canada from parents who had immigrated from Italy pointed out that such people prefer English as a language of communication, although their friendship networks consisted mostly of other second-generation Italians. These people still wish eventually to enter an Italian home for the elderly, yet in such a facility the Italian language might not be spoken or pasta eaten frequently. This point documents the need to understand cultural needs of ethnic seniors as a process, and to study and monitor them accordingly.

Existing institutions meet the cultural needs of seniors in two or three main types of settings: dominant culture facilities, and facilities serving seniors from a particular ethnic group. The prototype of a third possible type of a long-term care facility could be represented by the Dr. John and Paul Rekai Centre, a multicultural nursing home that was opened by Central Hospital in Toronto in 1988.

MacLean and Bonar (1983) point out that dominant-culture facilities appear as hostile to the ethnic elderly, and a lack of social and emotional supports. The three main issues are seen as the loss of family, loss of culture and loss of community. They discuss the seniors' loss of ability to communicate in their own language, which results in isolation, passivity and dependence, and a consequent physical and mental deterioration. In addition, the seniors lose the opportunity to interact with other people from the same ethnic background and may lose their sense of community.

In Canada, we do have a number of ethnic-specific long-term care facilities, such as Nipponia, the Japanese-Canadian home in Beamsville, Ontario, which was the first ethnic home to be established as such, in 1958. This was followed by the first Irvan-Franco residence for Ukrainian Canadians in Toronto. Across Canada, we do have homes that serve other ethnic groups such as the Chinese, Dutch, Estonians, Finns, Germans, Greeks, Jews, Italians, Latvians, Macedonians and Poles.

St. Michael's Extended Care Centre in Edmonton, Alberta, is a facility serving residents primarily of Ukrainian origin. Its publications, *Understanding Ukrainian Elderly* (1978) and *Ethno/Cultural Approach in Long Term Care* (1989), offer many valuable insights that are relevant to providing adequate services for seniors from this particular cultural background. The later publication presents "a conceptual framework [for enhancing residents'] quality of life in long term care facilities." This framework is based on a multidisciplinary care team. The publication stresses the importance of identifying cultural components necessary for the provision of "holistic care in a culturally-diverse society" (St. Michael's Extended Care Centre, 1989, iii).

Rowles (1980) points to the importance of elderly persons' feelings of identification with their surroundings and argues that taking people out of their community will deprive them of their sense of "autobiographical insidedness." Such a conclusion may not apply to some of the foreign-born elderly, who have perhaps never connected to the Canadian community but derive their feelings of "insidedness" from their presence in ethnic homes (Disman, 1987a).

The homogeneity of residents in regard to their cultural background (Keith, 1980; Disman, 1987b) and to their health status (Bowker, 1982) is important for community formation within a facility. Ukrainian residents in the Ukrainian Home for the Aged in Toronto scored higher in personal and social adjustments than their counterparts living in the community (Disman, 1987a). This tendency contradicts some research on mainstream seniors, among whom the respondents living in institutions tended to score lower in the two noted dimensions. These findings were interpreted as a consequence of institutionalization, which involves stresses such as relocation, the severing of social ties and a change in a diet. Perhaps ethnic homes can minimize some of these negative effects of institutionalization.

Disman (1987b) suggests that seniors' perceptions of their psychological well-being are centred on the continuity of what they see as the important features of their lifestyle. Consequently, although creation of community in a setting for seniors may somewhat harmonize inter-ethnic relationships, the main predictors for these relationships are relations and attitudes developed prior to institutionalization.

An example of strong ties shared by everyone in an institution is manifested in the Sephardic Home (Handel-Sebestyan, 1979), in which the continuity of social roles and relationships is universal. In this instance, an entire generation of an ethnic and religious community moved together into an institution. Thus, their participation in kinship and friendship was not interrupted. Such universal continuity of social roles and relationship as is present in the Sephardic Home makes the question of contradictions between past and present social organization almost meaningless (Keith, 1980,193). As aging is increasingly recognized as a cumulative process, housing supports for ethnic seniors should be designed to help people maintain continuity in their lives.

An ethno-specific facility may, in fact, be a most unsuitable home for a person who immigrated to Canada early in life and developed a multicultural friendship network. The Ontario Advisory Council on Senior Citizens (1989,87) points out "that seniors from cultural groups which have been established in Ontario for some time, tend to participate more frequently and in more cross-cultural activities." In addition, although the residents seem to be happiest when living in facilities with a highly homogeneous population, this solution may not always be practical. For example, in instances of small ethnic groups or particular localities with multicultural populations in which each different cultural background is represented only by a few individuals, a multicultural facility may answer their needs best. It is important to consider that the research favouring the homogeneous population implicitly compares facilities that are geared to mainstream seniors (e.g., from English and French backgrounds), but residents' populations of such institutions are de facto multicultural. However, while currently there are no programs for meeting these diverse cultural needs of seniors, a carefully planned multicultural facility may adequately meet the cultural needs of seniors from several ethnocultural groups.

For example, Lam (1985) compares the multicultural approach in long-term care facilities with the existing ethnocentric and monocultural patterns and points out the advantages of the multicultural approach for a comprehensive health care team.

Fresh Pond, a public housing complex in Miami, is the only ethnically heterogenous setting analysed in the literature reviewed. This housing complex is comprised of highly homogenous ethnic subcommunities, linked together by "culture brokers"—lay helpers from the clients' background, who convey norms, values, attitudes and expectations to the care-givers (Kandel & Heider, 1979). The ethnic subcommunities are homogeneous in terms of characteristics such as marital status, previous residence, religion and education (Keith, 1980,188).

In Canada, one example of a multicultural facility, which was planned as such, is the multicultural nursing home adjunct to Central Hospital in Toronto. There are 82 residents; the staff speaks 22 languages. This facility, as well as others that are ethnospecific, should be studied in order to identify what cultural needs of seniors have been identified and how they can be effectively met.

In the current climate of opinion, the institution provides the "last home" for the aged, where dying becomes a part of everyday life (Tobin & Lieberman, 1976; Gubrium, 1975). The fear of institutionalization is so strong that instruments for its measurement have been developed (Kuypers, 1969). This fear has detrimental effects on those who are waiting for admission to institutions (Tobin & Lieberman, 1976). Kleemeier (1961) and Shanas (1961) also address the common dread of institutionalization. Psychological decrements from "anticipation of the dreaded institutionalization" rather than the outcome of the institutionalization itself are identified by Lieberman and Tobin (1983,209) as an outcome of a cognitive appraisal that makes an event seem threatening (Lazarus, 1966).

Additionally, Lieberman and Tobin (1983) distinguish between relocation as a stress because of its symbolic properties compared with stress because of its adaptive demands. The major symbolic properties of relocation are identified as threat and loss. Consequently, according to this image of an institution, entering an institution is an "assistance move," an alternative where there is no alternative (Marshall, 1980). What kind of society are we, to institutionalize our elderly (ibid., 245)? Despite this, there is a one-in-four probability of institutionalization for persons 65 years of age (Kastenbaum & Candy, 1973) and demographic projections suggest the future rapid growth of the population most likely to be institutionalized.

In 1981, those aged 80 and over represented 19 percent of the Canadian population aged 65 and over; by 2001, they will make up over 24 percent of the over-65 age group (Ontario Gerontology Association, 1983).

In our opinion, the existing, very negative prevalent view of institutions has several roots: the historically grounded "poor house" image of an institution (Brody and Gummer, 1967); the traditional image of a family, which is supposed to take care of its elders; and the perception that an institution is a place that is excluded from the community. However, there is obviously a discrepancy between these negative perceptions of institutions and the demographic projections that suggest a growing need for the level of care that is presently associated with an institution.

In our view, it is inevitable that the traditional perceptions of institutions must change in order that their environments may be adapted to fit the needs of individuals. The image of a "poor house" does not hold as soon as people see the actual settings (and inquire about the costs). The traditional image of a family that takes care of its members is slowly changing as the roles of its members are being redefined, especially as more women are entering the labour force. The family will change even more with the increasing longevity of its members. Eventually, we may have five-generation families and the implication for care demands in that context is simply mind-boggling. However, if we insist on families continuing to take care of their own, achievements of women's liberation may well be cancelled out; women may once more be asked to be full-time homemakers.

The main suggestion that we make in this chapter is to bring the community, meaning the "outside world," into an institution as well as to place the institution within the community. The institution must be promoted as a community concern. The inquiry on attitudes to institutionalization that is reported on in this chapter is a step toward reaching the above goal.

EMPIRICAL STUDY: ATTITUDES TOWARD INSTITUTIONALIZATION: ETHNOCULTURAL DIFFERENCES

In an empirical study *executed in 1987 and 1988 we collected data dealing with effects of ethnocultural differences and other potential objective determinants on simply operationalized fear of institutionalization in three different ethnic groups living in Metropolitan Toronto. One of the goals of the study was to create a plausible model of genesis of fear.

Research Design and Data Collection

Research was focused on the target population drawn from the two largest ethnic groups in Metropolitan Toronto: Italian and Portuguese immigrants who were aged 65 and over and were living in Metropolitan Toronto. A control group was composed of Canadian-born, English-speaking elderly of British descent (referred to hereafter for the purposes of this study as "English"). The Italian-born community is served by a well-established network of services that includes a home for the elderly; the Portuguese community lacks such a facility and is not as well served.

The construction of the sample as well as of the field interviews was performed by Institute for Social Research (ISR) at York University. Sampling of the population under scrutiny represented a complex problem: 11% of the population of Metropolitan Toronto is 65 years of age or over, and of those, 62% are Canadian-born, 6% are Italian-born and only 1% are Portuguese-born. To obtain the required number of 100 Portuguese elderly by area-probability sampling would have been prohibitively expensive. Therefore ISR used an alternative method: the sampling frame was made up of school support lists for each of six municipalities within Metropolitan Toronto. From this base were created three independent samples: approximately 500 English-sounding names, 600 Italian names and 650 Portuguese names were selected. In a brief telephone interview the eligibility of potential respondents was tested. Data were collected in standardized face-to-face interviews, one per respondent, lasting an average of one hour. The interviews were conducted in English, Italian or Portuguese according to the respondents' wish. The data collection was completed in August 1988 and resulted in 311 completed interviews (104 from the English population, 109 from the Italian and 98 from the Portuguese). Only a fraction of data obtained from this project is discussed here.

Differences Between Populations as Background for Analysis

Data analysis was strongly influenced by the fact the differences between our three subpopulations are so dramatic that virtually all steps of analysis had to performed within the group. Analysis on a pooled sample was used only exceptionally. Our three subpopulations obviously differ in those dimensions for which they had been selected: ethnic culture and presence or absence of ethnic institution for elderly. However, since ethnic membership is heavily correlated with variables that potentially influence attitudes toward institutions, it was also possible that, by selecting a member of a particular ethnic group, we were also selecting a person who was significantly different in his/her socio-economic status (SES), demographic characteristics, lifestyle or even in the scale on which he/she would verbalize attitudes.

The lower SES of most ethnic minority groups in North America is an expected fact in any study. However, the results of our study reveal that the differences between the English on one hand, and the Italians and Portuguese on the other, are much greater than we had expected. The differences in education are dramatic; the average education (measured in years) of English subjects was 11.8 years, and is approximately four times higher than that of the Italians (4.2 years) and six times higher than that of the Portuguese (2.1 years). Even the difference between the Italians and Portuguese is statistically significant. Two-thirds of our Portuguese sample lacked any formal education and may be functionally illiterate. The same is true for one-tenth of the Italians, while no person from the English sample belongs to this category. The groups differ strongly also in regard to occupational status before retirement: with the exception of one person, all the Italians and Portuguese worked as unskilled or skilled manual workers.

The institution of the extended family in the Italian and Portuguese sample is prominent. The English lived alone more frequently than those in the other two groups. Italians and Portuguese lived much more frequently than did the English with members of their family other than their spouse. Thus it is not surprising that the groups differ significantly in type of dwellings: the English lived approximately seven times more frequently in apartments than did the other two groups, who had a predominantly rural background.

The command of English was of crucial importance for our study. The Italians were significantly better educated than the Portuguese, but they had also lived in Canada much longer than the Portuguese. Average length of stay in Canada was 31.6 years for Italians and only 20.7 years for the Portuguese. This may explain the significant differences in command of English: more than one-half of the Portuguese elderly are not able to communicate in English at all. This applies only to one-seventh of the Italian elderly. Close to one-third of the Italians are able to communicate "quite well" or "very well"; only less than one-tenth of Portuguese belong to the same category. It is obvious that communication in the language of the host society represents a serious problem for both non-English subsamples of elderly.

A serious methodological problem is represented by ethnocultural differences in reporting: each of the three groups depict a different response set. The analysis of questions presented in the form of an ordinal scale suggests systematic differences in the distribution of answers between the English on the one hand and the Italians and Portuguese on the other. English tended to use extreme positive alternatives more frequently than the others. They also tended to avoid systematically the extreme negative alternatives. Italians seemed to be more conservative in the selection of the extreme categories on both ends of the scales than the other two groups.

This phenomenon is well visible, e.g., in the distribution of reported health (see Figure 1).

The English reported "very good health" much more frequently than any other group (39% as compared with 10% for Italians and less than 8% for Portuguese). None of the English reported "very poor health," while this category in the Portuguese sample was represented by a considerable proportion of the respondents. The distribution for the Italians has basically a normal shape. The shape of the distribution for the Portuguese is also normal, skewed in direction of the negative values. The distribution for the English subsample is basically L-shaped.

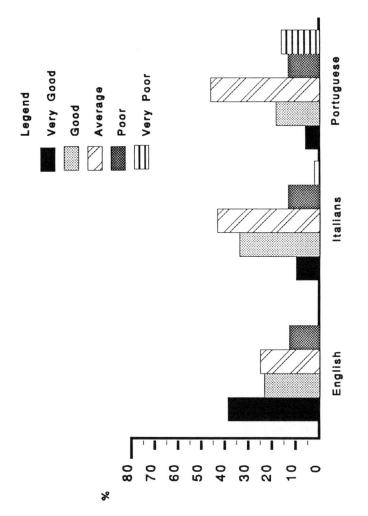

Figure 1: Reported Health in Target Population

The described pattern is very consistent across the variables: the same statement and the same verbal category may be attached in different cultures to different values. Mechanical comparison across ethnocultural borders may be misleading. However, tests of concurrent validity in all three subsamples confirmed that the indicators are valid within each ethnic group.

Fear of Institutionalization and its Determinants

The working hypotheses for our project dealt with more than 60 variables that may affect the level of fear of institutionalization. Here we will deal only with some of them: those which are theoretically the most important, and those that have a more important effect on the fear. The fear as discussed in this paper was measured by the question "If you were about to move into a senior rest home or nursing home, how happy or unhappy do you think you would feel?" The respondents chose an answer on an ordinal scale from "very unhappy" to "very happy."

1. Degree of Reported Fear among Groups

We hypothesized that fear would be present in all three ethnic groups. However, due to the factors of the different cultural traditions, differences in the systems of values of rural and urban societies, and the presence or absence of extended family, some differences in the frequency of reporting of fear were expected. In addition, the significant differences between groups discussed above should have contributed considerably to differences in the report level of fear. The data do not confirm this expectation. The differences between groups are not at all statistically significant. In all three ethnic groups, close to three-quarters of the respondents chose the "unhappy" alternative. The fear of institutionalization seems to be a universal characteristic for all three ethnocultural groups.

The differences in reported fear may be influenced by the general trends in a respondent's personality: persons who are very satisfied with living in general may evaluate potential institutionalization differently than those who are dissatisfied. A strong correlation between general satisfaction with life and reported fear would suggest that our indicator of fear is spurious.

Our results do not support this expectation (see Figure 2). In our graph, the variable "satisfaction with life" was used in a dichotomized form. Only for the English sample can we observe the expected tendency. However, the observed differences are so slight that the Chi-square suggests—after Yates correction—the perfect independency. In the Portuguese and in the Italian subsample we may observe an opposite tendency: among those Italians who are in general satisfied with life, 82% reported fear of institutionalization, while among those who are rather dissatisfied with life this proportion is 79%, clearly, if not significantly, lower.

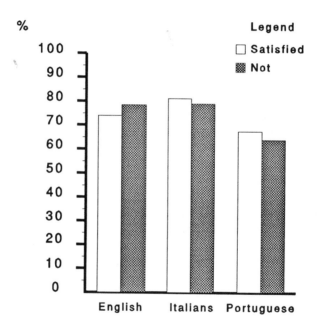

Figure 2: Proportion of Unhappy Respondents compared to those satisfied with Life.

For the Portuguese the corresponding numbers are 68% and 63% respectively. In both minority groups persons who were satisfied with life tended to report fear more frequently than did dissatisfied respondents. This tendency may reflect the fear that respondent may lose the lifestyle he/she likes as a result of institutionalization. We may conclude that the differences in reported fear are not significantly influenced by the general personal orientation of the respondents. The data do reject the hypothesis that our indicator of fear is a spurious function of general personal orientation of the respondent.

2. Socio-economic Status

It is plausible that socio-economic status may have an effect of fear of institutionalization. We hypothesized that persons in the higher social strata are better able manage their future and therefore their fear of institutionalization may diminished. People with a higher level of education may be intellectually more flexible and thus may report fear less frequently. This was not confirmed: none of the five analysed components of SES had a significant effect on the level of fear. Thus, we have to accept that SES has no significant effect on the level of fear in our populations.

3. Bonds with Neighbourhood

The next set of working hypotheses dealt with the respondents' bonds with the neighbourhood. We proposed that elderly who were closely linked with their neighbourhood would perceive the institutionalization as more threatening. Respondents who were satisfied with the neighbourhood or who had relatives or friends in the neighbourhood would exhibit negative attitudes toward institutionalization more frequently. This was not at all confirmed by our data: satisfaction with the neighbourhood does not have any significant effect on the frequency or reported fear. The distribution of data on the relation between friends living in the area and fear directly contradicts our hypothesis: those who had friends living in the neighbourhood reported negative attitudes toward homes for elderly slightly less frequently than others. However, none of the coefficients is significant. We did receive the same structure of data for relatives living in the neighbourhood: the Italian and Portuguese respondents with relatives living within the area were "unhappy" less frequently than the others. It seems that within the subcultures with a strong tradition of helping involvement of the extended family, the presence of relatives represents security and shelter and reduces the stress of potential institutionalization. We have to conclude that the strength of respondents' links with the present neighbourhood does not have significant effect on reported fear.

4. State of Health

We hypothesized further that with the increased probability that the respondent would have no choice other than to enter to an institution for the elderly, the level of fear would increase. The respondents reporting poor health, who needed help with their activities of daily life (ADL) and who lived alone would exhibit fear more frequently than those who did not. The data analysis did not find any significant effect of reported state of health on the level of fear.

5. Living Alone

In a case of illness or disability, persons living alone have less access to support than those living with spouse and/or family. The probability of entering an institution is high for such persons and we expected that the occurrence of fear would be higher. Our data totally refuted this hypothesis. For the English and Italian sample, the fact of living alone and fear are perfectly independent (p=1.000); only two Portuguese respondents lived alone. Living alone does not have any effect on frequency of fear.

6. No help with ADL

Further, we hypothesized that the elderly who need help in ADL and do not receive it will perceive the possibility of institutionalization as very real. Therefore we expected that among these respondents frequency of "unhappy" answers would be high. The data analysis offers interesting results (see Figure 3).

In all three subpopulations the data have a distribution contradicting the hypothesis: elderly who are not able to perform activities of ADL without help and are not getting this help, reported fear of institutionalization less frequently than other respondents. Our basic hypotheses that the increasing probability of institutionalization would increase fear must be rejected. The data seems to suggest a different hypothesis: if the likelihood of the institutionalization is very high, the attitudes towards homes for elderly will improve. If an unpleasant alternative becomes inevitable, persons seem to try to reinterpret this alternative in more positive terms.

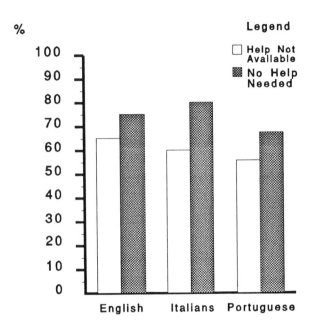

Figure 3: Proportion of Respondents who were Unhappy because of Lack of Help in ADL

7. Command of English

Our next hypothesis dealt with the command of English. For elderly members of minority ethnic groups, the notion of living in an institution with persons who did not speak their language might be very threatening. We hypothesized that persons without command of the majority language would exhibit fear more frequently. The differences between those with command and those without command of English should be more pronounced among the Portuguese than among the Italians, who have access to a well-reputed ethnic institution for elderly. However, no dependency between command of English and attitudes toward institutionalization was found in any of the minority ethnic groups.

For the Italians, the relationship between both variables is reversed from the one that was expected: among Italians able to communicate in English we received 82% of "unhappy" answers, while among those not able to communicate in English we received only 72%. The respondents with command of English reported the negative attitudes distinctly (also if not significantly) more often than elderly who are not able to communicate in the dominant language. The following explanation may be plausible: more acculturated individuals are better able to envision more negative aspects of institutionalization, and therefore exhibit more fear.

8. Lifestyle Variables

The effect of more than 20 lifestyle variables on reporting of fear was tested. Only in one instance, which we will discuss presently, did we find a significant relation. For all remaining variables the relation to fear was insignificant. Attendance at religious services has a special position among all lifestyle variables. It significantly reduces the frequency of reported fear for the English, visibly but not significantly for the Italians; it has no effect on the Portuguese. The relation between attendance and attitudes is virtually not testable for both minority groups; only eight Portuguese and three Italians did not attend church regularly. There is no variance in the independent variable.

The significant effect of attendance at religious services may thus be important for the minority groups too.

Our data do not include information about the respondents' church affiliation. Thus we are not able to estimate whether this effect is associated with certain denominations only. At the very least, the results suggest that the philosophical system that is consciously or subconsciously accepted by a person and his/her internalized system of values may significantly influence the occurrence of fear. We believe that this avenue should be followed in future research.

Also if education, intellectual activities and knowledge in general seem to have a slight negative effect on attitudes toward institutionalization, one type of knowledge seems to play a very specific role: concrete knowledge about institution based on contact with it. Contact with an institution was operationalized as a knowledge of someone who lives in a home for elderly.

9. Contact with Institution

Contact with an institution has a selective effect: for the Italians, it improves significantly attitudes toward institutionalization, it has distinct but not significant positive effect on the English and a very distinct negative effect on the Portuguese (see Figure 4).

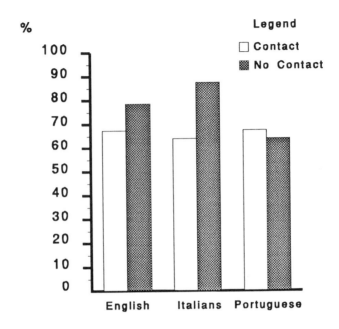

Figure 4: Proportion of "Unhappy" Respondents by contact with an institution

The interpretation of these differences is not difficult: Italians in Toronto have access to Villa Colombo, a very good and popular ethnic home for elderly. A contact with satisfied inhabitants of such an institution may help to overcome some preconceived negative notions about institutionalization. On the other hand, there is no corresponding institution for Portuguese elderly in Toronto. Regardless of the institution in which the contacted elderly had lived, this institution was strange to the Portuguese.

The contacts of the English respondents were obviously the inmates of general institutions belonging their own culture. The threatening effect of a strange culture is absent here. However, some of these institutions could have been of mediocre quality and thus some contacts may have also had a negative effect. This may explain that the positive effect was not as pronounced as it was in the case of the Italians.

The existence of an institution that is satisfactory for its potential clients (e.g., a good ethnic institution) is a necessary but not a sufficient condition for diminishing fear. (Italians, with the prestigious Villa Colombo, reported fear more frequently than any other group.) Only after the respondent was in an actual contact with an institution did the fear decrease.

A contact with a home for the elderly may significantly influence the attitudes of the elderly toward institutionalization: this influence may be positive or negative, depending on the quality of the institution as perceived by the culture of the respondent. If these findings are confirmed in a broader context, they may result in interesting possibilities for an effective social intervention.

DISCUSSION AND CONCLUSIONS

We were dealing here mostly with the factors that may influence, create or diminish the individual fear of institutionalization as viewed by the elderly from outside prior to institutionalization. Not many factors are significant in this respect.

In some instances this lack of influence may be simply the function of interplay between the structure of the general population and the size of the sample: there are only a few (if any) well-off, well-educated elderly in the minority ethnic groups. All of the respondents from these groups are religious. The overwhelming majority were socialized within a poor rural environment. Most of them live within the extended family: hardly any live alone. Very few of the Portuguese are able routinely to communicate in English. Small variance in the independent variables prevented discovery of any statistically significant dependency in our sample or if such a dependency exists in the population.

In all other instances the absence of statistically significant dependency seems to have an objective meaning and suggests the universality of fear of institutionalization. Fear of institutionalization is evidently present on the same prominent level in the rural cultures of southern Europe as in post-industrial urban Canada.

Fear of institutionalization is not even significantly influenced by respondents' health and their proficiency in ADL. The increasing level of acculturation does not improve the attitudes of elderly members of the minority ethnic groups. The hypothesis that persons closely linked to their neighbourhood will more frequently exhibit fear from relocation to the institution had to be rejected. Furthermore, the level of reported fear is not at all related to the respondents' general satisfaction with the quality of their lives.

The findings strongly confirm the universal character of fear of institutionalization. However, the fear is not inert. At least 2 of more than 60 tested variables have a significant effect on the frequency of reported fear: concrete knowledge about homes for elderly and a vivid experience of contact with someone living in an institution may have a meaningful effect on fear. The effect may be positive if the institution corresponds to the culture of contacted person, negative if not.

Further, the English elderly who attend religious services are significantly less unhappy than others. (For both minority groups attendance at services is rather a constant than a variable.) The internalized system of values and the consciously or subconsciously accepted ideology may influence the respondents' fear.

The sensitivity of fear to personal ideology and to a contact with an institution, together with invariability of the fear in regard to most of the environmental variables, suggests that fear is a multidimensional phenomenon.

The discussed data hint distinctly (but not significantly) that the objective factors are transformed, probably by the defensive mechanism of respondent's personality. From the universal character of fear it would be reasonable to expect that with the increasing probability of institutionalization, the fear will increase. The data suggest an opposite tendency. The immediacy of the event seems to trigger a defense: the respondents start to reinterpret the image of an institution in more favourable terms. In the analysis of the relation between frequency of thinking about homes and fear, the presence of an avoidance mechanism is clearly visible. Those who are afraid of institutionalization think about homes less frequently than those with positive attitudes. This relation is very significant for the pooled sample.

The "knowledge" may produce contradictory effect. More awareness about the mainstream institution is reflected in an increase of fear in members of the minority groups. However, concrete knowledge of a good ethnic home may produce a significant decline in the fear.

Multidimensionality of fear has important consequences for the methodology of research in this field. It points to the necessity of multivariate analysis. This, together with the high level of homogeneity of the minority samples requires research on big samples; a very unpleasant requirement in the present condition of funding.

The results also seem to stress the importance of the content of fear. While ethnocultural differences do not influence the level of fear, the cultural differences in content of fear are striking. Our analysis in progress found even differences between both minority groups in sets of items constituting content of fear. The factor analysis, however, isolated identical factors for these groups and different factors for the subsample of elderly from the host society.

Even this early results may be consistent with the following model of the genesis of fear: historical experience with the homes for elderly of the past created the image of homes as "poor-house." This image is then carried from generation to generation, from one social environment to another, as a constant stereotype. Only if confronted with a vivid experience of an institution of today and/or of the institution of the present social and cultural environment, will it change. The fear is thus accessible to social intervention.

This reseach was supported by a grant from the Social Sciences and Humanities Research Council of Canada (#410-86-0344). Manuscript preparation was supported by funding to the first author from North York Community Health Promotion Research Unit (NYCHPRU). The NYCHPU is a collaboration of the North York Public Health Department and the Centre for Health Promotion, University of Toronto and is funded by the Ontario Ministry of Health.

REFERENCES

Bowker, L.H. (1982). *Humanizing Institutions for the Aged*. New York: Lexington Books.

Brody, E.M., & Gummer, B. (1967). Aged applicants and non-applicants to a voluntary home: An exploratory comparison. *The Gerontologist*, 7(4), 234-43.

Disman, M. (1986). Pilot research interviews in Villa Colombo, Toronto, Ontario.

——. (1987a). Ethnicity and Its Impact on Subjective Perceptions of Well-Being in Later Years. A paper presented at the Canadian Association on Gerontology. October.

— —. (1987b). Explorations in ethnic identity, oldness and continuity. In D.E. Gelford & M. Barresi (Eds.), *Ethnicity and Aging: New Perspectives* (64-74). New York: Springer.

Gubrium, J.F. (1975). *Living and Dying in Murray Manor*, New York: St. Martin's Press.

Hendel-Sebestyen, G. (1979). Role Diversity: Toward the Development of Community in a Total Institutional Setting. In J. Keith (Ed.), *The Ethnography of Old Age*. Special Issue of *Anthropological Quarterly, 52,*19-28.

Kalish, R.A. (1986). The Meanings of Ethnicity. In Hayes, C., Kalish, R., & Gruttmann, D. (Eds.), *European-American Elderly-A Guide for Practice* (16-34). New York: Springer.

Kandel, R., & Heider, M. (1979). Friendship and Factionalism in a Tri-Ethnic Housing Complex in North Miami. In J. Keith (Ed.), *The Ethnography of Old Age*. Special Issue of *Anthropological Quarterly, 52,*2-38.

Kastenbaum, N., & Candy, S. (1973). The four percent fallacy: A methodological and empirical critique of extended care facility population statistics, *International Journal of Aging and Human Development, 4,* 15-27.

Keith, J. (1980). Old age and community creation. In Christine Fry (Ed.), *Aging in Culture and Society* (170-97). New York: J.F. Bergin Publishers.

Kleemeier, R.W. (1961). The use and meaning of time in special settings. In R.W. Kleemeier (Ed.), *Aging and Leisure*, New York: OUP.

Kuypers, J. (1969). Elderly persons en route to institutions: A study of changing perceptions of self and interpersonal relations. Unpublished doctoral dissertation, University of Chicago.

Lam, L. (1985). Multicultural Long-Term Care Facilities—Idealistic Dream or Practical Possibility. Presented at Canadian Association on Gerontology Meetings, Hamilton, Ontario.

Lazarus, R.S. (1986). *Psychological Stress and the Coping Process*, New York: McGraw Hill.

Maclean, M., & Bonar, R. (1983). The ethnic elderly in a dominant culture long-term care facility. *Canadian Ethnic Studies, 15*(3), 51-59.

Marshall, V. (1980). *Aging in Canada*, Don Mills, Ont.: Fitzhenry and Whiteside.

Ontario Advisory Council on Senior Citizens. (1989). *Aging Together: An Exploration of Attitudes Toward Aging in Multicultural Ontario.* Toronto: Ontario Advisory Council on Senior Citizens.

Ontario Gerontology Association. (1983). *Fact Back on Aging in Ontario.* Toronto: Ontario Gerontology Association.

Rowles, G.D. (1980). Growing old "inside": Aging and attachment to place in an Appalachian community. In N. Datan & N. Lohman (Eds.), *Transitions of Aging.* New York: Academic Press.

Shanas, E. (1961). Family relationships of older people. Health Information Foundation Research Series, No. 20, Chicago National Opinion Research Centre, University of Chicago.

Snyder, P. (1982). Creating Culturally Supportive Environments in Long-Term Care Institutions. *The Journal of Long-Term Care Administration* (Spring), 19-28.

St. Michael's Extended Care Centre, Edmonton, Alberta. (1989). *Ethno-Cultural Approach in Long-Term Care* (Paper #3). Contributor: A. Semotiuk, Edmonton, Alberta.

— —. (1987). *Understanding Ukrainian Elderly*, A. Morris (Ed.). (Paper #1). October.

Tobin, S.S. & Lieberman, M.A. (1976). *Last Home for the Aged,* San Francisco: Dossey-Bass Publishers.

Section 4

Research

Introduction

As with many aspects of social change there is often an absence of research on what needs to be done, on what Effect the change is having, and even on which responses are effective and which are not.

Research is being done on multicultural plural societies in relation to government and governing; educators are examining what policies should exist and what kinds of education are appropriate and effective in a plural or multicultural contexts.

There have also been research studies done on equity and the lack of equity. Lawyers and social workers as well as bureaucrats have paid increasing attention to equity, since not only women's groups but ethnic and racial groups have pointed out inequities or have done studies demonstrating inequities.

In health, social demands and even action have often preceded research into the extent of inappropriate care, facilities, and treatment. While the relationship of some diseases to particular groups has recognized, much research remains to be done. Similarly in treatment, research is still at the basic level in many areas, such as the metabolism of persons from various backgrounds to particular drugs and dosages.

How the diversity in Canada relates to nursing or medical care, how it relates to institutions and systems, and how it should or can be integrated into the totality of health care is still an area that needs attention.

Professor Joan Anderson in her article points out that in health research, the factor of pluralism is often overlooked. It is as if social class, poverty, gender and women's issues are disregarded.

In research, the most difficult aspect may be in formulating the research questions. The disregard of pluralism in formulating research questions in relation to health research in Canada cannot but result in biased analysis.

We hope that the articles in the two volumes will help all researchers to include pluralism or diversity as a factor in their research.

- 19 -

Ethnocultural Communities as Partners in Research

Joan M. Anderson

GAPS IN KNOWLEDGE: THE NEED FOR RESEARCH FROM A MULTI-ETHNIC PERSPECTIVE

Given that in the past few decades Canadian society has become increasingly pluralistic, and that health professionals are being called upon to provide care to people from ethnocultural and linguistic groups that are different from their own, one would expect to see an increase in health research that addresses ethnic and cultural pluralism. Yet, a review of studies conducted in English-speaking Canada reveals that this is not the case. In many instances people unable to communicate in English are excluded from the research that is being done.

One can speculate on the reasons for this exclusion. First, it is difficult to conduct research with people who are unable to communicate in the language of the researcher, and, for the most part, those who conduct research are either English- or French-speaking. Also, interpreter services are costly. Second, when language and cultural differences have to be considered, the complexity of the research process increases. Third, researchers might assume that the findings from research conducted with one ethnocultural group (e.g., Anglo-Canadian), can be generalized to other groups; hence it is unnecessary to conduct research that includes people from other ethnocultural groups. The fourth reason, I believe, is closely related to the third. There may be an ethnocentric bias amongst researchers, who fail to perceive the issues pertaining to health care in a multicultural society as warranting investigation. In fact, some health professionals may even be unaware that there are issues that need to be considered, because the models for clinical practice and research are, for the most part, drawn from an Eurocentric perspective (Anderson, 1992).

While research that deals with some types of phenomena might produce knowledge that is not context-dependent, this is not the case with research that deals with issues that are central to the delivery of health care in a multi-ethnic society. Such issues are highly complex, and have to be understood within the historical, socio-cultural, political and economic contexts of people's lives. Knowledge produced in one context may not be generalizable to another. The paucity of research that attends to the ethnic, cultural and linguistic diversity within Canada means that there are gaps in the knowledge that is being produced, as findings from research dealing with middle-class Anglo- or French-Canadians, do not inform us of the lives of people from other ethnocultural and social backgrounds. The circumstances of the lives of such groups are different, and are shaped, not just by the cultures from which they come, but also by the economic and social conditions under which they live. There is a need, therefore, to conduct research so as to build a knowledge base for clinical practice that will reflect the diversity within the country (Anderson, 1992).

This is no small feat, as research that attempts to be inclusive of different ethnic, linguistic and cultural groups brings into focus a number of issues. In this chapter, I draw upon my own experience in conducting research in the area of cross-cultural health care over the past ten years. I will identify some of the issues that I have come to consider important, and examine how we might move toward a paradigm of research that will make visible the health care needs of all Canadians.

THE ISSUES

Identifying The Research Question—From Whose Perspective?

Wilson (1985) points out that identifying the research question is one of the earliest steps of the research process. She goes on to outline the following conditions for formulating important problems: the systematic immersion of the researcher in the subject by first-hand observation, studying the existing literature, talking with people who have practical experience in the field, and maintaining a curious frame of mind.

While this approach to identifying research questions is undoubtedly sound, what seems to be missing is the inclusion of the consumer as a partner in identifying the kinds of research questions that need to be addressed by health professionals. For, from Wilson's perspective, it would appear that this is the prerogative of professionals. In fact, this is a perspective that is rooted in the "culture of professionalism" - it is often taken for granted that, through rigorous reviews of the literature, and experience gleaned from clinical practice, professionals will come up with the "right" research question. It is also believed that the possibility for doing so is heightened when clinician and researcher work in collaboration with one another. In fact, the idea of the "multidisciplinary team", that includes clinicians and researchers from different professions seems to be gaining in popularity in the health field. For not only do different professionals bring substantive knowledge from their respective disciplines; they may also bring different kinds of methodological expertise that allow researchers to tackle questions that require both "qualitative" and "quantitative" methods of inquiry. The combination of these two methods in research is gaining in popularity as qualitative methods are seen to allow researchers to "get the patient's point of view", and to inquire into the person's subjective experiences.

The "multidisciplinary professional team" undoubtedly provides the expertise required for carrying out complex studies. However, it is open to question whether a team of health professionals can come up with research questions that are relevant to the lives of those whom they serve. The issues, I believe, transcend competence in the methods of conducting research.

I contend that what requires examination is the process by which research questions are identified. First, it is necessary to ensure that the issues pertaining to health care in a multicultural society are addressed, given that such issues may be overlooked. Second, we have to ensure that when the issues are indeed addressed, the questions selected for investigation are derived not only from the theoretical and clinical perspectives of health professionals, but also from the life experiences of the people being served. They need to be involved, as partners, in the formulation of research questions and in the conduct of research, so that the issues that are relevant to different

ethnocultural communities are addressed. I raise this point, not
to cast doubt on the ability of professionals to formulate relevant
research questions, but rather to draw attention to how we come
to see certain questions as meriting investigation.

We need to recognize that professionals bring an explanatory
framework to their practice, and that research questions are
usually formulated from within this explanatory framework. It
should not be taken for granted that the questions that may seem
relevant to the professional discourse—the ·culture of professionalism,· so to speak—mirror those that are actually relevant
to the patient or the ethnic community from which the patient
comes. Furthermore, the interpretation of certain phenomena
that manifest themselves in clinical practice may not necessarily
coincide with the contextual realities of the patient's life. I will
use the concept of "non-compliance" to elucidate this point.

Discussions with health professionals over the past years
about key issues in their practice reveal that what is perceived
as the patient's "non-compliance" with prescribed care is of
central concern to professionals, regardless of the discipline
from which they come. Health professionals are in possession of
specialized, scientific knowledge; they prescribe treatment which,
they believe, is in the patient's best interest. They expect patients
to follow these treatments (such as taking medications, following dietary regimens, and the like). Patients who fail to do what
is expected of them are usually seen as "non-compliant". To deal
with the "problem" of "non-compliance", professionals usually
seek explanations for this behaviour.

When patients come from an ethnocultural group different
from that of the health professional, "non-compliance" quite
often is seen as enmeshed in cultural meanings. It is understandable that, in their attempts to improve the outcome of care,
health professionals may stress the importance of understanding the cultural beliefs of their patients, so as to negotiate care
that will be culturally acceptable, while at the same time, meeting the requirements of Western biomedical practice. If one
subscribes to this perspective, it is possible that research questions might be formulated to address the cultural beliefs of
patients. Such questions might deal exclusively with the patient's culture.

Yet, the definition of the situation from the patient's perspective may yield an entirely different explanation for the behaviour that is labelled as "non-compliant." The patient may believe
in the efficacy of the Western treatment but may be unable to

comply because of lack of funds to buy medications, or because of lack of time to carry out treatments. Or, quite possibly, the patient may have failed to understand the instructions given by the health professional. This misunderstanding may be due, not just to the patient's difficulty in understanding English, but to the fact that the instructions may have been too complex, and the language used by the health professional too technical. The professional may not have verified the patient's understanding of what was taught. In this case, it may be the professional who is "non-compliant" with the patient's expectations and needs.

Not following the prescribed medical treatments may have nothing to do with a patient's beliefs, but may result from pragmatic issues in everyday life. The real barriers to managing treatment may be located in a health care system that is organized to accommodate people who are English-speaking, and who have the financial means to carry out the prescribed treatment. What could be attributed to "cultural beliefs" may be understood instead within a complex web of social and economic relationships. However, this will only be ascertained if the research question directs us to the issues that are of central importance to the patients themselves.

The use of this example is not meant to suggest that non-compliance is explained in the same way by all health professionals. Nor is it implied that inquiry into people's cultural beliefs is not a legitimate area of study. Far from it. Rather, the point here is that research questions may often be grounded in a priori notions that are part of the professional discourse. All health professionals have a way of making sense of the situations they face in their practice because as individuals we all use theories, implicitly or explicitly, to interpret our world. For example, when we inquire into the "beliefs" of a given ethnocultural group, there is usually an implicit notion that people's "beliefs" make a difference in health and illness management. There may also be the notion that people from a given ethnic group share "beliefs" about illness and its management that may get in the way of "compliance" with Western biomedical treatments. This perspective may guide not only the formulation of research questions, but also the kinds of data collected, and the interpretation of these data.

The issue is not simply whether the research question asked requires the use of qualitative or quantitative methods. Too often, researchers focus attention on research *methods* to the exclusion of other issues. What also needs to be addressed is *who* defines the area of investigation and identifies the research question. A key consideration is whether the research enterprise is structured to accommodate the perspective of the professional or the consumer and whether the questions will bring into focus the issues that are relevant to those being served.

I contend that to conduct research that will have relevance to clinical practice, the participation of consumers in decisions about what is researched is essential. Too often the approach to research, and to health care delivery, for that matter, is from the "top down." The health professional, as the "expert," decides on what is to be studied, and the members of the ethnocultural communities are seen as the sources of data. When this happens, it is highly likely that the researcher will miss data that inform of the contextual meanings of everyday life. This not only may lead to the production of knowledge that has little relevance to clinical practice, but it may also misinform about key issues.

What is proposed here is a model for doing research that includes the community being served in both the process of the research and the ownership of the product. Such a model would ensure that the goals of a particular community-based group are being served (see, for example, the model described by Singer, Irizarry, & Schensul, 1991). A collaborative model of research should go beyond collaboration amongst professionals to a partnership that includes the consumer. The questions that are asked should be embedded within the life context of those being served, so that the research that is produced will be relevant to them. This would involve researchers and the ethnocultural communities they serve in seeking a common ground, and in working toward collective action.

Reconsidering the Deterrents to Research in Ethnocultural Communities

How would the proposed collaborative model amongst researchers, clinicians and consumers facilitate the conduct of research? How would such a model alter the process of doing research?

In the introduction to this paper, I suggested that several factors might account for the lack of research within different ethnocultural communities in Canada, one being the complexity of the research process when language and cultural differences exist. Even when these difficulties can be overcome (e.g., by hiring interpreters), the researcher may find that there are several other obstacles. First, access must be gained to participants for the research study. However, merely gaining access to a community does not guarantee that people will participate in the research. They may be reluctant to contribute time and energy to an enterprise that may not be fully understood. The benefits from the research may not be obvious; it may not be clear how the study relates to their lives. Usually there are concerns about how data will be used, even when assurances are given about confidentiality. Signing of consent forms may be a source of distress to people unaccustomed to such bureaucratic procedures.

Other difficulties may also have to be overcome. Even when interpreter services are available, working through an interpreter to collect data is less than ideal when the researcher requires indepth interviews in order to grasp the contextual meanings of situations and events in the participants' lives. In addition, analysing the data is in itself a complex process. Interpreters serve a key role in this process, as their own experiences and interpretations are usually reflected in the data (Lynam & Anderson, 1986).

However painstaking the process, when researchers enter an ethnic community as "experts" to carry out research from "their perspective," the relevance of the issues selected is open to question. Perhaps one of the most critical issues here pertains to the knowledge that is produced, and whether it accurately portrays people's life situation. Even when the research is relevant, there is no guarantee that it will actually be applied to clinical practice, if no mechanism is in place for ensuring that this will happen.

At issue also is the fact that the researcher usually has control over the final product, and may choose not to share the research findings with the study participants. A primary incentive for conducting the research may be that it is intended for scholarly publication; the researcher or practitioner may believe that he or she has met any obligations by communicating the research findings in scholarly journals, or at meetings attended by other researchers and practitioners. In such cases, it could justifiably be argued that the researcher has appropriated the participants' knowledge, and that the latter receive no clear benefits.

To what extent will this situation change if researcher, clinician and consumer collaborate to identify the research question and to conduct the research study? First, consumers will have a voice in articulating the issues that are important in their lives.

Ethnocultural communities —the "grassroots"—will enter into the definition of the research problem and the conduct of the research. This will ensure that the direction of the research will be from the standpoint of the ethnocultural community being served, thereby increasing the possibility that questions relevant to the community are being asked. In such a model, language differences may not be an issue, as members of the ethnocultural groups are actively involved in the conduct of the research, and in interpreting research data. They too, are the researchers, with a stake in the research, and are not merely collecting data for the health professionals.

In such a model, the relations among researcher, consumer and practitioner will be drastically altered, as the knowledge of the consumer is recognized as legitimate and valid. The notion of who is the expert becomes redefined, as the expertise of all parties is acknowledged. The researcher may, in fact, become more of a consultant to the members of the ethnocultural community, and may assist people in the development of research that they have defined as important to them. All share in the ownership of the research, and all take responsibility for making sure that it gets done (Anderson, 1992). As a team, they can work together on strategies for communicating findings, and for implementing recommendations. The key here is for practitioners, researchers and consumers to work together as a team to produce knowledge that is relevant within a multicultural and multi-ethnic society, and to examine ways of using this knowledge to bring about changes in health care delivery.

CONCLUSION

In presenting a practitioner/researcher/consumer "collaborative" perspective for conducting research with ethnocultural communities, it should be clear that it is not intended as a panacea, but as an exploration of a way to do research to ensure that the voices of all consumers are heard. I have argued that the issues pertinent to conducting research within a multicultural society transcend debates about research methods. They relate, instead, to more fundamental concerns of who asks the research questions, and how decisions are made about what questions to ask. I have alluded to the fact that such processes are not free of ethnocentric biases. Indeed, the paucity of research that takes into account the ethnic and cultural diversity in Canada may be a reflection of who conducts research, and who has control of the discourse pertaining to clinical practice and research.

The conduct of research that recognizes the ethnic composition of Canada will require, first of all, sensitivity to the health needs within different ethnocultural communities. It will also require a willingness on the part of health professionals (researchers and clinicians) to engage in a process of collaboration with members of different ethnocultural communities - not just the "professionals" within these communities but also those who are from the "grassroots".

What will this mean for the concept of "professionalism," and for the notion that the professional is the "expert"? The collaborative model or community-based model recognizes the "consumer as an expert"; the professional is expert, but is also a learner. The model therefore shifts the power relations to a more equitable distribution among the parties that are involved in the process of conducting research.

At a more pragmatic level, one must get down to the basics of how consumers and professionals will come together to identify research questions. Surely, this will require a lengthy process where each gets to know the other. The mechanism for this process may depend on the group with whom collaboration is sought.

While I cannot provide a recipe for collaborative research between health professionals and consumers, I would offer a word of caution. Too often health professionals come to encounters with consumer groups with rigid agendas. Unable to shed the mantle of professionalism, meetings emulate the structure of the corporate boardroom, thereby alienating those unaccustomed to Western bureaucratic practices. What is valued, under such circumstances, is what is valued amongst Western health professionals. Qualities such as being articulate, dynamic or assertive are seen as "good qualities." Furthermore, health professionals usually want to accomplish tasks in a given time frame. Not only must the agenda for a meeting be adhered to so that the "business" can be completed, but also, the project, whatever it might be, has to be accomplished in a specified time.

People who do not have and/or value the qualities that the health professional values may be judged as "incompetent." They may be seen as not having the "skills" to get the "job" done. Topics of discussion that do not comply with the health professional's agenda may be seen as "getting away from the topic." Health professionals may not recognize their ethnocentric biases, and the dynamics that are at play when they come together with people from backgrounds different from their own. It should not be overlooked that many people coming from Third World countries bring a history of European colonization and imperialism. Encounters with Euro-Canadian health professionals whose attitudes are interpreted as imperialistic may be a harsh reminder of colonial oppression. Hence, the encounter between health professionals and consumers may end in failure.

If health professionals wish to deliver "culturally sensitive health care" they must recognize their ethnocentric biases, and learn to work with people who do not share their values. What is called for, I believe, is a new sensitivity on the part of health professionals that will enable them to engage in interactions with those whom they seek to serve. Health professionals need to learn "to become learners," rather than the voices of authority. In the same vein, consumers from different ethnocultural communities are also learners - learning about life in Canada - and teachers, teaching the health professional about their culture and their way of life. It is only when there is dialogue between consumer and health professional that there will be hope of conducting research relevant to the issues of the day.

REFERENCES

Anderson, J.M. (1992). Using Research to Change Social and Health Policy. Talk. Canadian Council on Multicultural Health Second National Conference. Multicultural Health II: Towards Equity in Health Care. Whistler, B.C.

Lynam, M.J., & Anderson, M. (1986). Generating knowledge for nursing practice: Methodological issues in studying immigrant women. In P.L. Chinn (Ed.), *Nursing Research Methodology: Issues and Implementation* (259-74). Rockville: Aspen.

Singer, M., Irizarry, R., & Schensul, J. (1991). Needle access as an AIDS prevention strategy for IV drug users: A research perspective. *Human Organization, 50*(2), 142-53.

Wilson, H.S. (1985). *Research in Nursing.* Menlo Park, CA.: Addison-Wesley Publishing.

Contributors

Joan M. Anderson, is a professor of nursing, holds a Ph.D. in Sociology. She has been conducting research with different ethnocultural groups. Her areas of special interest include migration and health, the psychosocial aspects of chronic illness, women's health, and the political economy of health care.

Heather Clarke, B.A. has been the Coordinator of the Multiculturalism Programme at the Montreal Children's Hospital since 1986. Her particular interests are cross-cultural staff development and institutional change in the health care sector. She is president of the Conseil Canadien de la santé multiculturelle: filiale du Québec.

Enid Collins, R.N., M.S. M.Ed. is a professor in the Nursing Faculty at Ryerson Polytechnical University. She has previously worked for the Royal Victoria Hospital in Montreal, the City of Toronto Department of Health and the Hospital for Sick Children in Toronto. Her areas of interest include maternal child health, leadership and organizational change, multicultural health particularly the impact of chronic illness and ethical issues.

Marcel Danesi, Ph.D. is a professor and the director of the Programme in Semiotics, Victoria College, University of Toronto. He recently co-authored *Heritage Languages* with Jim Cummins. The book details the debate on multicultural education in Canada.

Milada Disman, Ph.D., a sociologist, is an assistant professor in the Department of Behavioural Science at the University of Toronto and a principal investigator in multicultural issues in the university's Centre for Health Promotion . Her interests include ethnicity and aging, cross-cultural issues in health, multicultural health promotion and qualitative research methodology.

Miroslav Disman, Ph.D. is an associate professor in the Department of Sociology at York University. His principal interest is the methodology of sociological research, namely in the problems of cross-cultural comparative research. He is currently involved in comparative research of effects of historical changes on private lives of families in post-communist countries of Europe.

Gloria Dubeski, M.D., was a resident in the Community Medicine Program, Faculty of Medicine, University of Toronto. At the time of her untimely death, she was working as a Community Health Physician to McGill Ethiopia Community Health Project.

Maria Herrera, is Multicultural Health Coordinator, Toronto Department of Public Health. She is one of the founding members of the Multicultural Health Coalition and is actively involved in health promotion activities. She is involved in efforts toward achieving equity in health for racial and cultural communities.

Barry Kinsey, Ph.D., is professor of sociology with interests in medical sociology, especially in the areas of chemical dependency, health policy, and gerontology. He teaches at the University of Tulsa.

Magdalena Krondl, Ph.D., R.P.Dt., Professor Emerita, University of Toronto, Department of Nutritional Sciences. Her research areas are the dietary status and influencing factors of selected populations in Canada and in Czechoslovakia.

Audrey Kobayashi, Ph.D. is an associate professor of Geography at McGill University. She has published widely in the areas of immigration, racism, gender, human rights and public policy. She has a forthcoming book on the geography of racism in Canada and Britain.

Lawrence Lam, Ph.D., is an assistant professor of Sociology at York University in Toronto.

Daisy Lau, Ph.D., R.P.Dt., P.H.Ec. is a Community Health Researcher funded by the Seniors Independence Research Program, (SIRP), Health and Welfare Canada with the Ontario Community Support Association. Her research interests are food patterns, food perceptions, geriatic nutrition and nutrition programs.

Maria Lee, M.S.W. is a professional social worker. She has supervised health promotion programs relating to multicultural access, smoking and alcohol prevention. She is a community activist on multicultural, poverty and social issues and is an intercultural trainer.

Margaret Lock, Ph.D. is a professor of medical anthropology in the department of Social Studies of Medicine and Anthropology at McGill University. She is the author of *Encounters with Aging: Mythologies of Menopause in Japan and North America*, University of California Press, together with four other books and numerous articles. She is the recipient of the 1993-1995 Isaak Walton Killam Research Fellowship.

Basanti Majumdar, M.Sc.N., M.Ed., M.Sc(T), is an associate professor with the Faculty of Health Sciences, McMaster University. Her field of experience includes community mobilization, cultural sensitivity training and implementation of participatory and experiential learning. Her research areas are in transcultural nursing and in teaching-learning methods.

Ralph Masi M.D., C.C.F.P. is a family physician who has been actively involved with community groups over the past fifteen years on issues of community health, especially as they relate to ethnoracial communities. Dr. Masi is an assistant professor in the Department of Behavioural Sciences, Faculty of Medicine, University of Toronto, and is the recipient of the 1991 Ontario College of Physicians and Surgeons "Excellence in Medical Care" Award.

Lynette Mensah is a health professional in the discipline of nursing. She is of Carribbean origin and a community activist. Professor Mensah has been the president of the Canadian Council for Multicultural Health.

Keith A. McLeod, Ph.D. is an educator who has been directly involved in ethnoracial or multicultural issues for over twenty-five years. He has worked particularly in the fields related to schooling, teacher education, community development, social services and health.

Harry K. Nishio, Ph.D. is a professor of sociology at the Kibi University in Okayama, Japan.

Marion Poliakoff, M.S., M.S.W. has been a medical social worker at the British Columbia Cancer Agency (BCCA)-Vancouver Clinic, and a social work consultant for the North Health Unit, Vancouver Health Department. She is active in the Multicultural Concerns Committee of the B.C. Association of Social Workers which she co-founded in 1977, and she was a founding member of the B.C. Chapter of the CCMH. She is a graduate of the U.B.C. School of Social Work (M.S.W. 1975) and the Columbia University School of Journalism (M.S., 1945).

Mark W. Rosenberg, Ph.D. is an associate professor in the Department of Georgraphy at Queen's University. His research is concerned with access to health care services, the changing demography of elderly persons and persons with disabilities and the implications for public policy.

Chandrakant P. Shah, M.D. is a professor in the Department of Preventive Medicine and Biostatistics and Co-ordinator for the Program Visiting Lectureship on Native Health, Faculty of Medicine, University of Toronto. He is also appointed as active staff, The Hospital for Sick Children, Toronto.

Amarjit Singh, Ph.D., M.P.H., is a professor in the Faculty of Education, Memorial University of Newfoundland with interest in sociology of education, multiculturalism, modernization, gerontology, and the theories of the self.

Hope Toumishey, R.N., S.C.M., B.N., M.Sc. (comm.med) has been a practising nurse for 45 years. She retired as an associate professor of nursing at Memorial University in Newfoundland in August, 1989, and now works as an independent health consultant.

K. Victor Ujimoto, Ph.D. is a professor of Applied Sociology with the University of Guelph and a research associate with the Canadian Aging Research Network.

John R. Williams, Ph.D. is the director of Ethics and Legal Affairs of the Canadian Medical Association. As well, he is an adjunct professor in the Faculty of Medicine at the University of Ottawa and was formerly the principal research associate with the Center for Bioethics, Clinical Research Institute of Montreal.

Paul T.P. Wong, Ph.D. is a professor of psychology at Trent University.

Index

The subject of these volumes is health care in multicultural settings. So, even when not explicitly indicated in the index, the context of most terms and practices is multicultural.

Terms like "cross-cultural" and "transcultural" are used too often to justify indexing their every use. They are indexed for sections of articles where they are defined or distinguished.

So too with words like "religion" and "belief." Most frequently they are associated with particular communities of immigrants, which are identified here by their culture, language, region, or country of origin.

I refers to Volume I, II refers to Volume II.

Aboriginal communities I:71-91, 261, II:66-73, 131-49, 198-99
training health care workers II:131-50
barriers to care I:87-88
concepts, traditional I:74-77
health care guidelines I:90, II:133-40
health status I:84-86
Abortion I:19, 100-101, 105, 258, 260, II:283
Acculturation II:88, 272-73
dietary I:187-93
Action Committee for Torture and Trauma Survivors II:324
ACTTS II:324
ADL I:305

Adolescents I:97, 191-92, II:26, 29-31, 83, 90-92, 101-102, 104-106, 198, 211, 233, 237-39, 264, 273, 281, 287
Adoption of native children I:78-79
Africa I:12, 21, 98-100, 126, 147, 188, 272, II:95, 255, 267, 277, 295
Aged, the See Seniors
AIDS I:105, 249, 271, II:43, 221, 224-25, 281, 287, 290, 324
Alberta Multicultural and Native Health Association II:324
Alberta Social Services Child Welfare Services I:90
Alcoholism I:83-86, 198, II:65, 84, 132-33, 190, 229-44, 299, 301

Alienation II:29, 64, 70, 73, 84,
    105, 213
Alzheimer's disease I:259,
    II:162
AMNHA II:324
Amyotrophic lateral sclerosis
    II:43
Anaemia I:14, II:298, 311-12,
    314
Analytic approach I:139-42, 149
Anigawncigig Institute II:137,
    140, 142
Anishnawbe I:74
Anishnawbe Health Toronto
    I:89
Anthropology I:37, 114, 153-55,
    197, 200, 251, 265-66, 268,
    II:11-13
Anxiety I:85-86, 143, 233-34,
    276, II:86, 98, 101, 105, 163,
    257-58, 290, 311, 313
Apartheid I:98
Appendicitis II:312
Argentina I:97, II:83
Arthritis I:170, 175, II:296-98,
    312
Asian communities I:229-38,
    II:28
    See also Cambodian, Chinese,
    Japanese, Korean, South
    Asian, Southeast Asian,
    Vietnamese
Asian-Pacific islands I:191, 277,
    285, II:65, 93
Assimilation I:72, 74, 148, II:88,
    241, 272-73, 315-16
    definition I:148
Asthma II:312
Atlantic provinces I:201-217,
    II:157-58, 272
Authority, attitude to I:34-35

Bafa Bafa I:163, 165

Bantustan I:98
Barriers to care I:87-88, II:158-
    60, 278-84, 319-22
BCCA I:272
Beamsville I:294
Beliefs I:118-21, 197-224, 273-87,
    II:11-14
Bereavement practices I:282-84
Biomedical ethics I:255-69
Bipolar disorder II:188
Black communities I:12, 14-15,
    18, 21, 98, 100, 147, 170,
    176, 178, 182, 285, II:54, 65,
    93, 101, 106, 166, 220
Blepharospasm II:312
Blood
    pressure, high II:256, 258,
        296-98, 302
    significance of I:280-81,
        II:127
    transfusions I:19, 265
Breastfeeding II:288
Bronchitis I:174, II:298

Calgary I:89, II:254, 257, 293-
    294
Cambodian communities I:190,
    281, II:69-70, 72-73, 100,
    171, 201, 290, 295, 308-309
Cambrian College II:142
Cancer I:15, 84, 175, 179, 184,
    191, 249-50, 263, 271-87,
    II:36, 43, 47, 51, 59-75, 121-
    30, 298
    control strategy guidelines
        II:74-75
    coping with pain I:277-79
Carotenoids I:191
Case studies
    chronic illness I:182-85
    Hong Fook II:180-84
    refugees' illnesses II:257-58
Cataracts II:312

CCS II:61
Chi I:281, 303, 126Chicken soup
    I:279, II:127
Child developmental
    psychology II:96-99
Child-bearing I:76, II:25-26, 145,
    277, 290
Childbirth I:251-52, II:26-27,
    282, 289
Children II:29-31, 79-109, 222-
    24
  special needs II:82-83
  stress of migration II:85-88
  mental health issues II:88-95
  refugee problems II:95-109
Chinese communities I:15, 42,
    60, 126, 150, 171, 176, 178,
    180, 188-91, 200, 229-38,
    263, 272-83, 286, 294, II:54,
    65-66, 104, 121-30, 163,
    169-84, 188-90, 200-201,
    218, 231-41, 311-12, 319,
    324, 290
Cholecystitis II:312
CHR II:132
Chronic illness I:169-85, 209,
    II:128
  case studies I:182-85
  definitions I:171-72
  ethical dilemmas I:183-85
  mutual participation model
    I:182-83
Circle of Life I:77, II:71
Circulatory system diseases
    I:84
Cirrhosis I:86, II:312
Ciskei I:98
Clarke Institute of Psychiatry
    II:171
Cleft palate II:312
CMHA II:175
Colombia I:97, II:217, 222-23

Communications needs I:39,
    50, 59-60, 62, 66, 87, 121-
    22, 150, 164, 167, 184, 230,
    275, 278, 293, 300, 306,
    307, 309, 319, II:38, 82, 164,
    233-36, 285, 310, 318, 320
Communities see under specific
    cultural groups:
  Aboriginal, Black,
    Cambodian, Chinese,
    Dutch, Eastern European,
    German, Greek, Hispanic,
    Italian, Japanese, Korean,
    Middle Eastern,
    Philippine, Portuguese,
    South Asian, Southeast
    Asian, Ukrainian,
    Vietnamese, West Indian
Community
  definition I:7
  issues I:15-17, 23-26, 29-30,
    59-60
Compliance with instructions
    I:285-86, 322-23, II:28, 32-
    33
Confucianism II:93
Conjunctivitis II:312
Constructs comparisons of
    health systems I:127
  table I:128-31
Contagion, fear of I:281-82
Contexting II:267-68
Contraception I:258, 262, II:280-
    81, 288
Coronary disease I:191
Cross-cultural care
  characteristics of I:17-18, 37,
    II:48-49, 310-11
  participants in (chart) I:133
  ethics in I:255-69
  learning model I:164-66
CSAC I:50
CSSSRMM I:49

Cultural awareness I:39, 83, 87-88, 90, 160, 162, 167, II:64, 75, 144-45, 179, 261
Cultural isolation II:273-75
Cultural sensitivity I:20, 49, 50, 152, 159, 163-64, 166-67, II:39, 74, 216-25, 274, 304
Culture I:16, 21, 33-36, 116-18, 140-53, 180, 199, 203, 213, 220, 224, 234, 245-47, 257-61, II:11-19, 50-54, 216, 267-68, 288
   definitions I:7-8, 21, 33-36, 143-45, 150, II:7-8, 48, 80
   ethics and I:256-57
   food habits and I:187-93
Culture shock II:217-18
Curanderismo I:174
Cystic fibrosis I:170

Deafness II:312
Deformities II:312
Demographics I:4, 12, 63, 80-81, 83, 170-71, 230, 297, II:4, 42, 131, 155-56, 159, 189, 263, 267, 295
Dental problems I:85, 258, 275, II:255-56, 260, 296, 311-12, 314, 317, 258
Depression I:85-86, 143, 206, 233-34, II:30, 82, 83, 90, 98, 100, 105, 126, II:217-19, 267, 311, 313
Developing countries, health care I:98-100
Diabetes I:84, 169-70, 175, 182, 191, II:43, 298, 312
DIAND I:87
Diarrhea II:98, 128
Dietary
   acculturation I:189-92

factors I:15, 25, 50, 134, 140, 174, 198, 205, 213, 280, 285, 294, 322, II:28, 63, 84, 126, 289, 296
Disabilities, physical I:83, 85-86, 99, 171-72, 198, 305, II:34, 83, 173, 180, 260
Disease See Illness and specific diseases
Discipline of children II:29-30
Disclosure of diagnosis I:262-63, 273-75, II:50-51
Drug abuse I:198, II:133, 231, 237-39
   prevention programs II:239-44
Dutch communities I:292, 294, II:65, 155
Dying I:180, 263, 275, 282-84, II:31, 36, 41-56, 68, 73, 128-30
   care guidelines II:48-56
   needs II:44-46, 129-30
Dynamic approach I:149

Ear See Hearing impairment
Eastern European communities I:146, 148, 178, 273, 294, II:42, 54, 65, 92, 255, 267, 295
Edmonton I:89-90, 294, II:307-308, 311, 319, 322, 324
Edmonton Public Health Department II:319
Edmonton Society for the Assistance of Newcomers II:308
Education of clients I:284-86, II:32-33, 174-75, 194-95, 220, 287-88
   for Professionals see Training

EL I:97, 160-66, II:42, 69, 72-73,
    95-96, 288
Elderly I:201-224, 229-39, II:31
    See also Seniors
Empowerment I:102, 161, II:74,
    205, 215-16
Endogenous factors II:65
Enryo I:236-37
Epilepsy II:183, 296-98
Ethics I:255-69
    definition I:256
Ethiopia II:54, 95
Ethnicity I:33-36, 117-18, 142-
    49, 189, 199, 203-204, 293,
    II:64, 157, 161
    definition I:8, 35, II:8, 155
    research I:298-309
    substance abuse and II:229-
    39
Ethnocultural communities
    problems if lacking II:271-73
    research partners I:319-28
    residential patterns II:268-
    69
    value of II:270-71
Ethnospecific
    approaches II:171, 195, 198-
    99, 131-50, 231, 239-40, 242
    institutions I:294-96
Euthanasia I:258, 260
Evil eye I:266
Exogenous influences II:65
Experiential learning I:159-67,
    II:145
Eye *See* Vision impairment

Families I:153-54, 262-63, 297,
    II:29-36, 44-56, 163, 235-43,
    267-68, 270, 272-73, 282,
    300
Aboriginal I:76-79, 83
Asian, I:231-37, II:73
    childbearing II:26-28

children and II:81-109
Chinese I:176-78, 273-87,
    II:122-23, 126-28
Italian I:299-304
nuclear I:104, 143
refugee II:300-305, 307-326
Fear of
    contagion I:281-82
    institutionalization I:302-303,
    305
Fetal alcohol syndrome I:86
Finns I:294
First Nations *See* Aboriginal
Folk care I:126, 128-31
Folk medicine, defined I:200-
    201
Food I:15, 34, 80, 100, 140, 144,
    170, 187-93, 245, 272, 279-
    81, 287, 292, II:28-29, 36,
    72, 122, 126, 162, 208, 265,
    270, 287
    acculturation I:189-92
    combinations I:188-89
    habits I:187-93
    perceptions I:189
    See also Nutrition
Foodways I:187
Foucault, Michel I:104-105
Fractures II:312
France I:273

Gaman I:236-37
Genetic diseases I:14, 147, 170,
    176, II:65
German communities II:155
Gerontology I:199, 291, 297
Gonococcal endometritis I:71
Graves disease II:312
Greater Vancouver Mental
    Health Service II:187-202
Greek communities I:152, 176,
    188, 244, 256-57, 276, 294,
    II:54, 92-95, 218

Guidelines
  Aboriginal health care I:90,
    133-40
  cancer control strategies
    II:74-75
  care of the dying II:48-56
  children's mental health
    II:107-108
  health promotion programs
    II:210-12
  health, universal right to
    I:96-105
  multicultural health care
    I:23-31, 48-53, 65-70, II:15-
    18
  seniors' health access II:165-
    66
  training of professionals
    I:55-57, 113-36, 153-55,
    159-67, 267-69, II:140

H.J. Kaiser Foundation II:210
Halifax II:162
Hallucinations I:179, II:180
Hawaiians I:191, 277, II:65
Health
  definition II:310
  perceptions of I:35, 74-76,
    104, 120-24, 151, 205-206,
    229-39, 243-52, II:27-28, 36-
    38, 217, 309
  right to I:95-106
  semiotic representation of
    I:243-52
Health care
  access to I:97-101
  beliefs of laity I:197-224
  comparison of types (table)
    I:128-31
  developing countries I:98-
    100
  ethics in I:255-69
  folk I:126, 128-31

multicultural guidelines
    I:23-32, 48-53, 65-70, II:15-
    18
  options I:124-35
  orthodox I:127-35, 139-42
  popular I:126, 128-31, 205-
    206
  self care I:125, 128, 198-99,
    206, 213-17
  training professionals I:55-
    57, 113-36, 153-55, 159-67,
    267-69, II:131-50, 288-90
  unorthodox I:126-31
Health education (of clients)
    I:284-86, II:205-226
  definition II:212
  PRECEDE model II:212
Health promotion I:67, 198,
    311, II:27, 172, 205-226
  community development
    approach II:207-209
  culturally sensitive II:216
  definition II:205
  H.J. Kaiser Foundation
    approach II:210
  health services approach
    II:207
  medical approach II:207
  Morehouse approach II:211
  Rifkin's approach II:207
  Rothman's models II:209
  sample programs II:221-25
  teaching methods II:220
Hearing impairment I:15, 85,
    II:255-56, 260, 296, 311-12
Heisenberg, Werner I:246
Hepatitis II:281, 287, 311, 312,
    314
Herbal remedies I:74-75, 176,
    280, II:38, 123, 309
HF II:180
Hindu religion I:179, 278, 283,
    II:92, 237

Hispanic communities I:97,
    100, 147, 152, 174, 279,
    285-86, II:42, 65, 69-73, 84,
    90-96, 100-102, 106, 188-90,
    197, 201, 231-41, 255, 257-
    59, 267, 277, 288-90, 295,
    303, 324
Home remedies I:174
Hong Fook model II:169-80,
    198
    cases II:180-84
    definition II:171
Hong Fook Mental Health
    Association II:171-72
Hookworm II:311
Hopkins Symptom Checklist-25
    II:313
Hospitals I:47-61, 78, 87-89,
    100-101, 208-209, 223, 258-
    59, 263, 269, 273, 276-78,
    283-84, 286, 293, 296, II:27,
    36, 51-52, 73, 127-29, 131,
    160, 172-77, 181-84, 255-58,
    278, 287, 289, 295, 319-22,
    324
Human rights I:101-106
Humour I:252
Hypertension I:15, 85, 169-70,
    175, 182, 191, 285, II:296,
    312

Ideology
    I:102-106
Illegal drug use
    II:23-39
Illness, perceptions of I:35, 74-
    76, 104, 120-24, 151, 205-
    206, 243-52, II:27-28, 36-38,
    217, 309
Immigrants
    health problems II:295-98
Indo-Canadian See South Asian
    See also Refugees

Infant mortality I:84, 98-99, 101,
    105, II:66, 131
Informed consent I:261-62
Insomnia II:182, 317
Institutionalization, attitudes
    toward I:298-311
    fear of I:302-309
Integrated Settlement Program
    II:308
Integration I:148, II:34, 81, 88,
    94, 103, 106, 293-305
    definition I:148
Inuit I:73, 80-81
Irvan-Franco residence I:294
ISP II:308
Italian communities I:146, 176,
    178, 277, 291-309, II:54, 65,
    106, 155, 269
Italy I:188, 252, II:73

Jamaica I:97, 171, 175, II:42
Japanese communities I:104,
    188, 191, 229-39, 263, 272,
    277, 294, II:65, 73
Jehovah's Witnesses I:265
Jessakid I:74
Jewish I:14, 264, 277, 279, 292,
    295, II:54, 90, 269

Kidney diseases I:84, 192, 279,
    II:68, 127, 256
Kika-nisei I:230, 233
Kolb, D.A. I:162-63
Korean communities I:232-36,
    II:42

Lactose intolerance I:14
Learning, experiential I:159-67,
    II:145
Leprosy II:312
Lethbridge I:89
Leukemia I:275, 282
Leukorrhea II:317

Lifeways I:134
Liver diseases I:279, II:43, 312
London, Ontario II:62, 68-75
LRCC II:68
Lung
    cancer I:273, 282, 284, II:61,
        63, 68
    diseases II:43, 296-97

Macedonians I:294
Malaria II:311-12
Malnutrition I:86, 98, II:25, 98
Mandala of health
    I:63-64
Manitoba II:278
Margaret Chisholm Reception
    House II:254, 293
Mashkikiwinini I:74
MCC II:308
MCCIQ I:54
McGill University I:48
MCH I:99
MCN II:308
MCRH II:254, 293
Mecca I:283
Medellin II:217
Medical ethics I:255-69
Medical screening, overseas
    II:259
Mediterranean countries I:14,
    147-48, 172, 188, II:92, 309
Melting-pot ideology I:148, 260,
    II:64-65
Memorial University I:207
Mennonite Central Committee
    II:308
Mennonite Centre for
    Newcomers II:308, 311,
    318
Menopause I:143, II:281

Mental health I:13, 85, 88-89,
    148-49, 198, 232, II:79-109,
    132-33, 135, 141, 169-80,
    187-95, 197-201, 209, 230,
    264, 267, 272-73, 278, 304,
    319, 322-24
    children and youth II:79-109
    Hong Fook model II:169-84
    multicultural liaison
        program II:189-202
M.E.S.S. II:201
Metaphor I:144, 152, 248-49,
    271
Métis I:73, 80-81
Mexico I:99-100, 174, 247, 276
Miami I:176, 296
Middle East I:147, II:255, 277,
    295
Midewiwin I:74
Migration
stress of II:263-75
Minerals I:191-92
MLSI I:231
Mohawk College II:142
Montreal I:48-61
Morbidity I:15, 85, 98-99, 169-
    70, II:67, 80, 170, 223
Morehouse School of Medicine
    II:211
Mortality I:15, 84-85, 98-99, 101,
    105, 169-70, 272, 282-84,
    II:31, 59-70, 75, 128-30,
    131, 223
Mount St. Vincent University
    II:162
MSSSQ I:49
Multicultural health care I:11-
    31, 33-40, 48-61, 115-16,
    II:15-19
    definition I:38
    ethics in I:255-69
    learning model I:164-66

policy development I:17, 23-31

research problems I:319-28

Multicultural Mental Health Liaison Program (Vancouver) II:192-202

Multiculturalism, definition I:13-17, 148-49, II:14

Multiculturalism Act (1988) I:118, 148, II:64

Muslim religion I:283, II:54

Mutual participation model I:180, 182

Mythology I:104, 120, 200, 256, 271, 275, II:27, 82

NADAP II:133

Narrative reconstruction I:152-53

Native language importance of II:103-104

Natural rights I:102-103

NCC:CD II:134

New Brunswick II:158, 272

New York I:279

Newfoundland I:201-217

NIMH II:84

Nipponia I:294

NNADAP II:133

Non-verbal cues I:15, 121

Norms and values I:15-21, 25, 33-37, 75-78, 106, 118-21, 142-43, 178, 192, 200, 236, 238, 296, II:27-39, 41-44, 46, 48, 52, 60, 66, 71, 73, 225, 238, 241, 259, 265-67, 274, 304, 327-28

Nova Scotia II:157

Nuclear family I:104, 143

Nutrition I:85, 100, 170, 187, 191-93, 285, II:26, 28, 144, 222-23, 256, 281, 287, 296, 311
See also Food

O.A.S.I.S. health project II:221-22

Ojibway I:74-75

Oklahoma I:202-217

Oncology II:121-30
See also Cancer

Ontario First Nations' chiefs II:138

Opioid analgesics II:51

Orthodox health care I:127-35, 139-42

Osteoporosis I:191

Overeating I:198

Pain I:142, 150-51, 175-76, 182, 249, 251, 272, 277-78, 287, II:25, 45-51, 60, 73, 102, 108, 123, 127, 128, 258, 260, 296-97, 300, 302, 317, 325

Palliative care I:179, 283-84, II:41-56, 64, 73, 160, 163
definition II:41-43

Palpitations II:182

Pancreatic cancer II:71

Pankhyda II:54

Paranoia II:86-87, 180, 289, 313

Pathway to health I:124-25

Philippine communities I:201-203, 204, 207-210, 213, 216-17, 223, 275, II:42, 267

Planned Parenthood Manitoba II:277-78

Pneumonia I:84, 86, II:257, 297

Popular health care I:126, 128-31, 205-206

Portuguese communities I:298-
    309, II:28, 42, 54, 106
Post-traumatic stress disorders
    II:99-100, 311, 313-14, 323
Postpartum practices II:289
PRECEDE II:212
Pregnancy I:76-77, II:26-27, 100,
    211, 255, 257, 260, 283,
    287, 314, 317
Prenatal program II:26
Prescription drug misuse
    II:236-37
Prevention of illness I:284-86,
    61-63
Psychologization I:151-52
Psychosis I:84, 177, II:88, 94, 96,
    99, 101, 180, 188, 257, 311,
    313
PTSD II:99

Race I:25, 36, 38, 54, 61, 66-69,
    98, 102-106, 139, 143, 147-
    48, II:56, 64, 155
    definition I:147-48
Racism I:18, 66-67, 105-106,
    142, II:75, 159, 170
Refugees I:63, 68-69, 170, 190-
    92, 280, II:79-109, 122, 164,
    188, 191, 201, 218, 236,
    253-61, 277, 289-90, 293-98,
    300-305, 307-326
    barriers to care II:319-22
    case studies II:257-58
    children and youth II:95-109
    health care utilization II:298-
    99
    health studies II:253-61, 293-
    305, 312-17
    medical screening overseas
    II:259
    statistics of health II:256-57,
    295-303
Religion, definition of II:48

Reproductive health II:277-91
Research
    attitudes toward
        institutionalization of
        seniors I:298-311
    lay beliefs I:197-224
    problems of multicultural
        care I:319-28
    refugee health problems
        II:294-303, 312
    satisfaction of health I:229-
        39, 302-304
Resettlement II:263-75, 293-305
    adaptation to II:268-75
    problems of II:265-68
    process II:265
Residential school system I:78
Residential patterns,
        ethnocultural II:268-73
Respiratory diseases I:84-85,
        II:255, 256, 296, 312
Rheumatism II:296, 298
Rifkin S. II:207-209
Right to health I:95-106
Right to refuse treatment I:264-
        65
Ritual practices I:75, 179, 266,
        283, II:27, 49, 52, 54, 162,
        165
Rogers, C.R. I:162-63
Rothman J. II:209-210

St. Michael's Extended Care
        Centre (Edmonton) I:294
SALEP II:106
Satisfaction of health I:229-39,
        302-304
Schizophrenia II:79, 83, 181-82,
        188, 267, 313, 320
Scratching the wind I:19
Self care I:125, 128, 198-99, 206,
        213-17
Semiotics I:243-52

Seniors I:86, 202-203, 259, 291-
96, II:155-66, 194, 325
access guidelines II:165-66
attitudes toward
institutionalization I:291-
311
barriers to health care II:158-
60
definition II:156
institutionalization II:160-64
statistics II:156
Sephardic Home I:295
SES I:299
Sexually transmitted diseases
I:71, 99, II:287, 311-12
see also AIDS
Shaking Tent I:75
Shamans I:74-75, 126, 179
Sickle cell anaemia I:14, 147,
170-71, 182
Sikh religion I:180, 283, II:92,
233-37
Sikkema & Niyekawa I:164-65
Smoking I:85, 141, 198, 205,
213, 284, II:63, 65, 67, 84,
212, 299, 301
Social Planning Council of
Toronto II:284
Socialization I:150
Socio-economic status I:12, 20,
23, 27, 79, 83-84, 86, 96-97,
101, 146, 180-81, 207, 213,
220, 250, 299, 304, II:42, 72,
79, 81, 85, 89, 101, 107,
158, 170, 264, 294, 302-303
Somatization I:233
Sontag, Susan I:249-50, 271
South Africa I:98-100
South Asian communities
I:173, 180, 272, 283, II:54,
89, 92, 104, 157, 188-90,
218, 221, 231-42

Southeast Asian communities
I:12, 14, 19, 21, 170, 173,
175, 190, 192, 281, II:122,
169-75, 179-80, 188, 190,
231, 255, 259, 287, 289,
307-312, 321
see also Cambodian and
Vietnamese communities
Soviet Union (former) I:273
Spain I:188, II:92
Spirits I:19, 74-76, 96, 102, 266,
281, 283-84, II:71, 128, 309,
322
Spiritual I:74, 77, 169, 183, 265,
II:41, 49, 63, 72, 92, 145,
237
Spiritual leader I:183
Statistics
I:210, 213
health insurance I:100
mortality I:84
refugees' health II:256-57,
293-303
Status Indians I:73, 80-81
Stereotyping I:18, 55, 172, 181,
II:53-54, 91, 161, 288
Stress
in migration/resettle-ment
II:83-84, 85-88, 263-75
reduction in ethnic
community II:270-71
refugee children II:95-109
transactional model of
II:264, 270
Stroke I:191, II:298
Subordination II:266
Substance abuse/misuse I:34,
85-86, 89, 250, 260, 281,
II:201, 211, 229-44, 314
community needs
assessment model II:232
ethnicity and II:229-39

prevention programs II:239-
44
Suicide I:84-85, 184, 263, 282,
II:100, 123, 131, 133, 188,
315, 317

Tay-Sach's disease I:14, 170
Teens *See* Adolescents
Terminally ill I:262-63
Thailand II:309
Thalassaemia I:14, 170-71,
II:312
Therapeutic privilege I:263
Thyroid II:298
Tobacco I:85, 141, 198, 205, 213,
284, II:63, 65, 67, 84, 212,
299, 301
Toronto I:60, 89, 179, 202-203,
207, 209, 213, 216-17, 232,
234, 293-98, 308, II:83-87,
94-96, 102, 105, 121, 169-
71, 176, 180, 183
Public Health Department
I:52-70
School Board II:174
Training, health care I:55-57,
113-36, 153-55, 159-67,
267-69, II:165, 288-90
Transactional Model of Stress
II:264
Transcultural care
I:36-37, II:121-30
Transfusion I:265
Trent University II:140
Trinidad I:142, II:42, 54
Truth telling *See* Disclosure of
diagnosis
Tuberculosis I:85, 271, II:255,
296, 298, 311-12, 317
Tumours I:273, II:298, 312

Ukrainian communities I:144,
294, II:54, 155

Ulcers I:175, II:296-98, 312
Universal right to health I:95-
106
United States, access to health
in I:97-100
University of British Columbia
II:191
University of Manitoba I:202
University of Toronto I:90
Unorthodox health care I:126-
31
Urban Native Child Welfare
Interagency Committee
I:90

Values *See* Norms and values
Vancouver I:60, 176, 272, 274,
278, II:157, 162-63, 180,
187-202, 221, 233-35
Vancouver (Greater) Mental
Health Service II:187-202
Vancouver Association for the
Survivors of Torture
II:201
Venereal disease *See* Sexually
transmitted diseases
Venipuncture I:174-75
Vico, Giambattista I:247
Vietnamese communities I:63,
177-78, 190, 272, 277, 279,
281, 283, II:170-72, 175,
179-82, 189, 197, 218, 231-
40, 242, 258, 290, 302, 308-
326
Villa Colombo I:309
Vision impairment I:85, 182,
II:260, 296, 311-12, 317
Vitamins I:205, 191, 213, II:26,
300, 302
Voodoo I:266

Wabeno I:74

West Indian communities I:97,
        142, 171, 175, 178-79, 182,
        188, 284, II:42, 54, 89, 267
WHO I:95-96, 102
Winnipeg I:60, 89
Withholding treatment I:264-65
Women I:16, 24, 73-74, 81, 84,
        86, 96-101, 104, 105, 179,
        188-89, 234, 251, 262, 279,
        284, 297, II:26-27, 36, 52-
        54, 60-63, 66-69, 90, 92,
        100, 156, 161-62, 190-91,
        218, 221-22, 233-37, 240-42,
        260, 267, 278, 280-83, 287,
        289-90, 315

Yin and Yang 190, 265, 279-80,
        283, II:37, 123-27
    definitions II:123, 127
    table of categories II:124-26
York University I:298
Yukon I:282